ALLE · ZEIT · WACH · 1842

A. Valavanis O. Schubiger T. P. Naidich

Clinical Imaging of the Cerebello-Pontine Angle

With 148 Figures

Springer-Verlag
Berlin Heidelberg New York London Paris Tokyo

ANTON VALAVANIS, Professor Dr. med.
Abteilung für Neuroradiologie
Universitätsspital Zürich
CH-8091 Zürich

OTHMAR SCHUBIGER, Dr. med.
Privatdozent für Neuroradiologie,
Klinik im Park
CH-8027 Zürich

THOMAS P. NAIDICH, M. D., Professor
Section of Neuroradiology
The Children's Memorial Hospital
2300 Children's Plaza
Chicago, Illinois 60614
U.S.A.

ISBN-13:978-3-642-71206-7 e-ISBN-13:978-3-642-71204-3
DOI: 10.1007/978-3-642-71204-3

Library of Congress Cataloging-in-Publication Data. Valavanis, A. (Anton), 1952– .Clinical imaging of the cerebello-pontine angle. Includes bibliographies and index. 1. Cerebellopontile angle – Radiography. 2. Cerebellopontile angle – Tumors – Diagnosis. I. Schubiger, O. (Othmar), 1942– . II. Naidich, Thomas P. 1944– . II. Title. [DNLM: 1. Cerebellopontile Angle – radiography. WL 320 V137c] RC280.B7V35 1986 616.99'38107572 86-33838 ISBN-13:978-3-642-71206-7 (U.S.)

Softcover reprint of the hardcover 1st edition 1987

2127/3130-543210

Preface

The cerebello-pontine angle has always posed a challenge to the neurosurgeon, the otoneurosurgeon, and the neuroradiologist. Angle masses which are very small and difficult to detect frequently produce symptoms, but may remain silent while growing to exceptional size. The neuroradiologist must have firm knowledge of the clinical manifestations of the diverse angle lesions in order to tailor his studies to the patients' needs.

The majority of angle lesions are benign; thus successful surgery has the potential for complete cure. Angle lesions typically arise in conjunction with vital neurovascular structures, and often displace these away from their expected positions. Large lesions may attenuate the vestibulocochlear and facial nerves and thin them over their dome. Since the nerves often remain functional, the surgeon then faces the need to separate the tumor from the contiguous nerve, with preservation of neurological function.

Depending on the exact location and extension of the lesion, resection may best be attempted via otologic or neurosurgical approaches. The neuroradiologist must determine – precisely – the presence, site, size, and extension(s) of the lesion and the displacement of vital neurovascular structures as a guide to selecting the line of surgical attack. Since the arteries, veins, and nerves that traverse the angle are fine structures, the neuroradiologist must perform studies of the highest quality to do his job effectively.

This book represents our experience with 275 lesions of the cerebello-pontine angle. Most of these cases were operated on by our esteemed colleagues Professor M. G. Yaşargil and Professor U. Fisch. All of the cases were discussed in detail with the referring physicians to understand the patients' symptomatology, the exact anatomic relationships of the tumors to the surrounding bone foramina, cisterns, vessels, and nerves; and the criteria by which one surgical approach was deemed more favorable than another for successful resection with minimal morbidity.

Our experience teaches us that neuroradiology is one part of a team effort to detect pathology, to display that pathology usefully, and to determine its exact relationships to surgically significant structures. The effective neuroradiologist must be an amalgam of anatomist, pathologist, otologist, neurosurgeon, and radiologist. He must have a "working" knowledge of the brain and its coverings, of its diseases, and of the special traits that distinguish one lesion from another. He must be expert in applying multiple radiologic examinations to the display of pathology. Most important, he must be thoroughly familiar with the diverse surgical procedures used by his surgical colleagues, so that he can obtain for them the information they need to do their job. The neuroradiologist must understand what is done in the operating room, so that he can interpret correctly the postoperative and follow-up studies used to monitor the success of surgery.

We are deeply grateful to Professor S. Kubik, Professor of Anatomy, at the University of Zurich for helping us to understand the cerebello-pontine angle and for preparing the beautiful anatomic specimens illustrated in this book. We are also deeply grateful to Professor Yaşargil and Professor Fisch for their patience with us and their constructive criticism of our work and our manuscript. If we have become more effective in our work, it is because of the assistance given us by our colleagues.

We would also like to thank our coworkers in the Section of Neuroradiology of the University Hospital of Zurich: Dr. Werner Wichmann and Dr. Dieter Haller as well as Brigitte Hilfiker, Annemarie Hugh-Sang, Felicitas Meyer, Ursula Pohl, Miro Stanice and Remo Tinner. The book was made possible by the high quality of the studies they have performed.

A special thanks is due to Patricia Stadler, secretary of the Section of Neuroradiology of the University Hospital of Zurich, for preparing the manuscript and to Otto Reinhard, Chief Photographer of the University Hospital of Zurich.

Zurich, Spring 1987

Anton Valavanis
Othmar Schubiger
Thomas P. Naidich

Contents

Historical Overview 1

CT Examination: Techniques for Evaluation of the Cerebello-Pontine Angle 4

1 Standard CT Examination 4
2 High Resolution CT 5
3 Physical and Technical Limitations of CT Examination of the Cerebello-Pontine Angle 5
4 Water Soluble Positive-Contrast CT Cisternography 6
5 Gas CT Cisternography 7
6 Dynamic Contrast Enhanced CT 8

CT Anatomy of the Cerebello-Pontine Angle 10

Axial Sections 13
Coronal Sections 18
The Anterior Inferior Cerebellar Artery 21
The Internal Auditory Canal 22
The Jugular Foramen 24
The Tentorial Incisura 26

General Principles for the CT Diagnosis of Cerebello-Pontine Angle Lesions 27

Pathology of the Cerebello-Pontine Angle 30

Acoustic Neurinoma 32

1 General Considerations 32
   A. Nomenclature, Statistics and Pathology 32
   B. Clinical Presentation 32
   C. Clinical Laboratory Evaluation 34

2 Conventional Radiology 34
   A. Plain Radiography and Geometric Tomography 34
   B. Meatocisternography with Positive-Contrast Media 35
   C. Angiography 36

3 Computed Tomography 38
   A. Indirect Signs of Acoustic Neurinoma 38
   B. Direct Signs of Acoustic Neurinoma 42
   C. The Internal Auditory Canal on High Resolution CT 51
   D. The Small Acoustic Neurinoma 54

Meningioma of the Posterior Surface of the Petrous Bone 60

1 General Considerations 60
2 Conventional Radiology 61
3 Computed Tomography 61

Epidermoid Tumors 77

1 General Considerations 77
2 Conventional Radiology 77
3 Computed Tomography 78
4 Differential Diagnosis 86

Arachnoid Cysts of the Cerebello-Pontine Angle 89

1 General Considerations 89
2 Conventional Radiology 89
3 Computed Tomography 89
4 Differential Diagnosis 94

Trigeminal Neurinoma 95

1 General Considerations 95
2 Conventional Radiology 95
3 Computed Tomography 96
4 Differential Diagnosis 99

Chordoma of the Cerebello-Pontine Angle 100

1 General Considerations 100
2 Conventional Radiology 100
3 Computed Tomography 102
4 Differential Diagnosis 106

Chemodectomas of the Petrous Bone 107

1 General Considerations 107
2 Conventional Radiology 108
3 Computed Tomography 108
4 Differential Diagnosis 116

Neurinomas of the Caudal Cranial Nerves 117

A. Neurinomas of the Hypoglossal Nerve 117
1 General Considerations 117
2 Conventional Radiology 118
3 Computed Tomography 118
4 Differential Diagnosis 121

B. Jugular Foramen Neurinomas 121
1 General Considerations 121
2 Conventional Radiology 122
3 Computed Tomography 122
4 Differential Diagnosis 125

Neurinomas of the Facial Nerve 126

1 General Considerations 126
2 Conventional Radiology 127
3 Computed Tomography 127
4 Differential Diagnosis 130

Vascular Lesions of the Cerebello-Pontine Angle 131

A. Berry Aneurysms of the Cerebello-Pontine Angle 131

1 General Considerations 131
2 Conventional Radiology 132
3 Computed Tomography 132

B. Giant Cerebello-Pontine Angle Aneurysms 132
1 General Considerations 132
2 Conventional Radiology 132
3 Computed Tomography 133
4 Differential Diagnosis 137

C. Megadolichobasilar Anomaly 137
1 General Considerations 137
2 Conventional Radiology 138
3 Computed Tomography 140
4 Hydrocephalus 141

D. Vascular Malformations of the Cerebello-Pontine Angle 142
1 General Considerations 142
2 Conventional Radiology 143
3 Computed Tomography 143

Secondary Tumors of the Cerebello-Pontine Angle 147

Magnetic Resonance Imaging of the Cerebello-Pontine Angle 152

MRI Examination Technique 152
MRI Anatomy 153
MRI of Acoustic Neurinoma 156
MRI of Other Cerebello-Pontine Angle Masses 163

References 173

Subject Index 197

Historical Overview

Acoustic neurinoma is the most common tumor of the cerebello-pontine angle. Therefore, the radiographic techniques used to evaluate the cerebello-pontine angle were developed first for the diagnosis of acoustic neurinoma and were applied to the diagnosis of other cerebello-pontine angle lesions only later.

The first pathologic description of an acoustic neurinoma was by Sandifort of Leyden in 1777, who noted that the tumor occupied both the cerebello-pontine angle and the internal auditory canal (500). In 1853, Toynbee (566) described the first purely intrameatal acoustic neurinoma. Virchow in 1858 (597) and Gruber in 1888 (183) recognized that widening of the internal auditory canal is a characteristic feature of acoustic neurinomas.

In 1912, Henschen (214) provided the first precise pathological and topographical description of acoustic neurinomas and of other cerebello-pontine angle tumors. He clearly recognized that acoustic neurinomas originate from the intrameatal portion of the vestibular nerve and that they extend into the cerebello-pontine angle cistern late in their evolution. Henschen predicted that the radiographic diagnosis of acoustic neurinomas might be based upon detection of a widened internal auditory canal. He then became the first to diagnose an acoustic neurinoma using the radiographic projection described by Schüller (520). Henschen also predicted that early radiological diagnosis of acoustic neurinoma would lead to a decrease in the operative mortality, then as high as 67 to 84% (117, 275).

In 1917 Stenvers (541) introduced a new radiographic projection that displayed the internal auditory canal more clearly. Also, in 1917, Harvey Cushing published his monograph "Tumors of the Nervus acusticus and the Syndrome of the Cerebello-pontine Angle" (76). Cushing was the first to recognize that unilateral hearing loss and tinnitus were important early symptoms of acoustic neurinoma, present in 25 of his 30 cases. Cushing also introduced the subtotal intracapsular removal of large acoustic neurinomas, thereby decreasing the operative mortality from 80 to 20% (163).

During the twenties, Dandy, Sicard and Moniz introduced pneumoencephalography, pneumoventriculography, positive-contrast ventriculography and cerebral angiography for the diagnosis of brain tumors (81, 82, 362, 531). Surprisingly these valuable techniques were not immediately applied to the diagnosis of acoustic neurinomas or other cerebello-pontine angle tumors. Rather, they came into use for the diagnosis of acoustic neurinomas years later, following perfection of the techniques.

Throughout the 1930s and 1940s, diagnosis of cerebello-pontine angle tumors still depended upon conventional plain film radiography. In 1928, Stenvers (542) and Schüller (521) published the first systematic descriptions of the radiological changes in the internal auditory canal and at the apex of the petrous bone caused by acoustic neurinomas. Stenvers recognized individual variation in the size of the internal auditory canals and concluded that asymmetry of the two canals was more significant than the absolute size of either canal alone – a fundamental observation still valuable 60 years after its first description. Near the end of the 1920s, Lysholm and Schönander developed a special radiographic unit to help position patients for the special projections used to evaluate the temporal bone (328, 329). Application of the Lysholm-Schönander X-ray unit to pneumoencephalography and ventriculography permitted standardized examinations of the cerebello-pontine angle (297). These standard studies provided the first reliable estimation of tumor size.

In 1935, Brunner (45) described the rare "medial" acoustic neurinoma that originates within the cerebello-pontine angle cistern medial to the internal auditory canal. He recognized that the medial type of acoustic neurinoma was not associated with significant enlargement of the internal auditory canal.

Parallel improvements in radiological diagnosis and surgical technique then led to a decrease in the operative morbidity and mortality. Early diagnosis of smaller tumor led Dandy (83) to abandon the standard procedure of posterior fossa decompression with intracapsular enucleation of the tumor in favor of an unilateral cerebellar approach, that remained in use until 1961, when microneurosurgery was developed (79, 231).

The 1950s and 1960s saw additional improvement in the radiographic diagnosis of acoustic tumors. Hodes (221) described the radiographic characteristics of 183 acoustic neurinomas and other cerebello-pontine angle tumors and refined the criteria for correct differential diagnosis of these lesions. Liliequist (307, 308) described in detail the encephalographic features of acoustic neurinomas and other cerebello-pontine angle tumors, permitting detection of small neurinomas that protruded only a few millimeters into the cerebello-pontine angle cistern.

During this same period, the potential value of vertebral angiography slowly came to be recognized. Atkinson (12) studied the anatomy of the anterior inferior cerebellar artery and recognized that clipping of the anterior inferior cerebellar artery during surgical removal of acoustic neurinomas was often responsible for postoperative morbidity and death. Knowledge of the position of the anterior inferior cerebellar artery with respect to the tumor mass was recognized to be important; however, routine use of vertebral angiography waited until 1956, when Lindgren (316) introduced percutaneous catheterization of the vertebral artery via femoral approach. By this time, many authors studied the vascular displacements associated with cerebello-pontine angle tumors (179, 277, 279). In 1957, Yaşargil (625) emphasized the importance of using the capillary and venous phases of the angiogram to demonstrate the tumor capsule and thereby define the precise site and size of the acoustic neurinoma.

Introduction of complex motion tomography in 1959 greatly increased the ease and accuracy of evaluating the internal auditory canals and the entire petrous pyramid, leading to improved radiographic diagnosis of cerebello-pontine angle tumors (375).

In the 1960s a surgical renaissance led to the introduction of the translabyrinthine approach (227, 228), the transpetrosal approach (285) and microneurosurgical techniques (134, 140, 626, 629) permitting more nearly complete removal of tumor with lowered morbidity and mortality. In turn, need for improved radiographic diagnosis of small tumors led to the widespread use of complex-motion tomography, later combined with Pantopaque meatocisternography (19, 139, 219, 582, 588).

During the same period, introduction of direct magnification angiography and photographic subtraction gave new impetus to the angiographic diagnosis of large cerebello-pontine angle masses (233, 234, 386, 600, 610).

In 1973, computed tomography (CT), first permitted accurate non invasive detection of medium- and large-sized acoustic neurinomas, and accurate display of their site, size and anatomic relationships (5, 225). Within a few years CT completely replaced pneumoencephalography and partially replaced angiography for the evaluation of a suspected cerebello-pontine angle mass. First and second generation CT units detected moderately large acoustic neurinomas that protruded at least 1 to 1.5 cm into the cerebello-pontine angle cistern (182, 191, 259, 387, 388). Modifications in the CT examination technique, use of overlapping CT slices, continuous infusion of contrast medium, and positive gantry angulation, permitted detection of acoustic neurinomas that protruded less than 1 cm into the cerebello-pontine angle (515, 573, 574). However, Pantopaque meatocisternography remained necessary for detection or exclusion of intrameatal acoustic neurinomas and for neurinomas that protruded only a few millimeters beyond the internal auditory canal.

In 1974, Greitz and Hindmarsh (181) began to instill Metrizamide into the intrathecal space prior to performing CT scans (Metrizamide CT cisternography). By 1977 to 78, this technique was applied to detect even small *extra*canalicular neurinomas accurately (111, 478, 481). Despite initial enthusiasm, however, the technique proved inaccurate for the diagnosis of *intra*canalicular neurinomas and could not replace Pantopaque meatocisternography for the detection of purely intracanalicular tumors.

In 1978 Sortland (536) introduced the technique of air CT cisternography for study of the internal auditory canal. Accumulated experience now suggests that gas CT cisternography is the most sensitive radiographic technique for detecting or excluding small and purely intracanalicular neurinomas (281, 393, 536, 577, 612). Coupling gas CT cisternography with late-generation CT scanners and new, high geometric resolution computer algorithms provides a powerful radiographic tool for detailed investigation of the temporal bone (517, 527, 528, 577). With the use of these modern imaging techniques, the proportion of small tumors diagnosed has increased, with a corresponding decrease in the number of medium and large tumors detected (200).

Magnetic resonance imaging (MRI) is the latest development in the field of neuroradiology. This method has already proved valuable for detecting and defining posterior fossa pathology (349, 633). Accumulating evidence suggests that MRI is at least as accurate as CT for detecting even intracanalicular neurinomas and that MRI will become a completely non invasive alternative to CT in the diagnosis of cerebello-pontine angle lesions (87, 88, 267, 358).

CT Examination: Techniques for Evaluation of the Cerebello-Pontine Angle

In patients presenting clinically with a cerebello-pontine angle syndrome, the primary aim of the CT examination is to prove or exclude a mass lesion. If a mass is encountered, CT studies should also display the relationship of the tumor to such important neurovascular structures as the anterior and posterior inferior cerebellar arteries, the facial nerve and the vestibulocochlear (statoacoustic) nerve. Proper demonstration of these structures improves the safety of operative intervention and may lead to preservation of neurological function following surgery. If possible, the CT examination should also provide a preoperative histological diagnosis.

CT studies provide most of the data needed in most patients. In some cases however, methodological imperfections render the CT examination of the cerebello-pontine angle difficult (256, 387), so more sophisticated examination techniques must be employed.

1 Standard CT Examination

The standard CT examination of the cerebello-pontine angle includes multiple thin axial sections obtained prior to and then following the administration of iodinated intravenous contrast agent. The axial section is inclined between $+10°$ and $+20°$ to the orbitomeatal line. The thin sections should cover the whole of the posterior fossa from foramen magnum to incisura, and may be obtained as either continuous "thin" sections measuring 1.5 to 2 mm in the Z plane or as partially overlapping thicker (3 mm) sections. This detailed evaluation of the cerebello-pontine angle is completed with 5, 8 or 10 mm thick sections through the supratentorial compartment from the incisura to the vertex. The raw data from the posterior fossa sections should be saved, so that those CT sections that pass directly through the internal auditory canal may be reconstructed with high spatial resolution (i.e. "bone") computer algorithms.

All experienced workers agree on the need for contrast enhanced CT study, even if a prior non contrast CT scan is negative. There is however some disagreement concerning the necessity for performing the non contrast scan. Kazner et al. (257) feel strongly that a non contrast CT should be the initial study, and that that study should be followed by a contrast enhanced CT scan. Conversely Kricheff et al. (283) recommend performing the contrast enhanced scan first. If that is negative, non contrast CT is not performed. If the initial contrast enhanced CT is positive, a non contrast study is performed at a later time for evaluation of calcification and hyperostosis.

There is also disagreement concerning the best way to administer contrast medium for a CT examination. All agree that contrast administration should achieve a high iodine concentration in the blood and should maintain that high iodine concentration throughout the examination period. In our opinion the easiest way to achieve these goals in adults is to give an initial rapid bolus injection of 60% contrast medium in a dosage of 1.5 ml per kg body weight, followed by drip infusion of 100 ml of 60% contrast medium during the 10 to 20 min required to complete the scan. This technique always achieves good enhancement of the vessels and of any enhancing lesion present. In a child, a total dose of 4 cc/kg of 60% contrast medium is used with two-thirds of the total given as the initial bolus injection and the last one-third infused through a micro-drip infusion set during the remainder of the study.

When axial CT sections demonstrate pathology, an additional set of coronal sections is obtained through the cerebello-pontine angle. These sections may be obtained in the prone, hyperextended position or in the supine "hanging head" position. In adults, use of an inclined board and a gantry tilt facilitate rapid, motion free studies. In children, the hyperextended hanging head position is well tolerated, so no board is required. If direct coronal scanning is not possible, reformatted coronal images are also helpful.

2 High Resolution CT

High spatial resolution CT aids considerably in delineating osseous structures. In general, this high resolution technique is employed as a "post-processing" program in which the raw data obtained in the initial CT scan are reprocessed through a computer algorithm that provides edge enhancement and reduces the X and Y dimension of the pixels to 0.25 mm. Since the images are reconstructed from scan data already obtained, there is no additional radiation dose to the patient and no additional scan time. Optimal use of this feature requires very thin CT sections (to reduce the Z dimension) and wide windows to display the pathology most clearly (321, 470, 527, 528).

High resolution CT of the petrous bone has nearly completely replaced complex motion tomography for the diagnosis of the wide spectrum of pathology encountered in the petrous bone and in the cerebello-pontine angle (195, 321, 494, 517, 527, 528, 577, 590).

3 Physical and Technical Limitations of CT Examination of the Cerebello-Pontine Angle

a) Many structures in the cerebello-pontine angle are only a few mm in size. They can be obscured by adjacent structures that are included with them if the CT slices are 5 to 10 mm thick. This "partial volume" phenomenon prevents optimal demonstration of the anatomy of the cerebello-pontine angle (182). The difficulties caused by partial volume phenomenon are minimized by performing very thin slices (1 or 2 mm) or by deliberately overlapping thicker slices.

b) If radiation dose is kept constant, any decrease in slice thickness is accompanied by a decrease in the photon flux and a decrease in signal. As a result the signal-to-noise ratio decreases and the ever-present quantum noise produces a "grainier" image. To reduce this problem, photon flux must be increased by increasing the radiation dose or by using more efficient collectors to capture a greater percentage of the photons available. Because machine geometry and detectors are fixed for any particular CT scanner, in practice one must increase the mA and must use slow scan speed to increase photon flux to the range of 600 to 1100 mAs.

c) As an X-ray beam passes through a structure, the structure preferentially absorbs the "softer", less energetic part of the X-ray beam. The "harder", more highly energetic portion passes through relatively less attenuated. As a result, the characteristics of the beam that emerges from the structure are different from that that entered. This effect is called "beam hardening". Manufacturers compensate for this effect by writing computer algorithms that take into account the beam hardening expected to result from passage through the "normal" skull. The algorithms compensate far less well for the widely variable degree of hardening produced by the dense petrous pyramid (44). "Beam hardening" is responsible for the confusing hyperdensity commonly observed at the cisternal opening of the internal auditory canal (Fig. 5) (576). Improved computer algorithms now minimize this artifact.

d) The so-called Hounsfield artifact (226, 256) consists in one or more very dark lines that run horizontally between the two petrous pyramids. This artifact often prevents clear delineation of the cerebello-pontine angle cistern and may obscure small lesions. Use of very thin (1 to 2 mm) sections reduces, and in some cases completely eliminates, the Hounsfield artifact.

e) Patient motion is more critical in the cerebello-pontine angle than in other regions of the head. Due to the abrupt density differences between the high density petrous pyramid and the low density air within the middle ear cleft and the associated air cells, slight patient motion creates myriad radial streaks that seem to originate from any sharply angled surface. These streaks obscure the cerebello-pontine angle cistern and degrade image quality severely. Firm head fixation, and patient sedation help to minimize this problem.

4 Water Soluble Positive-Contrast CT Cisternography

Positive-contrast CT cisternography remains useful for excluding the presence of mass within the cerebello-pontine angle and for differentiating arachnoid cysts and epidermoid cysts from other lesions that appear similar on non contrast and contrast enhanced CT scans (107, 110, 335, 478, 491, 526, 623). Positive-contrast CT cisternography is not useful for demonstrating lesions within the internal auditory canal itself. Two examination techniques may be employed:

a) Lumbar route: 4 to 8 ml of an isotonic solution (170 mg iodine/ml) of Metrizamide or another water soluble non ionic positive-contrast medium are injected by lumbar puncture with the patient prone. The table is then tilted 50° to 60°

head-down for 1 to 2 min to bring the contrast into the intracranial subarachnoid space. Thereafter the CT examination is performed in the usual axial projection with the patient supine (337, 481).

b) Cervical route: The patient is placed in decubitus position with the side of clinical interest lower. Lateral C1-C2 puncture is accomplished with vertical beam fluoroscopy. The table is inclined head downward 20° to 30° and 3 to 4 ml of isotonic non ionic water soluble contrast agent are instilled via the needle. The contrast flows directly and preferentially to the dependent cerebello-pontine angle cistern. At times the head may be rotated slightly prior to instillation of contrast, in order to layer the contrast directly onto the posterior face of the petrous pyramid. The use of such small quantities of contrast medium lowers the side effects of positive-contrast CT cisternography as compared to myelography. Nevertheless, headaches, vertigo and vomiting are common side effects, occurring 2 to 4 h after contrast administration and lasting for the next 5 to 12 h (481). Epileptic seizures are very rare, since they seem to be related to the type and the total amount of contrast medium used (534). A history of seizures and recent use of a drug that lowers the seizure threshold (e.g. phenothiazine drugs) should be contraindications for the intrathecal use of Metrizamide.

5 Gas CT Cisternography

Gas CT cisternography and meatography have completely replaced Pantopaque meatocisternography and positive-contrast CT cisternography for the study of the internal auditory canal. Gas CT cisternography demonstrates, better than any other radiographic study, the arteries and nerves within the cerebello-pontine angle cistern and the intrameatal segments of the seventh and eighth nerves (243, 282, 334, 438, 444, 577, 612). Gas CT cisternography is indicated whenever

a) there is high clinical suspicion of an intracanalicular mass, even when other studies are negative,
b) the high resolution CT sections show possible abnormality of the internal auditory canal, even if the contrast enhanced CT scan is negative, or
c) the contrast enhanced CT scan reveals a small, predominantly intracanalicular lesion. In this circumstance gas CT cisternography is indicated in order to assess the relationships of the tumor to the surrounding structures.

Compared to Pantopaque meatocisternography and water soluble positive-contrast CT cisternography, the main advantages of gas CT cisternography are (393):

1. Absence of contrast toxicity and rapid absorption of gas from the subarachnoid space.
2. Absence of late sequelae such as arachnoiditis that are known to occur after intrathecal injection of positive contrast media.
3. Much lower surface tension of gas compared to Pantopaque, allowing entrance of gas into even small internal auditory canals.
4. Extreme density difference between bone and air, giving a high contrast CT picture.

Gas CT cisternography combines a very high diagnostic accuracy with a very low technical failure rate (7, 26, 69, 235, 302, 430, 438, 444, 471, 536, 574, 612). The failure rate of Pantopaque meatocisternography has been reported to be as high as 28% (139).

Examination technique: The gas is usually injected by lumbar puncture performed with the patient sitting on the CT examination table. It is helpful to sit the patient with his legs hanging over either the left or the right side of the table, so the ear to be studied faces away from the gantry. The patient is then in proper position for easy placement into the gantry. The body and the head of the patient are then tilted downward towards the normal side, so that the ear to be studied becomes the highest part of the body. Air is then injected rapidly and the patient is kept in this position for approximately 2 min to allow time for the air to percolate into the cerebello-pontine angle. The patient usually experiences a "bubbling" or a sudden stabbing retroauricular (rarely retroorbital) pain when the gas reaches the cerebello-pontine angle cistern. This indicates correct location of the gas (281). The patient is then lain over toward the gantry in lateral decubitus position, so that the ear to be examined points upwards. The patient is positioned carefully, so that the head is perfectly symmetrical despite the decubitus position. CT examination of the uppermost petrous pyramid is then performed with very thin slices and use of the high resolution "bone" algorithms (444, 577). If the opposite side also has to be examined, the patient is turned 180° rapidly through the *prone* position to bring the contralateral side uppermost. With such a manoeuvre, the air is retained within the posterior fossa and passes directly into the opposite internal auditory canal when that becomes the uppermost canal. The head is realligned into symmetrical position and the opposite side is scanned (302).

There is some disagreement about the proper volume of gas to inject for this study. Initial reports recommended use of as much as 10 cc (536). With further experience, the amount of gas necessary has decreased progressively to as little as 1.5 or 2 cc (7, 26, 235, 302, 336, 393, 430, 439, 444, 471, 536, 590, 612). The disadvantage of using extremely small quantities of gas is that only one side can be examined. Use of 4 cc of gas permits examination of both ears, if necessary (302, 577). The sole side effect of gas CT cisternography is headache. Such headache is present in perhaps 50% of patients and is severe in 11.5% (7, 69, 430, 444, 536, 577). It may be caused by the gas itself or by leakage of cerebro-spinal fluid following the lumbar puncture (243). The incidence of headache can be lowered dramatically (to 8%) by the use of oxygen or carbon dioxide, since these gases are absorbed more rapidly than air (444, 536, 577).

6 Dynamic Contrast Enhanced CT

Dynamic CT consists in the rapid successive scanning of the same plane during an intravenous bolus injection of contrast medium. The contrast medium that reaches the area of interest with the blood causes a rapid initial increase in density (the "wash-in"). This wash-in is followed by an equally rapid density loss, when non opacified normal blood replaces the contrast (the "wash-out") (104, 589). The contrast induced density changes are then plotted against time for a selected picture element and that plot is displayed as a time-density curve. Thus far dynamic CT has been performed most commonly for differentiating vascular lesions such as aneurysms or arteriovenous malformations from tumor (68). However, dynamic CT may also be used to assess vascular deficiency of the pons and the midbrain in cases of vertebro-basilar insufficiency (589).

CT Anatomy of the Cerebello-Pontine Angle

Knowledge of the normal anatomy of the cerebello-pontine angle and of the frequent artifacts occurring in this area is essential for correct interpretation of pathology in the cerebello-pontine angle.

The cerebello-pontine angle or pontocerebellar cistern is the subarachnoid space between the pons, the cerebellum and the posterior surface of the petrous

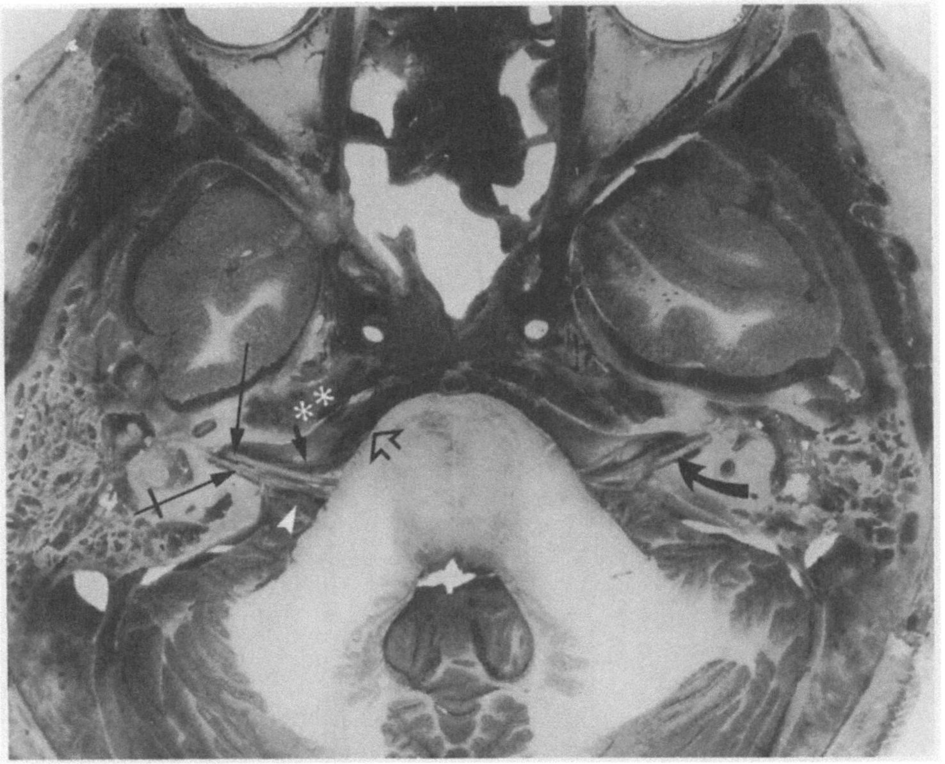

Fig. 1. Horizontal cryotomic section at the level of the internal auditory canal, showing the cerebello-pontine angle and its contents. The triangularly shaped pontocerebellar cistern is bounded medially by the lateral surface of the pons (*open arrow*), laterally by the posterior surface of the petrous bone (*white asterisks*) and posteriorly by the anterior contour of the flocculus (*white arrowhead*). The neurovascular bundle traverses the posterior portion of the pontocerebellar cistern and enters the internal auditory canal in an antero-lateral direction. Cochlear nerve (*arrow*), inferior vestibular nerve (*crossed arrow*), facial nerve (*curved arrow*) and anterior inferior cerebellar artery (*short arrow*). (Courtesy Prof. S. Kubik, Department of Anatomy, University of Zürich)

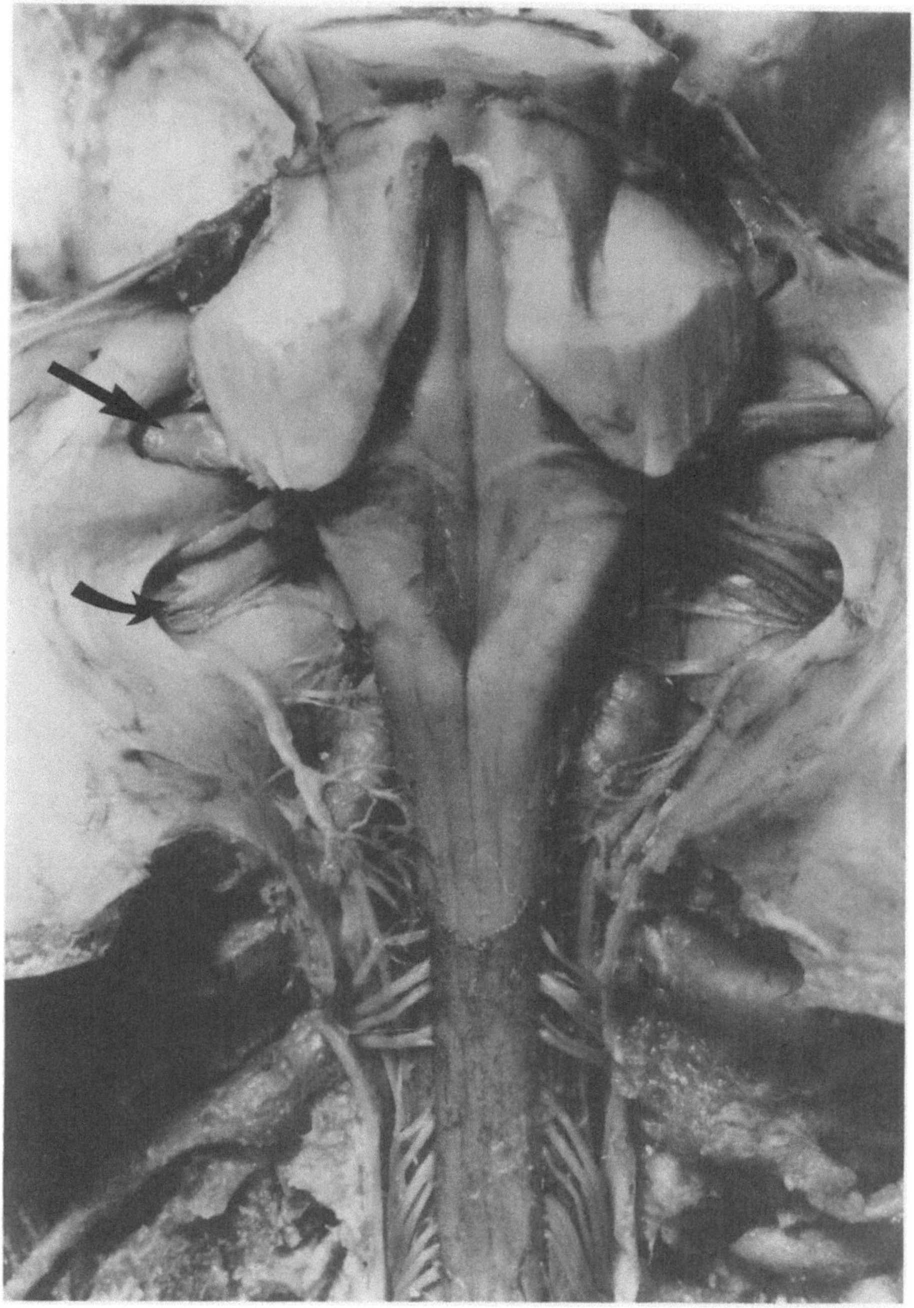

Fig. 2. Posterior view of the cerebello-pontine angle showing its close relationship to the inferiorly located lateral cerebellomedullary cistern. The cerebellar hemispheres have been removed. Neurovascular bundle (*arrow*), caudal cranial nerve group (*curved arrow*). (Courtesy Prof. S. Kubik, Department of Anatomy, University of Zürich)

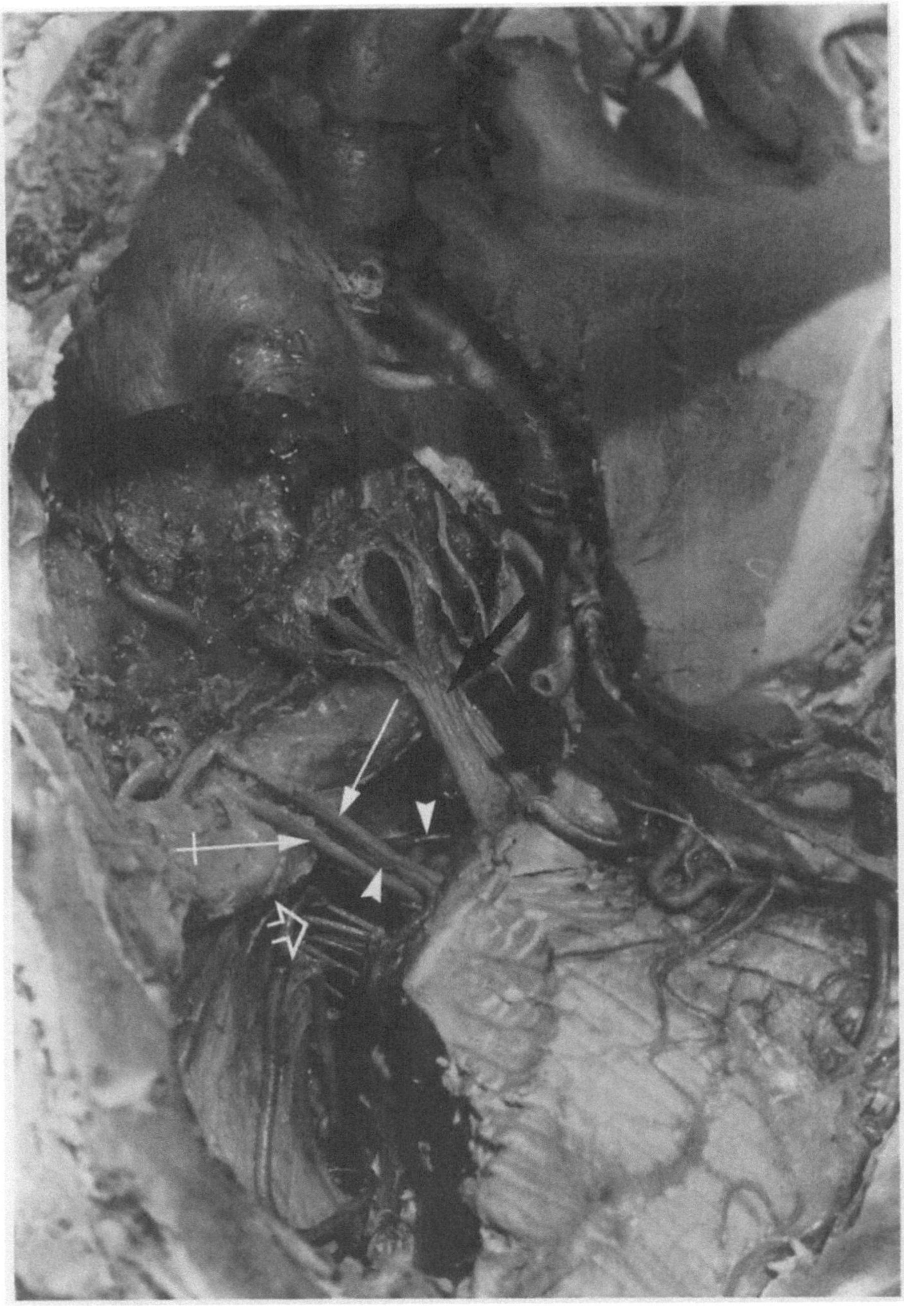

Fig. 3. Oblique view of the cerebello-pontine angle from posterosuperiorly. The tentorium and the upper part of the petrous bone have been removed. The trigeminal nerve (*thick arrow*) courses through the anterior part of the pontocerebellar cistern. Other structures visible: facial nerve (*white arrow*), vestibulocochlear nerve (*crossed white arrow*), AICA loop (*white arrowheads*), caudal nerve group (*open arrow*). (Courtesy Prof. S. Kubik, Department of Anatomy, University of Zürich)

bone (Fig. 1) (25). This cistern communicates basally with the lateral cerebellomedullary cistern, rostrally with the prepontine cistern and cranially with the infratentorial portion of the ambient cistern (Fig. 2) (629). The cerebello-pontine angle cistern extends directly into the internal auditory canal.

The pontocerebellar cistern contains the facial, intermediate and vestibulocochlear (statoacoustic) nerves, the peripheral loop of the anterior inferior cerebellar artery and the petrosal vein of Dandy (Fig. 1). The trigeminal nerve courses rostro-laterally in the anterior part of the cistern (Fig. 3) (629).

Axial Sections

On axial CT sections the pontocerebellar cistern has the shape of a triangle with its largest dimension at the level of the internal auditory canal (Fig. 4). It usually appears as a homogeneously hypodense triangle that is situated medial to the internal auditory porus. Its density is normally equal to cerebero-spinal fluid, but this may be obscured by beam hardening or Hounsfield artifacts (Fig. 5). The lateral border of the pontocerebellar cistern is formed by the medial part of the posterior surface of the petrous bone. The internal auditory canal is located in the posterior part of the cistern. The medial border of the pontocerebellar cistern is formed by the lateral surface of the pons, and appears slightly convex laterally. The posterior surface of the pontocerebellar cistern is formed by the flocculus. This border is convex anteriorly. The flocculus lies between the posterolateral cerebellar fissure

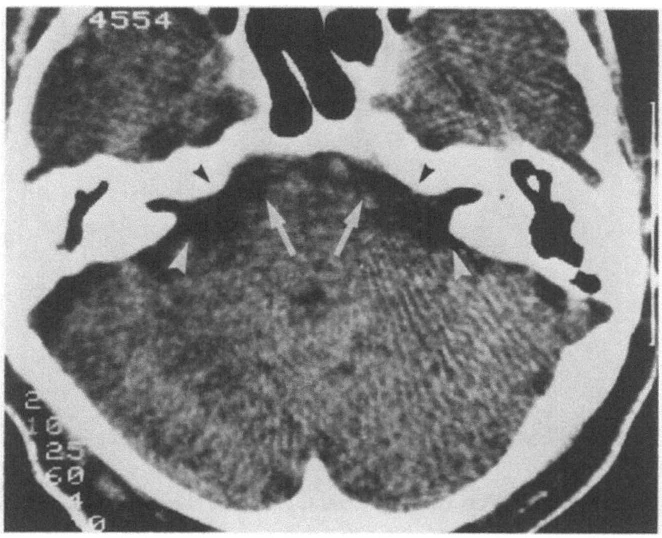

Fig. 4. Axial CT section at the level of the internal auditory canal. The pontocerebellar cistern appears as a triangularly shaped hypodensity, bounded medially by the pons (*arrows*), laterally by the posterior surface of the petrous bone (*black arrowheads*) and posteriorly by the flocculus (*white arrowheads*)

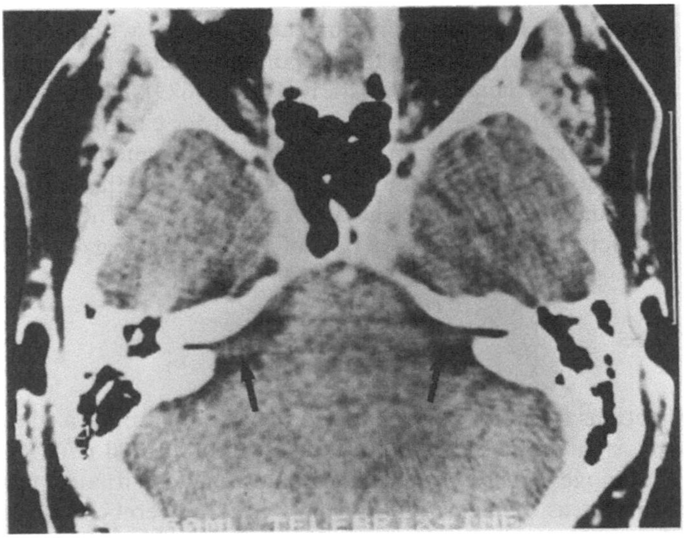

Fig. 5. Bilateral beam hardening and Hounsfield artifacts in the pontocerebellar cistern (*arrows*) should not be misinterpreted as pathology

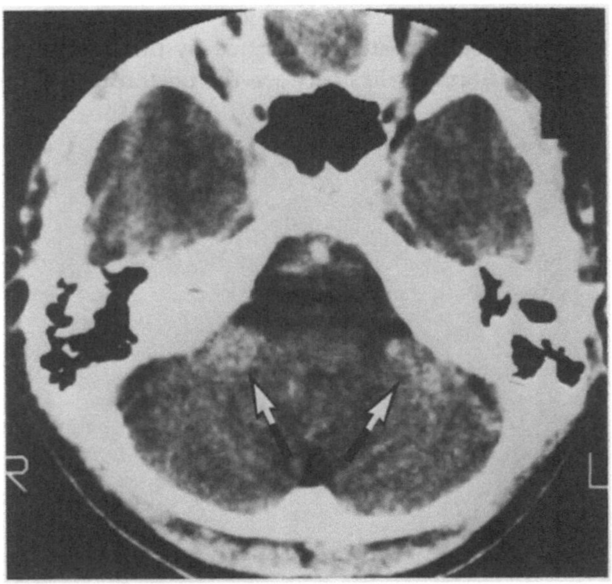

Fig. 6. Pseudotumor flocculi. Post contrast axial CT. Bilateral enhancement in the region of the flocculus (*arrows*)

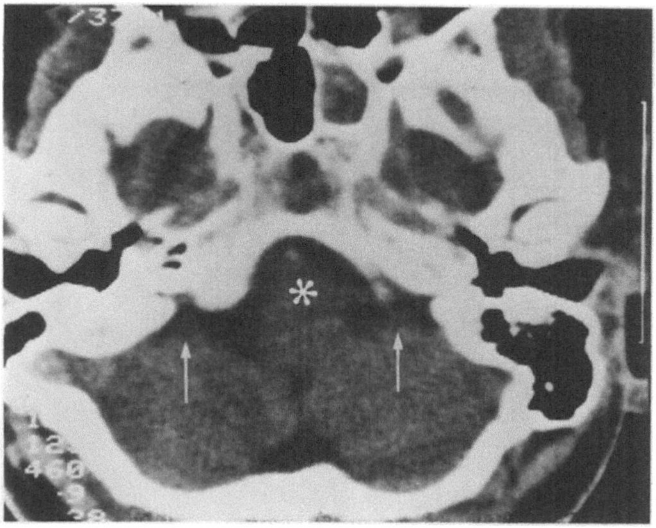

Fig. 7. Axial CT section through the lateral cerebellomedullary cistern. The cistern is bounded medially by the medulla (*asterisk*) and posteriorly by the cerebellum (*arrows*)

and the anterior cerebellar lobe (399). Axial CT sections display the flocculus between the brachium pontis and the cerebellar hemisphere (39). Like the vermis, the flocculus often shows more pronounced contrast enhancement than does the surrounding cerebellum (Fig. 6). The normal floccular blush or pseudotumor should not be misinterpreted as pathology (85, 274).

Inferiorly the triangular pontocerebellar cistern merges with the triangular lateral cerebellomedullary cistern. The lateral cerebellomedullary cistern is bounded laterally by the posterior surface of the petrous bone and the jugular foramen, medially by the medulla and dorsally by the cerebellum (Fig. 7). The lateral recess of the fourth ventricle empties into the lateral cerebellomedullary cistern between medulla and the cerebellum. The lateral recess contains enhancing choroid plexus that protrudes into the medial part of the lateral cerebellomedullary cistern and may overlie the flocculus (Fig. 8). Rarely the anterior inferior cerebellar artery is seen to course within the cerebellomedullary cistern (Fig. 9) (85). The glossopharyngeal, vagal and accessory nerves also run in the lateral cerebellomedullary cistern, but they are not visible on standard CT examinations.

The jugular tubercles are regularly seen to protrude upward into the inferior part of the lateral cerebellomedullary cistern (Fig. 10). These tubercles originate from the inferolateral clivus and lie medial to the jugular foramina (423). The tubercles are commonly asymmetrical in height, a finding best appreciated on direct coronal CT sections.

The upper portion of the pontocerebellar cistern is usually narrow, often slit-like. At this level, contrast enhanced CT scans often show a punctate density that represents the enhancing petrosal vein (Fig. 11).

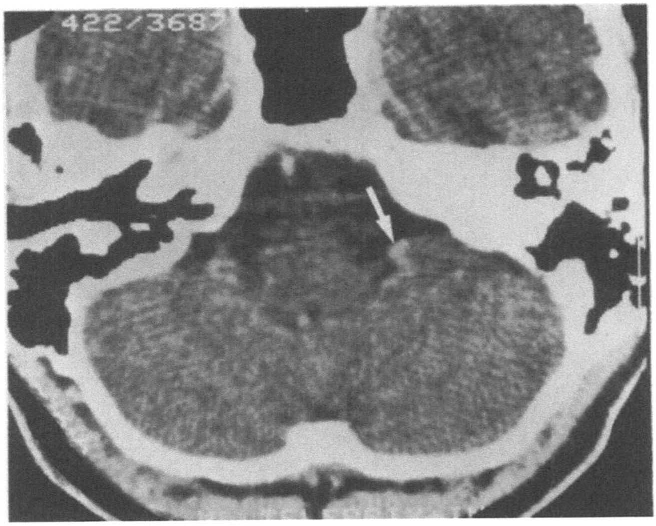

Fig. 8. Contrast enhanced axial CT section through the lateral recess of the fourth ventricle. The enhancing choroid plexus is seen as a curvilinear density (*arrow*) along the lateral recess, and protrudes into the lateral cerebellomedullary cistern

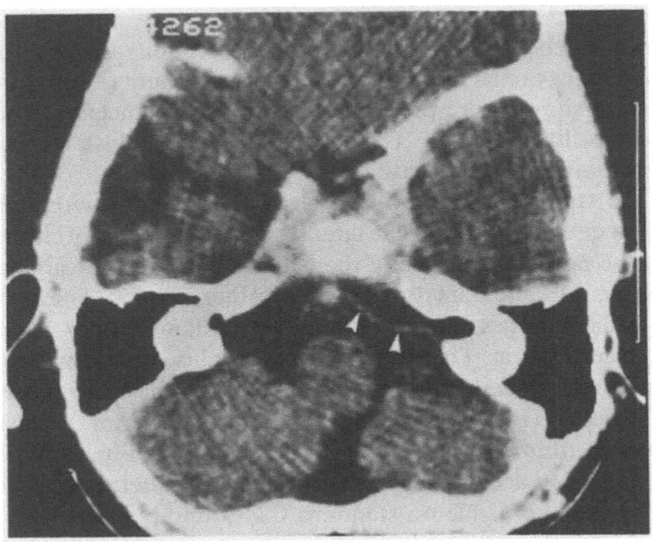

Fig. 9. Contrast enhanced axial CT section, showing the AICA (*arrowheads*) from its origin at the basilar artery to the internal auditory canal

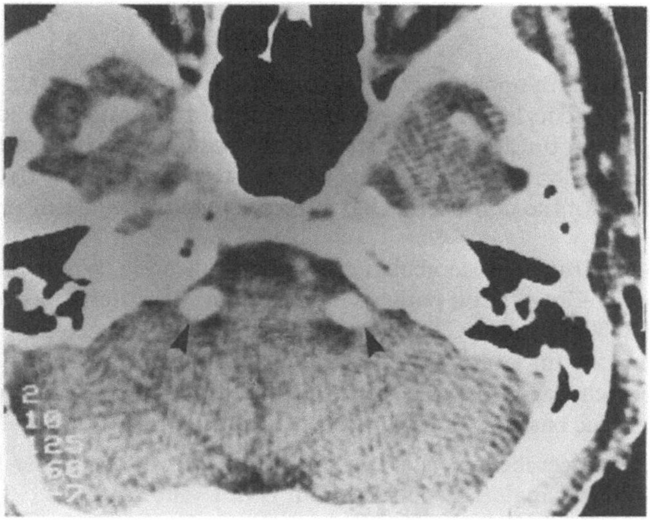

Fig. 10. Axial CT section through the lateral cerebellomedullary cistern. Symmetrical demonstration of the jugular tubercles (*arrowheads*) protruding into the cistern

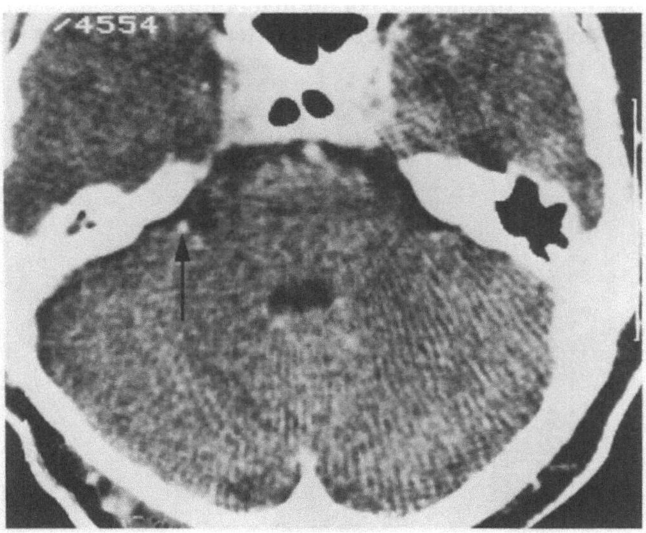

Fig. 11. Contrast enhanced axial CT section through the upper portion of the pontocerebellar cistern. The petrosal vein of Dandy (*arrow*) is seen as a punctate enhancement

Coronal Sections

In the coronal plane, the pontocerebellar cistern appears as a triangle with its tip pointing cranially and its largest dimension at the level of the internal auditory canal (Fig. 12). The lateral border of the cistern is the posterior surface of the petrous bone. Further cranially, the lateral border of the cistern is formed by the tentorium. The medial border of the pontocerebellar cistern is the ventro-lateral surface of the pons.

CT depiction of the pontocerebellar cistern depends upon the size of the cistern. Review of a large series of adult patients indicates that the cistern may be displayed successfully in 85% of routine CT studies, if special attention is given to this region and thin contiguous (or overlapping) sections are used.

The pontocerebellar cistern has been classified pneumoencephalographically into 3 groups on the basis of its size and the appearance of the petrosal vein (307):

- In 7%, the pontocerebellar cistern is small and ends at the upper level of the internal auditory canal. The petrosal vein is not visible.
- In 78%, the pontocerebellar cistern ends above the level of the internal auditory canal. The petrosal vein indents the superior margin of the cistern.
- In 15%, the cistern is large and the petrosal vein is completely surrounded by the cistern.

CT demonstrates similar findings: 5% of normal pontocerebellar cisterns are small and are visible on only one CT section. 80% of cisterns are of medium size, visible on

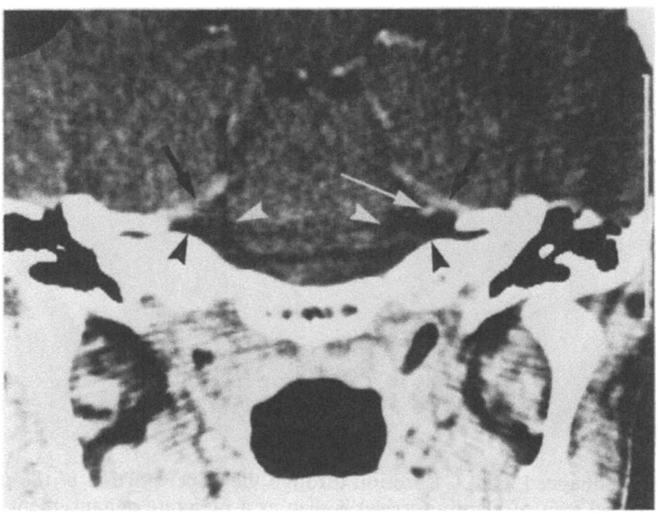

Fig. 12. Contrast enhanced coronal CT section at the level of the internal auditory canal. The pontocerebellar cistern has a triangular shape. It is bounded infero-laterally by the posterior surface of the petrous bone (*black arrowheads*), i.e. the internal auditory canal, medially by the pons (*white arrowheads*) and supero-laterally by the tentorium (*black arrows*). In the supero-lateral portion of the cistern punctate enhancement is seen, representing the petrosal vein of Dandy (*white arrow*)

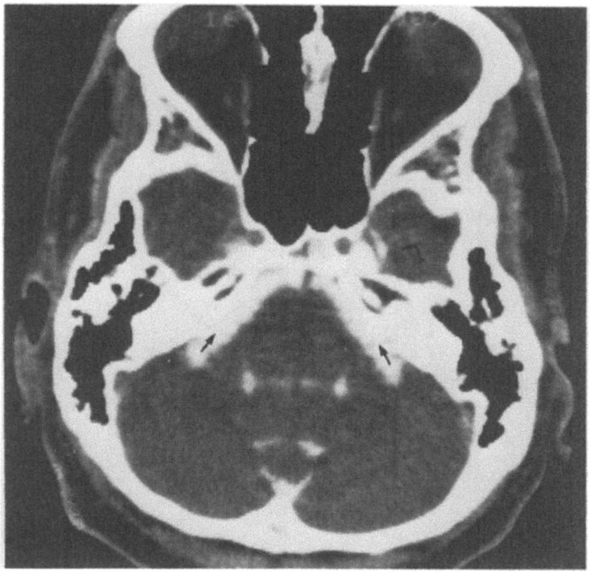

Fig. 13. Metrizamide CT cisternography. Axial section. The cisternal segment of the vestibulocochlear nerve is seen as a linear filling defect within the pontocerebellar cistern (*arrows*). The facial nerve is not discernible

3 contiguous sections and 15% are large cisterns, visible on more than 3 contiguous sections.

The petrosal vein may be visualized on contrast enhanced CT scans in approximately 65% of cases (Fig. 12). Visibility of the petrosal vein depends on the size of the cistern. The anterior inferior cerebellar artery is visible in 5% of the cases. The facial and vestibulocochlear nerves can not be visualized on standard CT scans.

Display of the anterior inferior cerebellar artery and of the fifth, seventh and eighth cranial nerves is improved by meatocisternography. Water soluble positive contrast CT cisternography demonstrates the cisternal segments of the facial and verstibulocochlear nerves as linear filling defects in the opacified cistern (Fig. 13). However, the intracanalicular segments of the facial and verstibulocochlear nerves are rarely demonstrated. The anterior inferior cerebellar artery is seen only occasionally on water soluble positive-contrast CT cisternography.

Gas CT cisternography provides more accurate delineation of the nerves and vessels coursing through the pontocerebellar cistern (Fig. 14) (444, 577). This technique has limited value when used in conjunction with second generation CT equipment (26, 281, 336). When combined with late generation CT equipment and high resolution algorithms, the technique can demonstrate the neurovascular bundle in approximately 90% of cases (439, 443, 444, 577). In 80% of these cases, the facial and the vestibulocochlear nerves can be demonstrated as separate structures. In 20% of these cases, both nerves form a single bundle. The facial nerve courses anterior to the vestibulocochlear nerve. The intermediate nerve that runs between

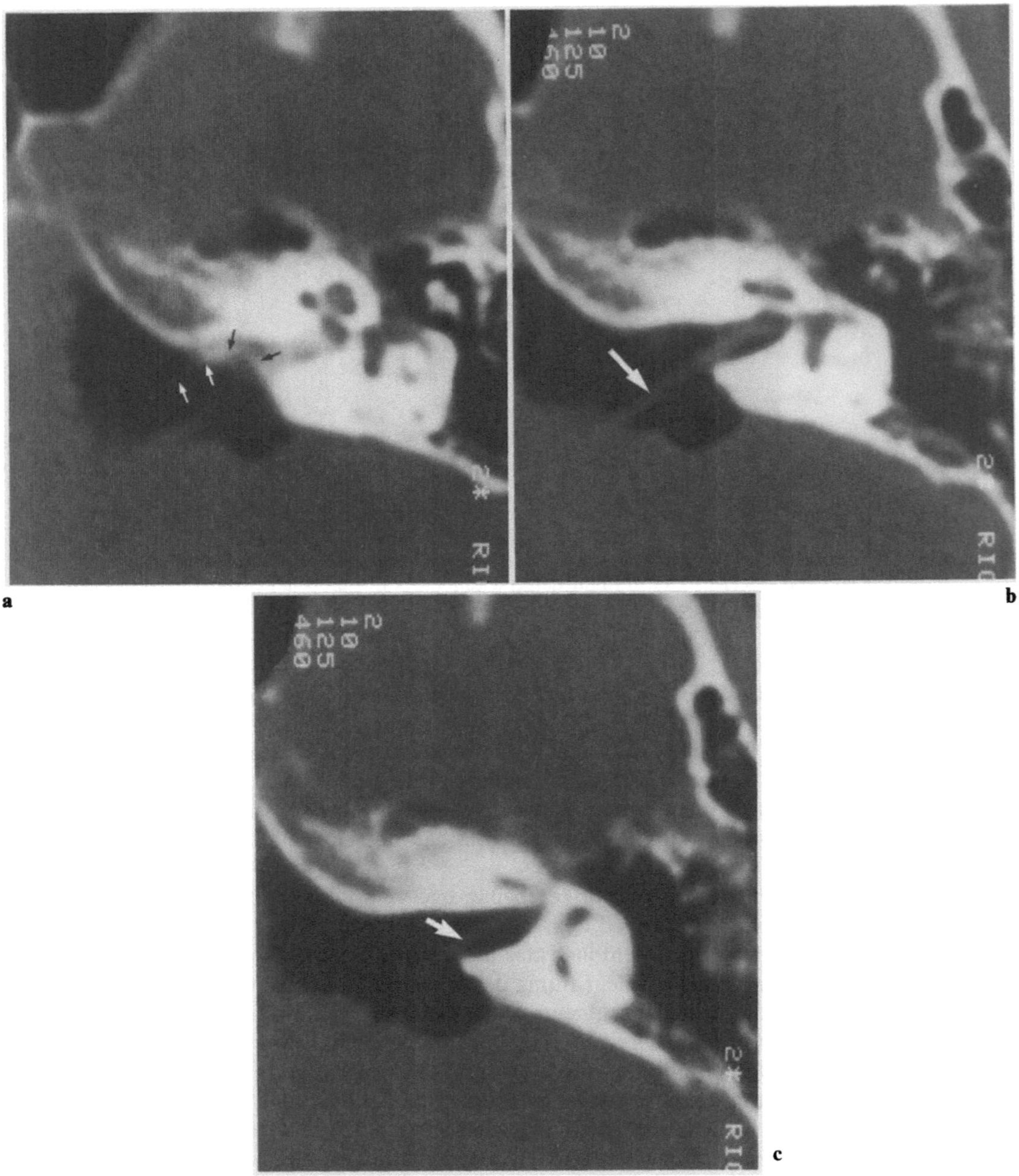

a b c

Fig. 14a–c. Gas CT cisternography. Axial CT. **a** Section at the lower level of the internal auditory canal demonstrates the AICA (*short arrows*), with its loop located at the porus, **b** section at the level of the vestibule demonstrates the entire course of the vestibulocochlear nerve (*arrow*) from its exit at the pons to the fundus of the internal auditory canal, **c** section through the upper portion of the internal auditory canal demonstrates the facial nerve in its intrameatal course (*arrow*) as well as its entry into the Fallopian canal the facial and vestibulocochlear nerves has not yet been demonstrated by gas CT cisternography. Even on macroscopic dissections, the intermediate nerve cannot be separated from the vestibular division of the vestibulocochlear nerve in 20% of cases (474).

The Anterior Inferior Cerebellar Artery

In more than 70% of cases the anterior inferior cerebellar artery (AICA) originates from the caudal or middle third of the basilar artery and courses caudo-laterally along the belly of the pons to reach the pontocerebellar cistern (385, 554). At this level it often divides into medial and lateral branches (554) which supply the flocculus and the biventral lobule respectively. The lateral branch of the anterior inferior cerebellar artery then forms a loop that runs rostro-laterally in intimate relationship with the intracisternal segments of the facial and vestibulocochlear nerves to approach, or enter, the internal auditory porus. Thereafter the artery loops back, medially, to reach the brachium pontis. The proximal portion of the arterial loop usually lies ventro-medial to the facial and vestibulocochlear nerves. The distal portion usually runs dorso-medial to the nerves en route to the cerebellum (554). The precise relationship among the anterior inferior cerebellar artery, the nerves and the internal auditory porus are detailed in other works (12, 36, 133, 185, 346, 380, 424, 496, 602, 609). In combined series the meatal loop of the anterior inferior cerebellar artery lies outside the porus acusticus in 53% of cases

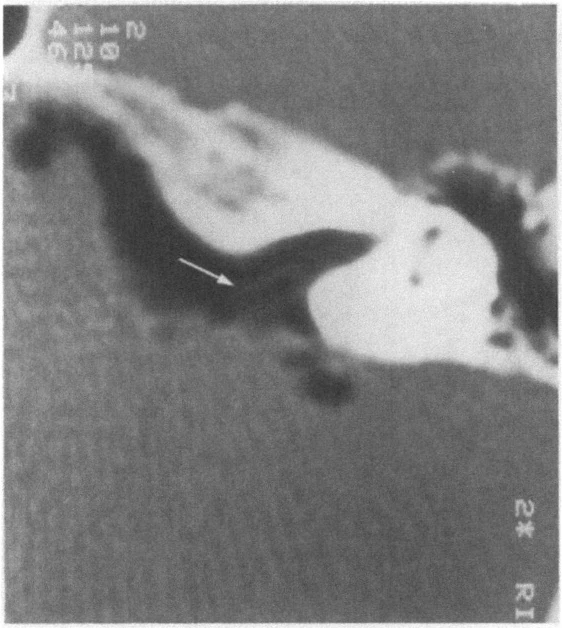

Fig. 15. Gas CT cisternography. Axial CT section demonstrates the loop of the AICA located at the porus acusticus internus (*arrow*)

(Fig. 15), at the porus acusticus internus in 25% of cases and within the porus acusticus in 22% of cases (36, 346, 424, 496). The relationship of the meatal loop to the seventh and eighth nerves has been studied by different authors (346, 424, 496). The loop is situated below the nerves in 45% of cases. It lies between the nerves in 41% of cases and above the nerves in 7% of cases. The anterior inferior cerebellar artery forms no loop within the cistern in 7% of cases.

Gas CT cisternography demonstrates the cisternal loop of the anterior inferior cerebellar artery in more than 50% of cases (Fig. 15) (26, 33, 439, 444, 577). Pulsations of the anterior inferior cerebellar artery cause "blurring" of the vessel and may be responsible for the low rate of visualization (472). Used together, intravenous contrast enhancement and gas CT cisternography demonstrate the anterior inferior cerebellar artery loop in approximately 80% of cases (577).

The Internal Auditory Canal

The internal auditory canal (synonym: acoustic meatus) is the conduit through which the facial, vestibulocochlear and intermediate nerves and the labyrinthine vessels course between the inner ear and the cerebello-pontine angle (Fig. 16). The canal lies along a coronal plane. Thus, the canal inclines 45° to the obliquely oriented posterior surface of the petrous pyramid. The lateral end of the canal, called the fundus, is formed by the cribriform plate of the bone. The intracranial opening of the canal, called the porus acusticus internus, is open to the pontocerebellar cistern. Because the posterior surface of the petrous pyramid is oblique to the canal, the ostium of the canal has an oval shape oriented with its long axis parallel to the long axis of the petrous bone.

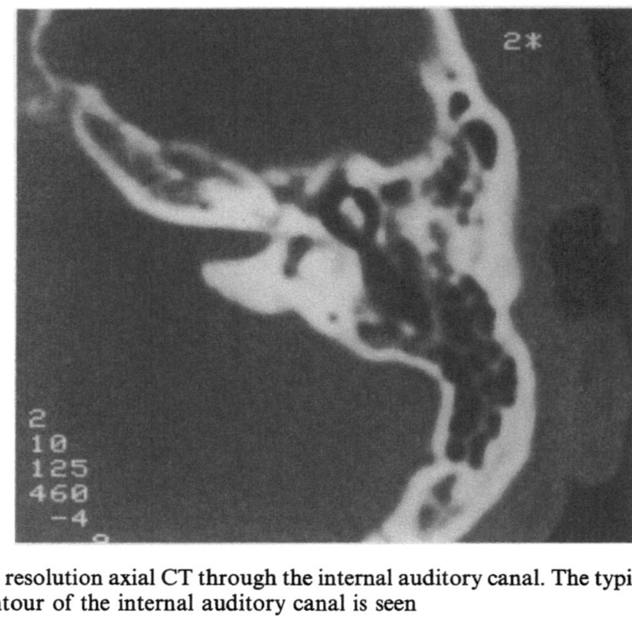

Fig. 16. High resolution axial CT through the internal auditory canal. The typical appearance of the bony contour of the internal auditory canal is seen

The porus is located in the antero-medial half of the middle third of the posterior surface of the petrous bone. The internal auditory canal is completely lined by dura and pia-arachnoid. The subarachnoid space extends laterally for the entire length of the internal auditory canal. At the fundus of the canal, the subarachnoid space communicates with the perilymphatic space of the epineurium. The nerves are covered by pia mater.

The posterior, lateral and inferior margins of the porus acusticus internus are formed by a dense bony ridge. The supero-medial end of the porus merges with the posterior surface of the petrous bone. At the fundus of the canal, the falciform crest of the cribriform plate divides the canal into a smaller superior and a larger inferior compartment. A very small crest – Bill's bar – subdivides the superior compartment into anterior and posterior portions. Similarly, the small inferior vertical crest subdivides the inferior compartment into anterior and posterior portions. Each of these four compartments contains a specific nerve: The antero-superior compartment contains the facial nerve. The antero-inferior compartment contains the cochlear nerve. The postero-superior compartment contains the superior division of the vestibular nerve, and the postero-inferior compartment contains the inferior division of the vestibular nerve.

The superior and inferior walls of the internal auditory canal are displayed most clearly in the coronal plane (Fig. 17). In this plane, the canal usually appears as a horizontal tube with nearly parallel superior und inferior margins (72%) (577). However, there is considerable normal variation. In 17.5% of our cases the canal exhibited central narrowing. In 10% of cases it had an oval or elliptical cross section in the coronal plane. In a single case (0.5%) the canal was narrow medially and wide laterally. Similar observations have been reported by Camp and Cilley (32) and Valvassori (588). The incidence of medial narrowing of the canal appears to vary.

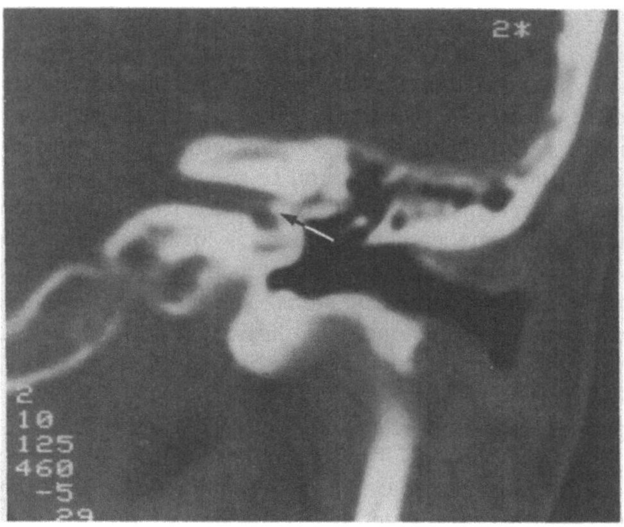

Fig. 17. Coronal high resolution CT through the internal auditory canal at the cochlear level. At the fundus of the internal auditory canal the falciform crest (*arrow*) subdivides the lateral portion of the internal auditory canal into an inferior and superior compartment

Table 1. Dimensions of the internal auditory canal: 200 high resolution CT examinations (577) (Measurements given in millimeters)

	Height (vertical diameter)	Antero-posterior diameter	Length of the posterior margin
Minimal	2.0	2.0	4.0
Maximal	6.0	7.0	15.0
Mean	3.9	4.6	8.2

Valvassori (588) found no instance in 300 canals studied, whereas Camp and Cilley (52) observed medial narrowing of the canal in 12% of 500 cases. These discordances may reflect differences in the techniques used to examine the canal. Based upon our own material, it seems probable, that the medially narrow canal can be a rare normal variant. A canal that is narrow medially and wide laterally is *not necessarily* abnormal.

The left and right internal auditory canals were asymmetrical in 13% of our material. Measurements of the diameters of the canals and of the lengths of the posterior surfaces of the internal auditory canals are given in Table 1. These measurements correlate well with the measurements previously published in the literature (52, 116, 177, 588).

The Jugular Foramen

The jugular foramen is the conduit by which the jugular vein and cranial nerves nine, ten and eleven pass through the skull base. The jugular foramen connects the lateral cerebellomedullary cistern with the upper paravertebral extracranial space. The endocranial opening of the jugular foramen is related to the cerebellum cranially, to the hypoglossal canal medially, to the petrosal sinus inferiorly and to the internal auditory canal supero-laterally. The exocranial opening is related to the floor of the middle ear cavity, to the stylomastoid foramen and styloid process laterally, to the carotid canal centrally and to the occipital condyle medially.

The jugular foramen is divided into two compartments by a fibro-cartilaginous or osseous bridge. The smaller compartment is located antero-medially and is designated the pars nervosa of the jugular foramen. This contains the glossopharyngeal nerve and the inferior petrosal sinus. The larger compartment is located posteriorly and is designated the pars vascularis. It contains the jugular bulb, the vagal and accessory nerves and the tympanic branch of the ascending pharyngeal artery (Fig. 18) (86).

In our experience the important relationships of the jugular foramen are displayed best by high resolution CT in the axial projection. Anteriorly, the vertical portion of the carotid canal is separated from the jugular foramen by a thin bony ridge. The canal for Jacobson's nerve lies postero-lateral to the carotid canal. Coronal views are most appropriate for depicting the thin hypotympanic bone plate that separates the jugular bulb from the hypotympanum and for displaying the hypoglossal canal that is situated medial to the jugular foramen.

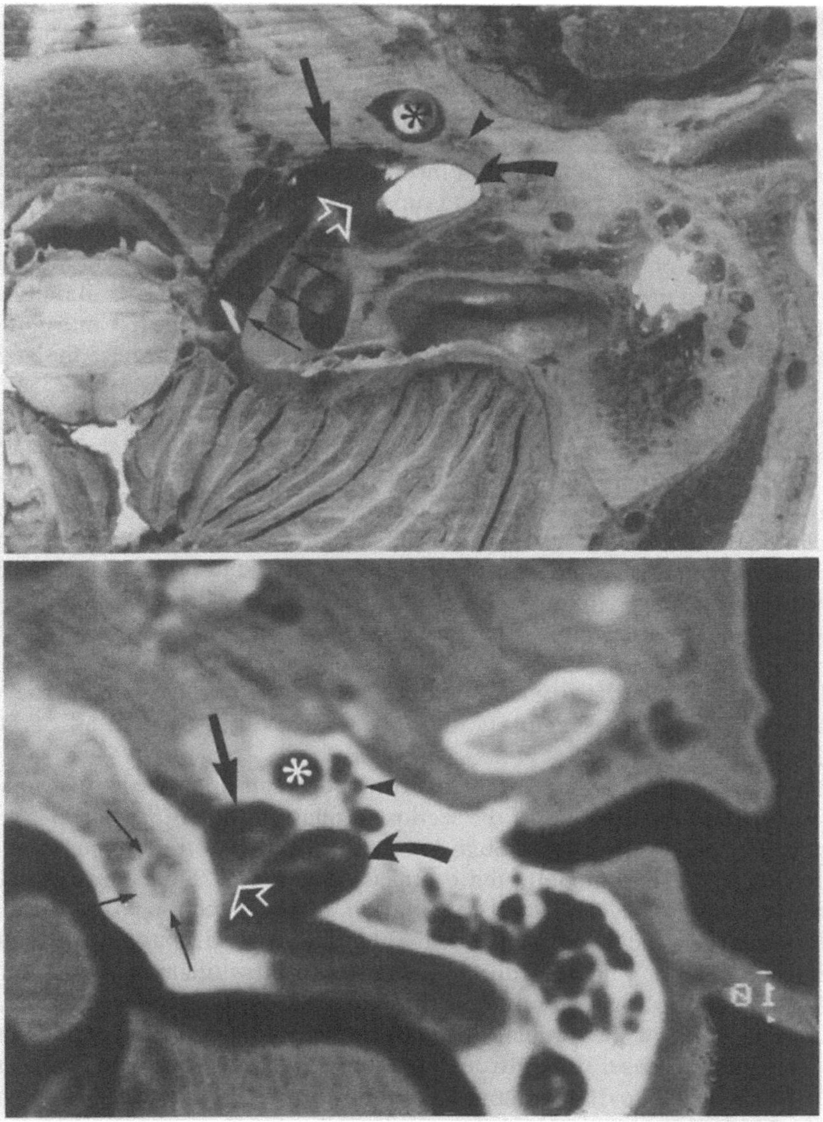

a

b

Fig. 18a, b. Jugular foramen, axial sections (different specimens). **a** Cryotomic section, **b** CT-section. Both portions of the jugular foramen, the anteriorly located pars nervosa (*thick arrow*) and the posteriorly located pars vascularis (*curved arrow*) are identified. They are separated by a fibrous band (*open arrow*). The hypoglossal canal (*small black arrows*) is visible medial to the jugular foramen. The carotid canal (*asterisk*) lies anterior to the jugular foramen. Jacobson's canal (*arrowhead*) is located postero-lateral to the carotid canal

The two jugular foramina are commonly different in size. In cases of asymmetry, the right foramen is usually larger than the left (13, 101). This asymmetry involves only the vascular part of the foramen and in general correlates with the size of the transverse and sigmoid sinuses.

The Tentorial Incisura

Synonyms: tentorial hiatus, tentorial notch, incisura tentorii

The tentorium is a double fold of dura that creates the tentlike roof of the posterior fossa (250). Laterally the tentorium inserts onto the occipital and petrous bones along the courses of the transverse and superior petrosal sinuses. Anteriorly the free medial margins of the tentorium insert onto the anterior clinoid processes, while the lateral margins of the tentorium continue from the petrous pyramids to the posterior clinoid processes as the petroclinoid ligaments. In the dorsal midline, the tentorium merges with the falx, enclosing the straight sinus. The free margins of the tentorium begin at the anterior clinoid processes, pass laterally around the midbrain and end posteriorly where the vein of Galen enters the straight sinus (47, 546). The laterally convex free tentorial margins define the tentorial incisura. In essence, the incisura tentorii is just the space or gap between the free medial margins. Through this gap the supratentorial compartment communicates with the infratentorial compartment. The tentorial incisura has the shape of a gothic arch, that stands on the clinoid processes and has its apex at the straight sinus (389). The anterior part of the incisura contains the mesencephalon. The posterior part contains the superior vermis (rarely the splenium of the corpus callosum instead) (47, 389, 546). The quadrigeminal plate cistern is located at the level of the tentorial incisura, between the mesencephalon and the superior vermis.

The tentorium is an extracerebral fibrous structure that lies outside the blood-brain barrier. It enhances regularly and is always seen on post contrast CT (156, 170, 389, 406).

On CT sections, the shape of the tentorium depends upon the angulation of the CT section and the position of the section in relation to the torcular (389). A CT section that passes directly through the incisura displays the full contour of the enhancing medial margin of the tentorium as a gothic arch. Such images are usually achieved only with negative gantry angulation. If the CT section passes through the tentorium above the torcular, but below the free tentorial margin, the tentorium resembles the letter V. If a portion of the posterior falx is included dorsal to the V, tentorium and falx together resemble the letter Y. If the CT section passes through the tentorium below the torcular, the tentorium appears as two diverging bands. If the CT section passes directly through the torcular, the tentorium may present as a letter M, created by partial volume superimposition of the V and the two diverging bands. In all such cases – V, Y, M and diverging bands – the anteriormost ends of the tentorial blush represent the free medial margins of the tentorium. Therefore the space between the anteriormost ends of the tentorial blush is the incisura.

The nature and extent of supratentorial growth is documented by the relationship of the tumor mass to the incisura. Any mass that passes between the anterior ends of the tentorial blushes is crossing the incisura. If the mass protrudes above (anterior to) the anterior ends of the tentorial bands, it has entered the supratentorial space. If the mass remains below (posterior to) the anterior ends of the tentorial bands, it remains infratentorial.

General Principles for the CT Diagnosis of Cerebello-Pontine Angle Lesions

Cerebello-pontine angle lesions are infratentorial extraaxial masses located within the pontocerebellar cistern. These must be distinguished from contiguous intraaxial lateral cerebellar and pontine lesions. The following signs have proved useful for differentiating the extraaxial cerebello-pontine angle lesions from intraaxial masses (387):

1. Continuity of the lateral tumor margin with the posterior surface of the petrous bone or with the tentorium. This sign is found in 72 to 100% of cerebello-pontine angle lesions. It has low specificity, since it may also be observed with intraaxial tumors located in the pons, cerebellar peduncle or lateral cerebellum (387, 574, 575).

2. The most reliable sign of an extraaxial tumor is "paradoxical" widening of the ipsilateral pontocerebellar cistern (Fig. 19) (387, 574, 575). This sign is well known from earlier pneumoencephalographic studies (308, 312, 313, 490). "Paradoxical" widening of the cistern results from medial displacement of the pons and cerebellum by the infratentorial mass. This "paradoxical" cisternal widening

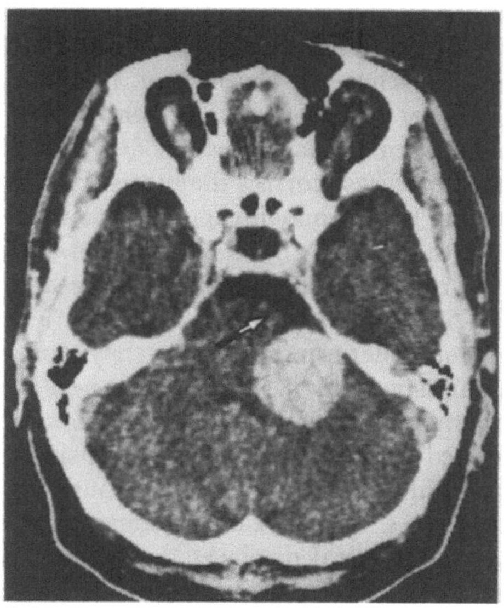

Fig. 19. Paradoxical widening of the pontocerebellar cistern in a case of acoustic neurinoma. Axial post contrast CT shows ipsilateral widening of the anterior portion of the pontocerebellar cistern (*arrows*)

occurs at the anterior and posterior portions of the pontocerebellar cistern, which are not filled by tumor. This highly specific sign is found in only 17 to 30% of the cases examined by CT and is most common with small to medium-sized cerebello-pontine angle tumors (387, 574). The low incidence of such widening is explained by the fact that voluminous tumors completely fill the cistern, obliterating it rather than widening it.

Pontocerebellar masses may also cause "paradoxical" widening of the infratentorial part of the ipsilateral ambient cistern. This sign indicates that the tumor has 1) displaced pons and midbrain medially, 2) rotated them and 3) displaced the cerebellum cranially and laterally, thereby widening the space between brainstem and cerebellum. This sign is found in 60 to 80% of medium- and large-sized acoustic neurinomas (308, 574).

For identical reasons, pontocerebellar tumors that displace the pons may also cause widening of the lateral cerebellomedullary cistern (308). The sign has been present in 67% of cases studied by CT in the authors' series and has been reported to be present in 90% of the cases studied by pneumoencephalography (308).

3. Bone changes. Bone erosion, infiltration and hyperostosis are observed commonly with extraaxial tumors (90%) and infrequently with strictly intraaxial tumors. Acoustic neurinomas, meningiomas and other tumors often produce nearly specific osseous changes, contributing to the correct histologic diagnosis.

4. Sharp margin of the tumor. This criterion is the least specific of the criteria for extraaxial tumor location, since many intraaxial lesions (e.g. hematomas, hemangioblastomas or metastases) also present sharp margins.

Each of the criteria above has its own specificity. The greater the number of criteria fulfilled, the more reliable the diagnosis of an extraaxial cerebello-pontine angle lesion becomes. Other criteria, such as configuration of the fourth ventricle, cisternal obliterations, presence or absence of peritumoral edema, and the configuration and degree of contrast enhancement proved to be unreliable for differentiating intraaxial from extraaxial lesions (387, 388, 391).

In a limited number of cases, correct diagnosis may be impossible. Primary *extra*axial, slowly growing lesions may invaginate into the adjacent cerebellum or pons and come to mimic the signs of an intraaxial lesion (357). Conversely primary *intra*axial lesions may grow into the extraaxial space and behave like primary extraaxial lesions (387, 574).

As extraaxial pontocerebellar tumors enlarge, they grow toward or through the incisura in fairly characteristic fashion. In most cases pontocerebellar tumors grow upward within the subarachnoid cisterns and remain confined within the cisterns. Such growth is designated upward transcisternal transincisural growth.

Initially pontocerebellar tumors grow large enough to reach, compress and rotate the pons. This causes "paradoxical" widening of the ipsilateral pontocerebellar cistern and contralateral displacement of the fourth ventricle. As the tumor enlarges further it begins to compress and elevate the cerebellum, separating it from the brainstem. This causes widening of the ipsilateral ambient cistern. At the same time that the tumor grows medially, it also extends along the lateral wall of the posterior fossa. Especially with acoustic neurinomas, the lateral margin of the

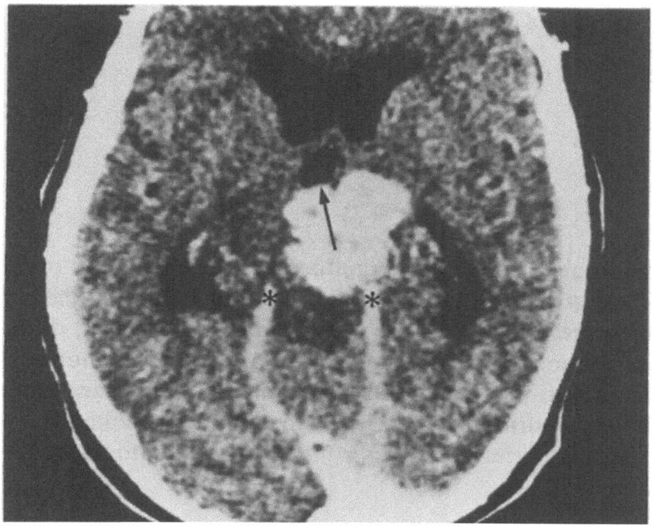

Fig. 20. Transcisternal, transincisural extension of left-sided cerebello-pontine angle tumor (acoustic neurinoma). The tumor extends through the incisura (*asterisks*) into the supratentorial space and causes angular cutoff of the posterior third ventricle (*arrow*)

tumor is initially confined to the posterior surface of the petrous pyramid. As the tumor enlarges, the posterior margin reaches and then flattens out against the undersurface of the tentorium. In long-standing cases, it may thin the tentorium and bulge it upward.

With further tumor growth, the mass begins to bulge upward toward or into the incisura. The lateral border of the tumor comes in contact with the ipsilateral free margin of the tentorium. The tumor now fills and obliterates the quadrigeminal plate cistern, rotates the midbrain, and displaces it superiorly. It compresses the aqueduct and may cause obstructive hydrocephalus. Further upward growth of tumors typically compresses and displaces the obstructed third ventricle producing a characteristic angular cutoff of the posterior third ventricle (Fig. 20) (558). The mass grows between the thalamus and the temporal lobe, causing supero-lateral displacement of the ipsilateral obstructed temporal horn.

Malignant and invasive tumors such as sarcomas and chemodectomas may extend supratentorially by infiltration of the tentorium and destruction of the petrous apex. This form of supratentorial spread should be called true transtentorial tumor extension (387, 390). Differentiation from transcisternal, transincisural extension may be difficult. If the tumor is visualized simultaneously both medial to the tentorial margin and lateral to the insertion of the tentorium at the petrous bone, this is a strong indication for the presence of true transtentorial extension. Thickening or splitting of the tentorium also indicates true transtentorial extension (390).

Pathology of the Cerebello-Pontine Angle

The most common neoplasms of the pontocerebellar cistern are primary tumors that originate from structures normally located in or bounding the cistern. These structures include the cranial nerves, vessels, arachnoid mater, dura mater and bone. The most common primary cerebello-pontine angle tumor is the acoustic neurinoma. The second most common is meningioma. All other primary tumors such as epidermoids, neurinomas of other cranial nerves, arachnoid cysts, primary melanomas etc. are very rare. The relative frequencies of pontocerebellar tumors are given in Table 2.

Table 2. Classification and frequency of cerebello-pontine angle lesions

	Revilla (1947)		Zülch (1956)	Yaşargil (1978)		Authors' material	
	No.	%	%	No.	%	No.	%
Primary tumors of the cerebello-pontine angle							
Acoustic neurinoma	154	75.1	79.2	164	66.2	275	60.5
Meningioma	13	6.3	6.7	24	9.7	31	6.8
Epidermoid	13	6.3	4.6	10	4	17	3.7
Arachnoid cyst	–	–	0.4	2	0.8	9	2.0
Neurinoma of the fifth, seventh, ninth, tenth, and eleventh nerves	10	4.9	–	9	3.6	18	4.0
Primary melanoma	1	0.5	–	2	0.8	1	0.2
Hemangioma	–	–	–	–	–	3	0.7
Secondary tumors of the cerebello-pontine angle							
Chemodectoma	1	0.5	–	2	0.8	47	10.3
Ceruminoma	–	–	–	–	–	1	0.2
Chondroma	–	–	0.4	1	0.4	2	0.4
Chordoma	–	–	–	2	0.8	8	1.8
Cerebellar and petrous bone tumors infiltrating the cerebello-pontine angle	13	6.4	1.9	16	6.4	6	1.3
Metastases	–	–	1.4	2	0.8	12	2.6
Vascular lesions							
Aneurysm	–	–	–	11	4.5	4	0.9
Arterio-venous malformation	–	–	–	3	1.2	4	0.9
Megadolichobasilar anomaly	–	–	–	–	–	17	3.7

Intraaxial and extraaxial tumors that originate outside the pontocerebellar cistern may invade the cerebello-pontine angle secondarily. This group of "secondary tumors" of the cerebello-pontine angle includes chemodectomas, chordomas, meningiomas of the tentorium and foramen magnum, intrinsic tumors of the petrous bone, medulloblastomas and ependymomas.

Metastases arising within or secondarily growing into the cerebello-pontine angle are rare. Vascular lesions of the angle such as aneurysms and arteriovenous malformations are also rare. However the megadolichobasilar anomaly is observed in a surprisingly high proportion of aged patients.

Acoustic Neurinoma

1 General Considerations

A. Nomenclature, Statistics, and Pathology

The acoustic neurinoma is a benign, slowly growing and encapsulated tumor that originates from the Schwann cell (74, 184, 327, 376, 441, 447, 492). The correct designation therefore is "Schwannoma". However, the term "acoustic neurinoma" is so widely accepted, it will also be used in this book.

Acoustic neurinomas constitute 5 to 10% of all intracranial tumors and 70 to 90% of cerebello-pontine angle tumors (230, 417, 473, 586, 629, 641). They occur most frequently between 30 and 60 years of age with a slight female preponderance (203, 641). The occurrence of an acoustic neurinoma may be an expression of von Recklinghausen's neurofibromatosis (252, 563). In such cases, the neurinomas tend to manifest far earlier and are predominantly bilateral (though not necessarily at the same time). Acoustic neurinomas arise at the transition zone where the glial cells of the nerve sheath change to Schwann cells. This transition zone is usually located within the internal auditory canal, so acoustic neurinomas usually originate within the internal auditory canal (25). In rare cases, the transition from glial to Schwann cells is located more proximally within the cerebello-pontine angle. Rarely, acoustic neurinomas may then originate medial to the internal auditory canal within the pontocerebellar cistern (25, 184).

For unknown reasons, the Schwann cells along the superior vestibular nerve exhibit an unusually high rate of turnover (so-called "over production"). Perhaps for this reason the commonest site of origin of acoustic neurinomas is along the superior vestibular nerve (25). Neurinomas originate from the cochlear nerve with the same low frequency as neurinomas of the other cranial and spinal nerves (98, 247, 381).

B. Clinical Presentation

The clinical symptomatology associated with an acoustic neurinoma correlates well with the size of the tumor, since the symptoms result primarily from the pressure exerted upon the neighbouring structures (202). The initial symptom of acoustic neurinoma is usually a slowly progressive sensorineural hearing loss, with or without tinnitus (138). In 5 to 15% of patients, the acoustic neurinoma presents as an acute hearing loss, apparently related to either intratumoral bleeding or acute compression of the internal auditory artery (25, 215, 344, 456).

Vestibular symptoms usually appear late, even though the tumor originates from the vestibular nerve. The first clinically detectable vestibular symptoms are gait disturbance and dizziness (203, 318, 344, 415, 510). Slow growth rate of the tumor and central compensatory mechanisms (202) appear to account for 1) the frequent, long delay between the onset of sensorineural hearing loss and the correct diagnosis of an acoustic neurinoma and 2) the late onset of vestibular symptoms.

With increasing tumor size and tumor extension into the cerebello-pontine angle, additional symptoms arise from compression of neighbouring structures (25, 143, 344, 530), including the adjacent cranial nerves, cerebellar hemispheres and ventricular system.

Compression of the trigeminal (fifth cranial) nerve produces palsy characterized by decrease or loss of sensation in the face. The most important clinical sign of trigeminal compression is loss of the corneal reflex. In exceptional cases trigeminal palsy may manifest instead as neuralgia. Cerebello-pontine angle tumors almost never cause palsy of the motor division of the trigeminal nerve, so atrophy of the masticatory muscles is almost never observed.

The facial (seventh cranial) nerve is the motor nerve of the facial musculature. Compression of the facial nerve causes facial palsy manifesting as weakness of the facial (mimic) musculature on the affected side. Partial paresis is easily diagnosed by difference in the closing force of the eyelid. In cases of peripheral facial palsy the whole territory of the facial nerve is affected, whereas in cases of central facial palsy, the forehead partially retains its motility.

The vestibulocochlear (statoacoustic, eighth cranial) nerve is divided into a vestibular and a cochlear division. Compression of the cochlear division by a cerebello-pontine angle mass usually causes slowly progressive sensorineural hearing loss. The patient himself may not be aware of the impaired hearing. Compression of the cochlear nerve may also cause tinnitus. In rare instances neural compression is expressed as an acute hearing loss. Involvement of the vestibular division of the eighth cranial nerve causes vertigo. This deficit may be compensated centrally. However, a lesion of the vestibular nerve is easily recognized by laboratory tests (caloric vestibular testing, electronystagmography).

For diagnostic purposes, the main functions of the glossopharyngeal (ninth cranial) nerve are sensory innervation of the posterior tongue, including taste, and motor innervation of the pharyngeal musculature. Glossopharyngeal palsy from compression of the nerve is diagnosed by loss of taste in the posterior tongue and loss of the gag reflex. Patients may complain of slight difficulties in swallowing.

The vagal (tenth cranial) nerve courses through the whole of the neck and thorax to reach the abdomen. Together with the glossopharyngeal, the intermediate and the accessory nerves, the vagal nerve forms part of the parasympathetic system. The pharyngeal, laryngeal and recurrent laryngeal branches of the vagal nerve are important for diagnosis. Palsies of the pharyngeal and laryngeal branches cause difficulties in swallowing. Palsy of the recurrent laryngeal branch causes hoarseness, since this branch is the motor laryngeal nerve.

The accessory (eleventh cranial) nerve is the motor nerve of the sternocleidomastoid and trapezius muscles. Palsy of the accessory nerve causes weakness in the sternocleidomastoid and trapazius muscles. Clinically, this manifests as diminished force when elevating the shoulder.

The hypoglossal (twelfth cranial) nerve is the main motor nerve of the tongue. Hypoglossal palsy is easily recognized by ipsilateral palsy and atrophy of the tongue.

The major function of the cerebellum is motor coordination. Large ponto-cerebellar masses cause cerebellar dysfunction that is easily recognized by ataxia. Various neurological tests allow recognition of more subtle functional disorders of the cerebellum. Compression of the fourth ventricle and aqueduct may cause impaired cerebro-spinal fluid circulation that leads to obstructive hydrocephalus, headache and papilledema.

The rare medial type of acoustic neurinoma that originates outside – medial to – the internal auditory canal, usually presents with the full clinical symptomatology of cerebello-pontine angle tumors (45).

C. Clinical Laboratory Evaluation

Patients with possible acoustic neurinoma undergo extensive otoneurological work-up prior to any radiographic evaluation of tumor size and location. This clinico-laboratory testing includes:

a) audiometry (164, 244, 344)
b) caloric vestibular testing (138, 317)
c) electronystagmography (160, 216, 248, 344, 568)
d) stapedial reflex testing (164, 216, 241, 244, 420, 525, 529), and
e) electric response audiometry (auditory evoked potentials) (66, 453, 525, 563).

In patients with acoustic neurinomas, audiometry provides evidence of a retrocochlear hearing loss in up to 95% of cases. Caloric vestibular testing is positive in up to 94% of cases. Electronystagmography is positive in 78 to 98% of cases, and the stapedial reflex is decreased or lost in 71 to 100% of cases. Brainstem electric response audiometry has a diagnostic accuracy of 98% and is the most sensitive non invasive test for patients with an acoustic neurinoma. Normal brainstem electric response audiometry nearly excludes an acoustic neurinoma (23, 202). Used as a screening survey, the combination of both brainstem electric response audiometry and contrast enhanced CT identifies up to 99% of acoustic neurinomas (23, 35).

2 Conventional Radiology

A. Plain Radiography and Geometric Tomography

In most institutions, several different radiographic projections are used for the initial evaluation of possible acoustic neurinoma. These include

1. transorbital view of the petrous bones, projecting each internal auditory canal into each orbit (521),
2. Stenvers' view (542), providing good delineation of both the fundus and porus of the internal auditory canal, and

3. anteroposterior pluridirectional tomography, providing the best demonstration of the osseous structures of the petrous bones (585).

Acoustic neurinomas usually cause erosion and widening of the internal auditory canal. Such erosion may take on different radiographic appearances including:

1. Enlargement of the full length of one internal auditory canal.
2. Enlargement of the middle third of one internal auditory canal (so-called ampullary enlargement).
3. Spherical enlargement of the porus of the internal auditory canal, and
4. non specific erosion of the petrous apex.

Ampullary and spherical enlargements are believed to be pathognomonic for acoustic neurinoma (55, 454). Funnel shaped enlargement of the porus signifies widening of only the medial portion of the canal, so the canal is narrow laterally and wide medially. Funnel shaped widening of the canal is a non specific sign found with large acoustic neurinomas that have grown secondarily into the cerebello-pontine angle. This sign is also observed with the medial type of acoustic neurinoma that grows secondarily into the internal auditory canal and with other tumors that extend secondarily into the internal auditory canal (454).

The changes seen on the conventional X-ray studies are demonstrated with greater frequency and precision by pluridirectional tomography (585, 586, 588). In addition, tomographic studies display erosion of the falciform crest and of the borders of the internal auditory canal that are difficult to detect on plain radiographs.

In collected series of acoustic neurinomas, pluridirectional tomograms provided evidence of tumor in 82% of cases, whereas plain radiographs provided evidence of tumors in only 72% of cases (29, 55, 60, 73, 80, 111, 116, 121, 193, 216, 220, 252, 291, 297, 305, 315, 320, 344, 408, 415, 417, 419, 422, 448, 449, 466, 467, 509, 510, 532, 563, 586, 590, 599, 634).

B. Meatocisternography with Positive-Contrast Media

Prior to introduction of CT, meatocisternography was the most sensitive and accurate radiographic test for the proof or exclusion of acoustic neurinomas (139, 587, 611). Pantopaque meatocisternography with pluridirectional tomography proved to be particularly useful (139, 217, 514, 590).

In these studies acoustic neurinomas typically appeared as medially-convex filling defects in the pontocerebellar cistern (Fig. 21) (20, 42, 75, 137, 139, 204, 217, 503, 586, 605, 607, 608, 611, 617). Different patterns of filling defects could be distinguished (137).

Pantopaque meatocisternography gave true positive results in 96 to 100% of cases (75, 111, 164, 191, 251, 344, 587). Rarely, false positive results were caused by arachnoiditis (136, 310, 587), abnormally narrow internal auditory canal (139) or inflammatory swelling of the vestibular nerve (310).

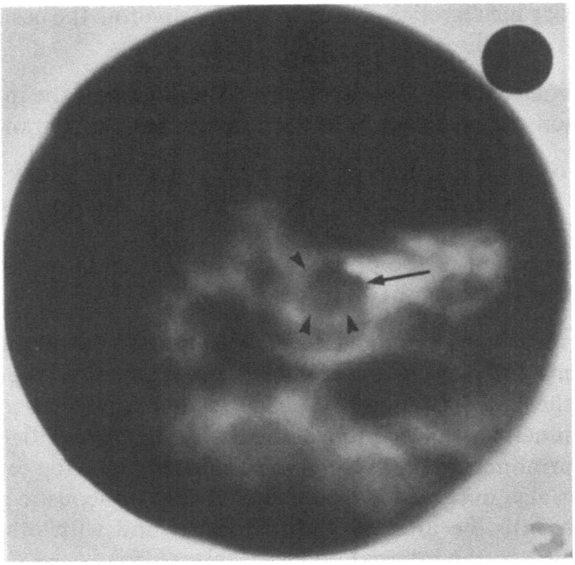

Fig. 21. Pantopaque meatocisternography in a case of acoustic neurinoma. Tomography in Stenvers projection. The anterior pontocerebellar cistern contains contrast medium. A round mass at the porus of the internal auditory canal causes a medially convex filling defect in the contrast column (*arrow*) and prevents entrance of Pantopaque into the internal auditory canal (*arrowheads*)

C. Angiography

Now little used for the diagnosis of acoustic neurinomas, angiography was previously widely employed for the diagnosis of tumors greater than 2 cm in diameter (111, 429, 530, 552). Small pontocerebellar and purely intracanalicular tumors were not displayed.

Angiographic diagnosis of acoustic neurinomas depends upon assessment of vessel displacement, hypervascularity, capillary blush, patterns of venous drainage and the specific source of vascularity (49, 179, 234, 277, 315, 386, 396, 421, 489, 551, 553, 554, 600, 625). In the arterial phase, large acoustic neurinomas cause stretching and bowing of the AICA loop with either upward (Fig. 22) or downward (Fig. 23) displacement of the AICA, depending upon the main direction of tumor growth. The proximal segment of the superior cerebellar artery is typically displaced superiorly, forming a curve that is convex superiorly above the mass. The posterior inferior cerebellar artery (PICA) is displaced caudally. The basilar artery and the vermian branch of PICA are typically displaced to the opposite side. With very large tumors that extend through the incisura, the posterior cerebral artery is also displaced superiorly (Fig. 22).

In the venous phase, acoustic neurinomas typically exhibit compression and/or elevation of the petrosal vein. The vein may be totally obliterated with large acoustic neurinomas. Dilatation of the ipsilateral petrosal vein by drainage of tumor

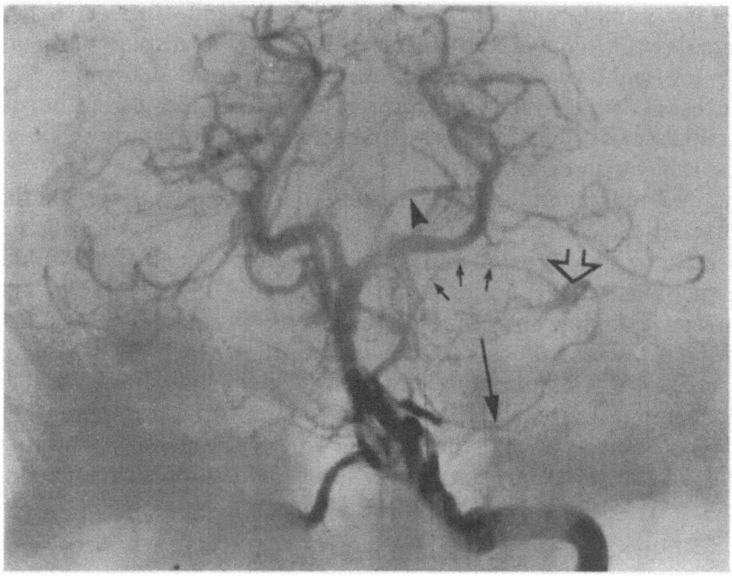

Fig. 22. Vertebral angiography in a case of large acoustic neurinoma. Arterial phase. Towns view. The anterior inferior cerebellar artery is elevated and stretched (*small arrows*), whereas the posterior inferior cerebellar artery is displaced caudally, marking the inferior border of the tumor (*arrow*). The basilar artery is displaced to the opposite side and the superior cerebellar artery bulges upward (*arrowhead*), indicating large size of the tumor. Note in this case early drainage through the dilated and elevated petrosal vein (*open arrow*)

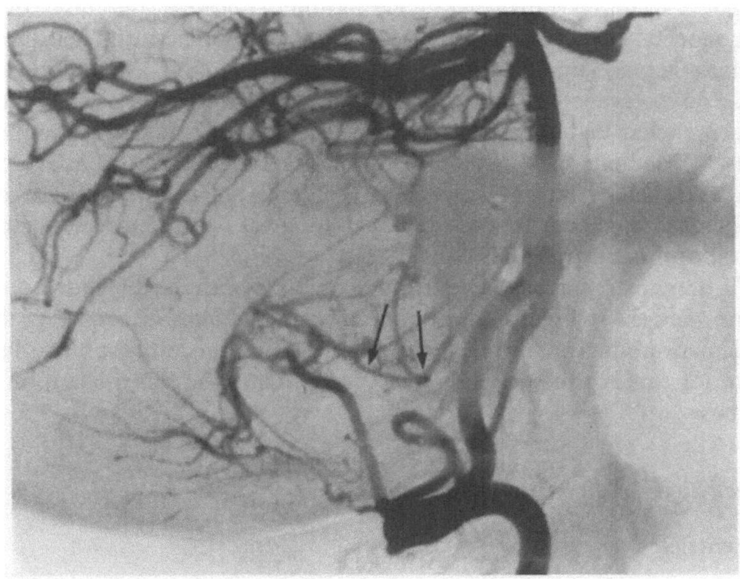

Fig. 23. Vertebral angiography in a case of medium-sized acoustic neurinoma. Arterial phase. Lateral view. The anterior inferior cerebellar artery is displaced downward (*arrows*)

vasculature is a reliable sign for acoustic neurinoma and other cerebello-pontine angle tumors (600). The precentral cerebellar vein is displaced upwards and posteriorly. It often displays a typical kink or "crows foot" deformity. The vein of the lateral recess of the fourth ventricle may delineate the medial border of the tumor, but this vein is often impossible to detect in the positive study. The vein of the lateral recess may also drain the tumor.

Subtraction and magnification techniques significantly improve the angiographic diagnosis of acoustic neurinomas. These techniques provide a better view of the displaced arteries and veins and often demonstrate a shell-like tumor blush. Homogeneous blush of the entire tumor is unusual (619).

Superselective angiography of the branches of the external carotid artery may show additional vascularization of acoustic neurinomas by branches that normally supply the cerebello-pontine angle (102, 561). These include the petrosal branch of the middle meningeal artery, the meningeal branch of the ascending pharyngeal artery and the mastoid branch of the occipital artery. The meningeal branches of the internal carotid and vertebral arteries may also provide supply to cerebello-pontine angle tumors.

3 Computed Tomography

The role of CT is to assist the surgeon in planning as safe and complete a resection of tumor as is appropriate to the case. Thus CT must detect the tumor, define its size and extension, display any cysts, hemorrhage or unusual internal feature of the tumor, demonstrate its relationships to the surrounding structures and document the presence of complicating factors such as obstructive hydrocephalus and ascending or descending transincisural herniation. At present, the choice of surgical approach depends largely on tumor size. For that reason acoustic neurinomas are usually classified as small, medium and large (229, 449). Small purely intracanalicular pontocerebellar tumors and tumors that protrude only a few mm into the pontocerebellar cistern are operated via a middle fossa, transtemporal approach (145). Medium-sized tumors with a diameter of 2.5 to 3 cm are operated upon via a translabyrinthine approach (145). Large tumors with a cisternal diameter greater than 3 cm are best operated upon via a combined suboccipital and transmeatal approach (627, 629).

The CT diagnosis of acoustic neurinoma relies on both the direct demonstration of the tumor and the indirect signs of bone erosion and mass effect. More than 60% of acoustic neurinomas are not *directly* visualized on non contrast scan. Successful recognition of tumor thus depends upon recognizing the more common *indirect* signs of mass.

A. Indirect Signs of Acoustic Neurinoma

Fourth Ventricle

Acoustic neurinomas are masses of the anterior compartment. As such they displace the fourth ventricle posteriorly, even if only slightly. The presence of posterior

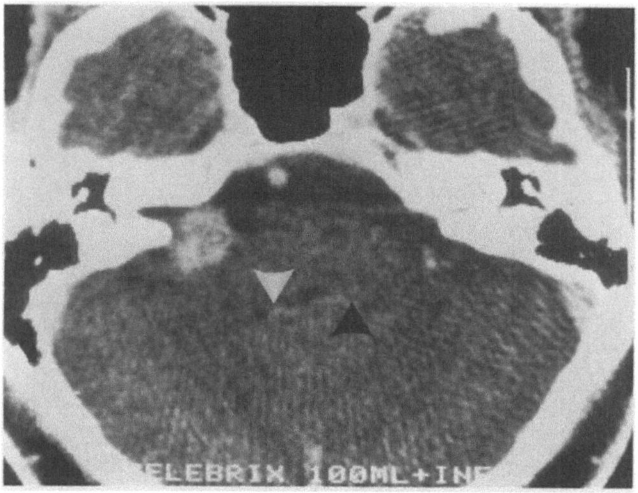

Fig. 24. Displacement and rotation of the fourth ventricle in a case of medium-sized acoustic neurinoma. Post contrast axial CT. The right lateral recess of the fourth ventricle is displaced dorsally (*white arrowhead*); the left lateral recess is in normal position (*black arrowhead*). The whole fourth ventricle is slightly rotated

displacement distinguishes cerebello-pontine angle tumors from cerebellar and posterior extraaxial tumors. Intrinsic pontomesencephalic tumors may also produce posterior displacement of the fourth ventricle, but the displacement is much more pronounced with pontomesencephalic tumors than it is with cerebello-pontine angle tumors (639, 573, 574, 638).

The degree of distortion and compression of the fourth ventricle depend upon tumor size. Compression and distortion are found in almost 100% of large neurinomas, and with decreasing frequency in smaller tumors (Fig. 24). The most subtle detectable deformation of the fourth ventricle is compression of one lateral ventricular wall. This may be detected with tumors only 1.5 cm in diameter (574, 596).

Obstructive hydrocephalus is a common finding in acoustic neurinomas (13 to 18.5%) but is seen only with large tumors that cause compression and displacement of the fourth ventricle (574, 596).

Cisternal Changes

Acoustic neurinomas characteristically deform the pontocerebellar cistern (387, 539, 573, 574). Small pontocerebellar acoustic neurinomas fill out the lateral portion of the cistern, but often do not affect the size of the cistern (Fig. 25). Modest acoustic neurinomas displace the adjacent brain stem just enough to widen the ipsilateral cistern (Fig. 26). Large acoustic neurinomas also widen the ponto-cerebellar cistern, but the tumor mass completely fills the widened cistern, so the cistern appears obliterated rather than widened (574, 596). In more than half of the cases, acoustic neurinomas also widen the infratentorial segment of the ipsilateral ambient cistern.

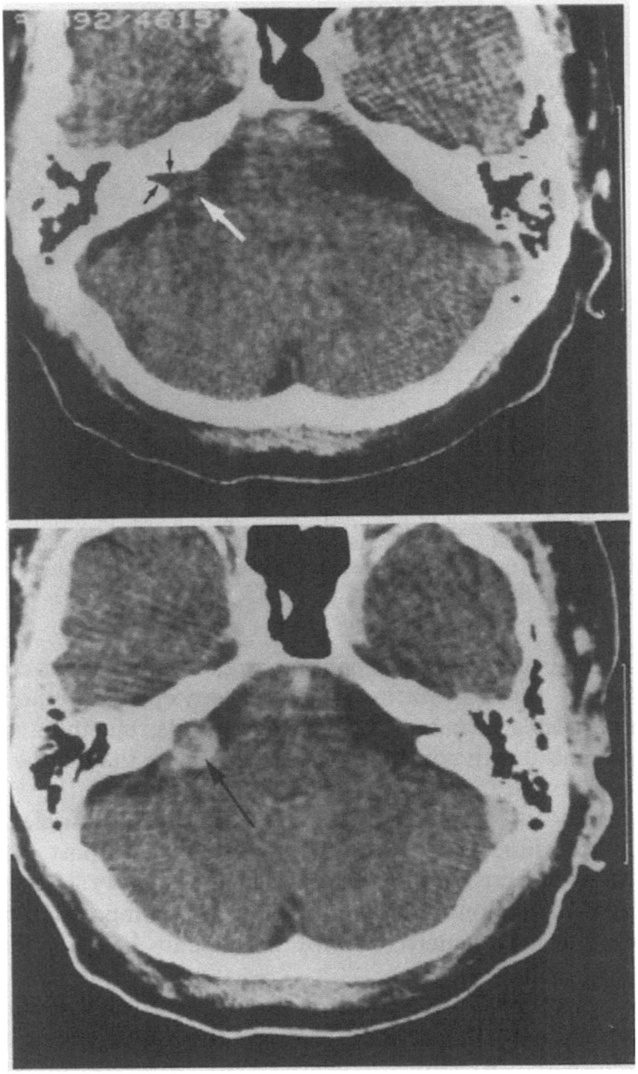

a

b

Fig. 25a, b. Cisternal obliteration in a case of small acoustic neurinoma. **a** Non contrast CT. Dilatation of the right internal auditory canal (*small arrows*). Note obliteration of the pontocerebellar cistern by an isodense mass (*white arrow*). The cistern itself is equal in size to the normal left cistern. **b** Post contrast CT. The enhancing acoustic neurinoma (*arrow*) fills out but does not expand the pontocerebellar cistern

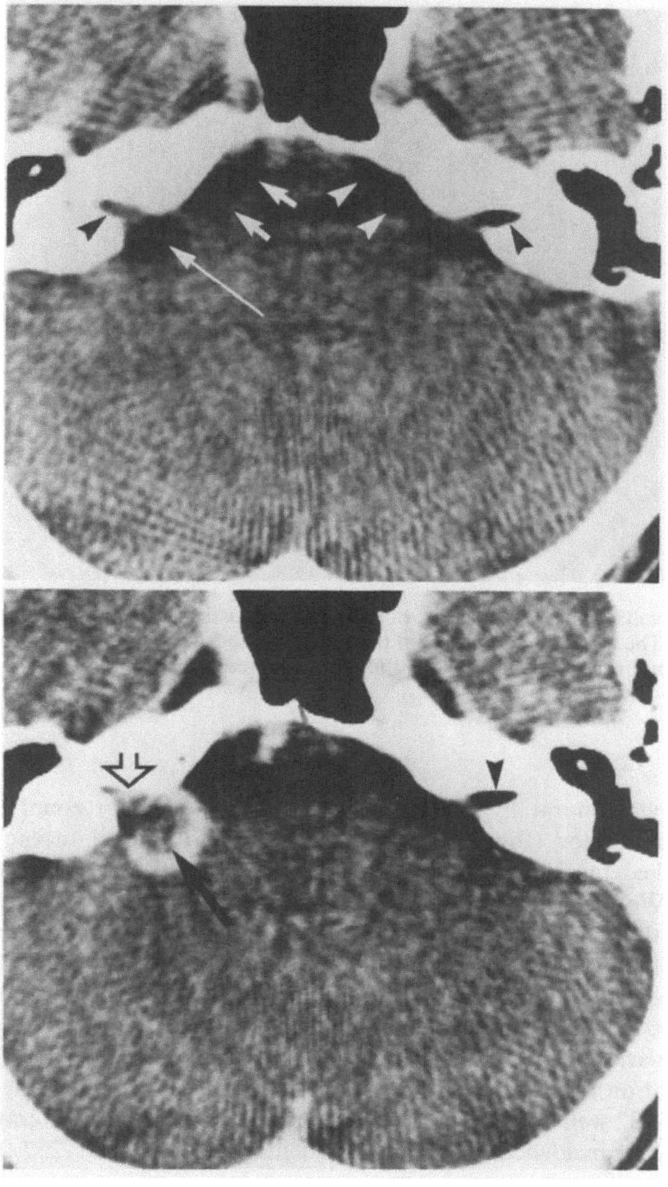

a

b

Fig. 26a, b. Medium-sized acoustic neurinoma causing slight cisternal dilatation. **a** Non contrast CT. The anterior compartment of the pontocerebellar cistern on the right side (*short arrows*) is dilated when compared with the normal left side (*white arrowheads*). The posterior compartment of the cistern is occupied by an inhomogeneous, partially hypodense mass (*long arrow*). Note the density difference of the contents of the two internal auditory canals (*black arrowheads*). **b** Post contrast CT. The acoustic neurinoma shows inhomogeneous enhancement (*arrow*). The intracanalicular tumor portion shows enhancement (*open arrow*), whereas the CSF-containing left internal auditory canal does not enhance (*arrowhead*)

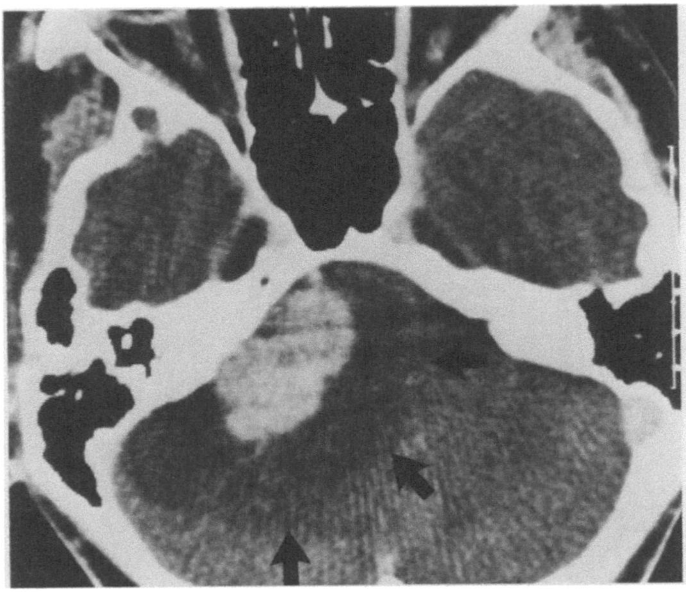

Fig. 27. Post contrast axial CT in a case of right-sided acoustic neurinoma with large peritumoral hypodensity. The whole circumference of this medium-sized acoustic neurinoma is encircled by a thick hypodense rim (*arrows*), which is thought to represent peritumoral edema

Peritumoral Edema

The term peritumoral hypodensity signifies a low density zone that partially encircles the tumor (Fig. 27). Most probably peritumoral lucency represents peritumoral edema, not pressure-related atropy (159, 191, 257, 259, 360, 387, 427, 540, 574). We have never observed persistence of hypodensity in postoperative follow-up studies as would be expected, if the hypodensity represented atrophy. Peritumoral edema is a non specific sign of mass. It occurs with diverse tumors, including acoustic neurinomas. The presence and degree of peritumoral edema appear to be related to tumor size; such edema is observed only with large tumors. Therefore, variations in the incidence of peritumoral edema (11 to 44%) probably reflect variation in the size of the tumors collected in different series (360, 427). Analysis of 432 well documented acoustic neurinomas from the literature suggests that the average incidence of peritumoral edema is 28% (159, 191, 257, 259, 360, 387, 427, 574).

B. Direct Signs of Acoustic Neurinoma

Density and Contrast Enhancement

The definitive diagnosis of acoustic neurinoma relies upon the morphologic analysis of the tumor itself. Only 36.7% of acoustic neurinomas are directly visible on the non contrast scan. The majority of acoustic neurinomas (63.3%) present as lesions that

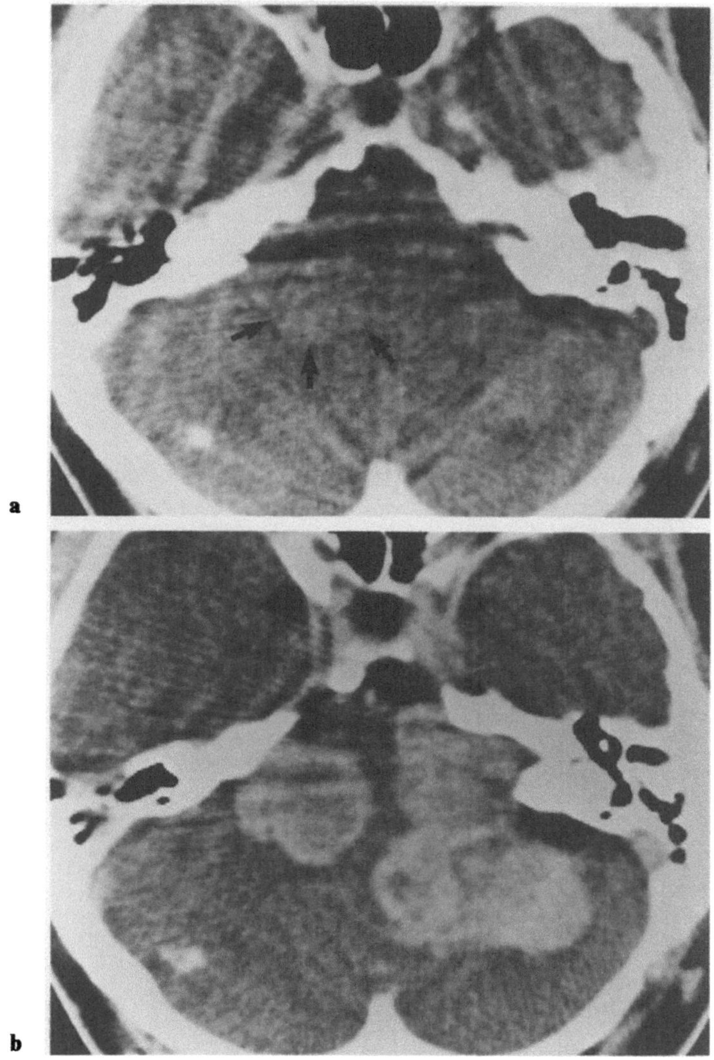

Fig. 28a, b. Bilateral acoustic neurinoma (Recklinghausen disease). **a** Non contrast CT. The pontocerebellar cistern is obliterated bilaterally. A slightly hyperdense mass can be delineated on the right side (*arrows*), whereas on the left side, the tumor is isodense and cannot be seen on the non contrast scan. **b** Post contrast CT. Despite their slightly different appearance on the non contrast scan, both acoustic neurinomas show intense enhancement

are isodense with the surrounding cerebellum and are therefore not directly visible on a non contrast scan (Fig. 28) (94, 159, 182, 191, 257, 259, 360, 427, 477, 563, 574, 596). 17.1% of acoustic neurinomas are hypodense (Fig. 29) and 14.6% hyperdense (Fig. 28). 5% of acoustic neurinomas present as mixed lesions composed of iso- and hyperdense components (Fig. 26).

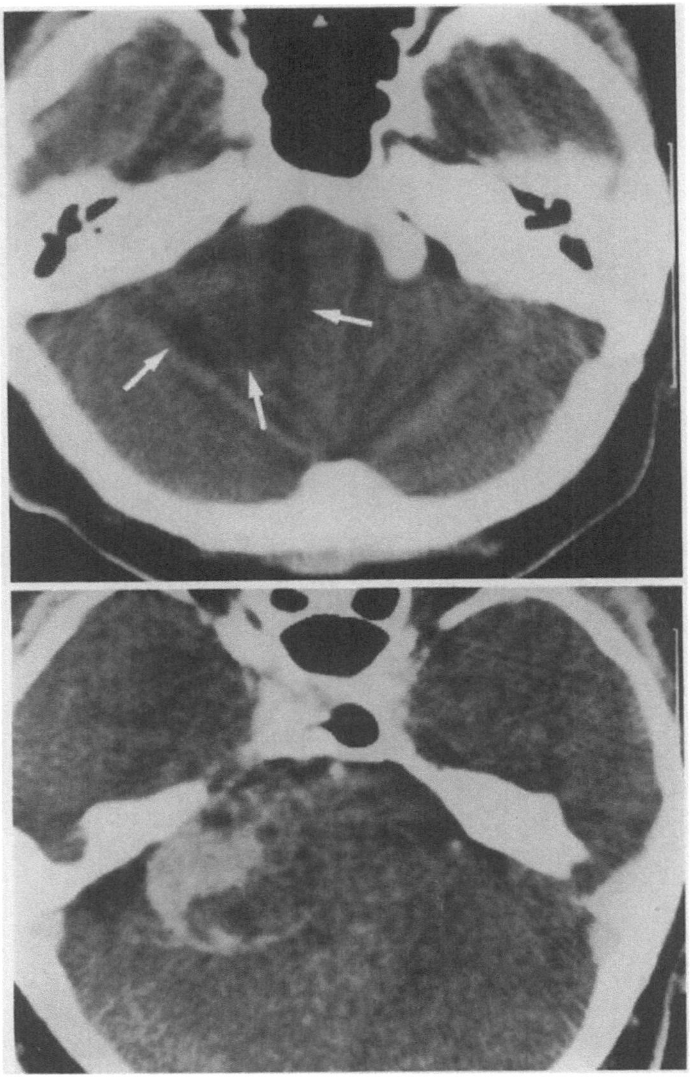

a

b

Fig. 29a, b. Right-sided large acoustic neurinoma. **a** Non contrast axial CT. The right cerebellopontine angle is filled and dilated by an almost homogeneous hypodense mass (*arrows*). **b** Post contrast CT. The hypodense tumor shows intense, but irregular enhancement

The vast majority of acoustic neurinomas show substantial contrast enhancement. Enhancement is reported to occur in 90 to 100% of medium-sized and large neurinomas (159, 182, 259, 387, 427, 539, 574, 596). The enhancement is homogeneous in 74% (Fig. 30), inhomogeneous in 16% (Figs. 31 and 32) and ringlike in 10%.

As a general rule, CT morphology correlates well with the size of the tumor (574). Medium-sized tumors typically appear isodense on non contrast CT scans,

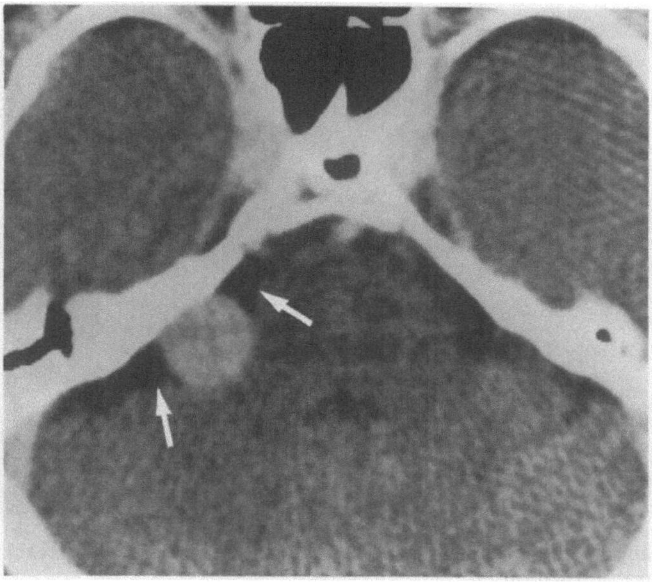

Fig. 30. Homogeneously enhancing right-sided acoustic neurinoma. Note the dilatation of the pontocerebellar cistern (*arrows*).

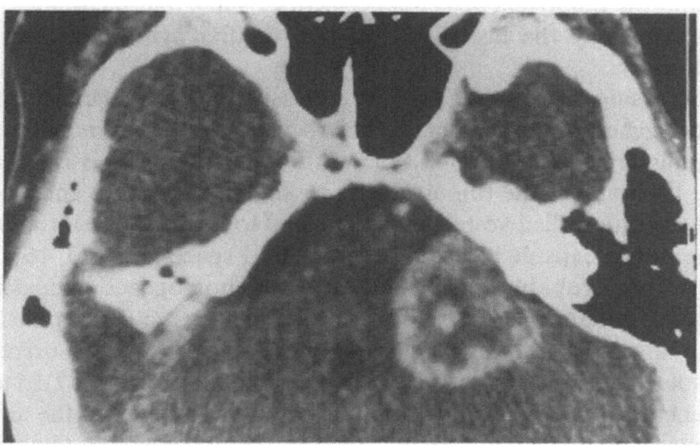

Fig. 31. Inhomogeneously enhancing left-sided acoustic neurinoma

whereas the proportion of hypo- and mixed density tumors increases with increasing tumor size. On contrast enhanced scans most medium-sized tumors exhibit homogeneous enhancement, whereas large tumors are more often inhomogeneous.

The morphology of the contrast enhancement also correlates well with the histoarchitecture of the tumors (574). Small and medium-sized neurinomas are composed of the Antoni-A tumor tissue with regularly bundled, spindle-shaped cells that give a regular appearance on the cut surface. The vessels in the Antoni-A

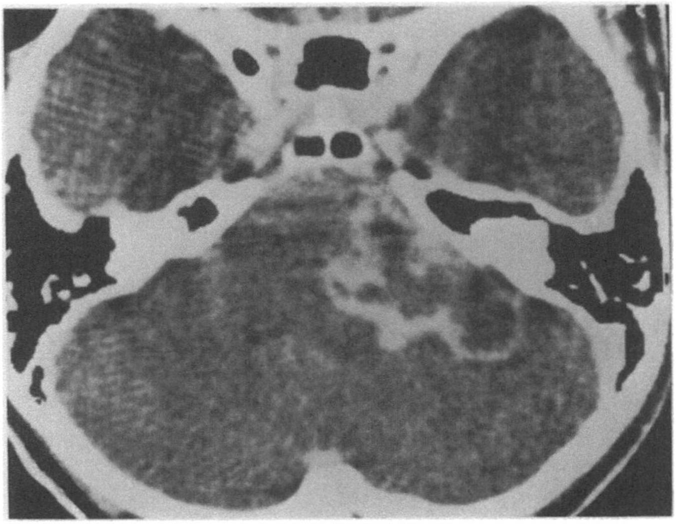

Fig. 32. Inhomogeneously enhancing left-sided acoustic neurinoma with irregular margins and central cystic transformation

type tumor show no regressive changes (61, 115, 184, 487). The homogeneous isodensity and the homogeneous enhancement of small and medium-sized tumors may be explained by the homogeneous and regular cyto-architecture of these Antoni-A tumors.

With increasing size of the tumor, regressive changes such as spongy and microcystic degeneration often lead to macrocystic degeneration. These regressive changes characterize the Antoni-B type of tumor tissue. Regressive changes may also reduce the walls of the tumor vessels to an extremely thin endothelial layer. Rupture of the thin walled vessels may then lead to hemorrhage into the tumor or through the tumor capsule into the subarachnoid space (58, 130, 165, 348, 383). Such changes are probably responsible for the inhomogeneous density and the inhomogeneous enhancement observed with large acoustic neurinomas (115, 184, 487, 574). In rare cases the entire tumor becomes a single large cyst surrounded only by the capsule. This appears on CT as a ring of enhancement (487). Tumors with cystic degeneration may exhibit layering of contrast within the cyst on CT examinations performed approximately 60 min after intravenous administration of contrast medium (Fig. 33).

In acoustic neurinomas, contrast enhancement results from iodine within the vascular compartment and from iodine extravasated into the interstitial space. The iodine index may be defined as the ratio of the iodine content of the tissue to the iodine content of blood. In acoustic neurinomas, it has been shown that the iodine index may be over 100% (197). This means that at a certain time the extravasation of contrast medium into the interstitial space causes a higher iodine concentration in the tumor than in the vessels. Since the blood vessels of acoustic neurinomas have no tight junctions, there is no blood-brain barrier in the tumor. Contrast medium reaches the interstitial space in the same way as in all normal tissues, with the exception of brain tissue (272, 286).

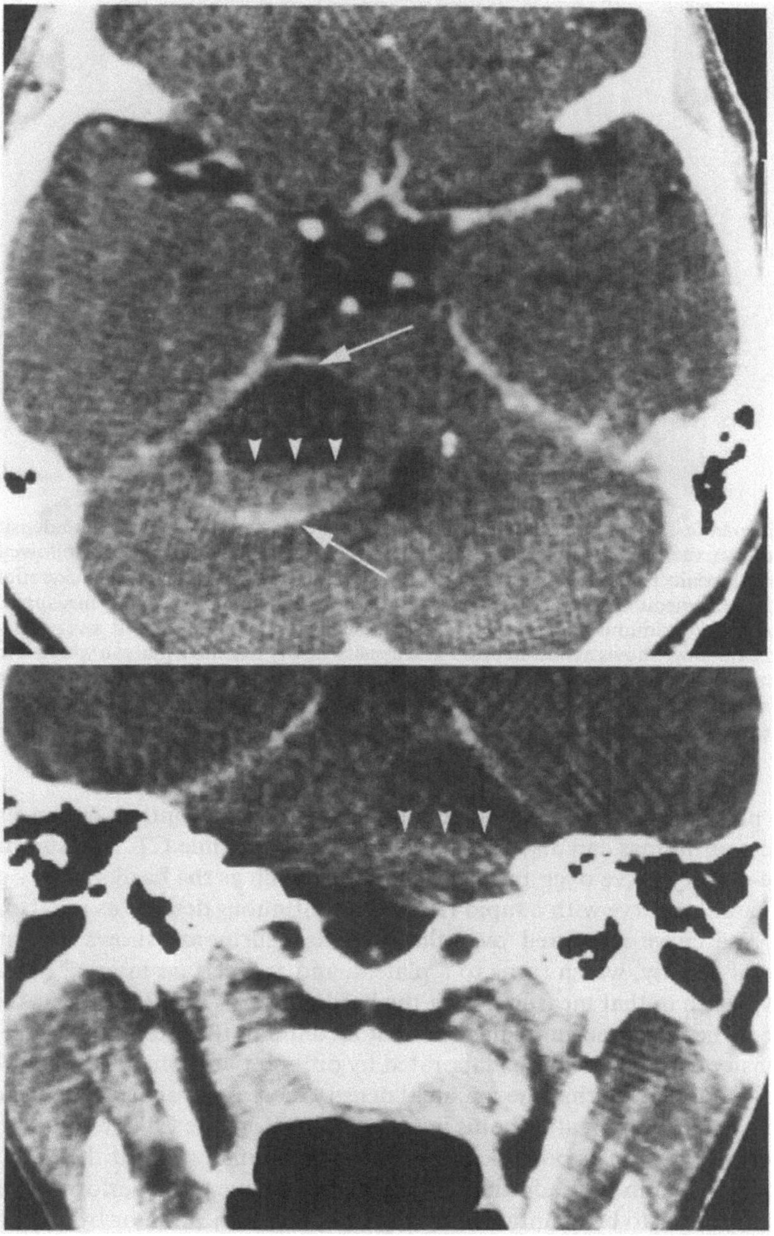

a

b

Fig. 33a, b. Ring-like enhancement in a medium-sized acoustic neurinoma. Post contrast CT. **a** Axial scan. The mainly hypodense acoustic neurinoma shows ring enhancement (*arrows*). Note the contrast layering (*arrowheads*), indicating the cystic nature of the tumor. **b** Coronal scan with the patient in supine position. Note again the contrast layering (*arrowheads*)

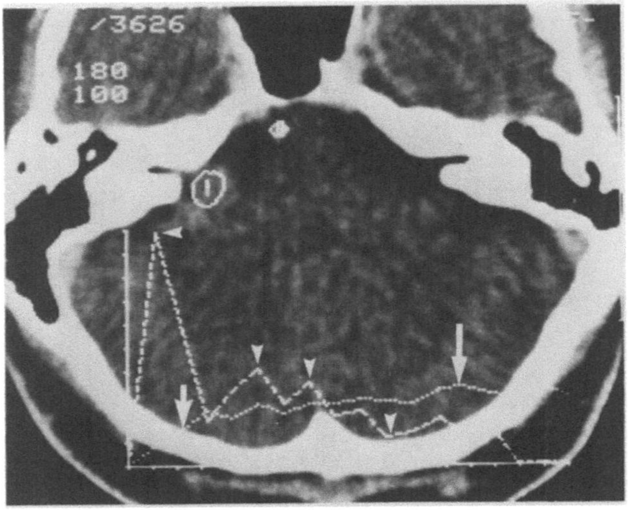

Fig. 34. Dynamic CT in a case of a small right-sided acoustic neurinoma. The time-density curve, measured over the basilar artery (*arrowheads*) exhibits an initial density peak followed by two further small peaks (rebound-phenomenon). With increasing time, when renal excretion begins and the contrast medium has partially escaped into the interstitium, the density measured over the basilar artery continuously decreases. The time-density curve measured over the acoustic neurinoma (*arrows*) shows no initial peak. The density slowly reaches a plateau which is much less high than the maximal peak over a vessel. However, the tumor density still increases when the density in the vessel already decreases. This type of curve evidences poor tumor vascularization. The increase in density results primarily from contrast accumulation in the interstitial space

The presence of an extravascular compartment of the contrast enhancement in acoustic neurinomas can also be demonstrated by dynamic CT. Measurements of the time-density curve over an arterial structure such as the basilar artery give the typical vascular curve with a rapid rise and a continuous descent as renal excretion begins. The curve measured over the acoustic neurinoma shows a continuous increase of density, which turns to a plateau and at a certain interval has an even higher value than that measured over the basilar artery (Fig. 34). This can only be possible if the tumor accumulates contrast medium in the interstitial space. These time-density curves have been elaborated by different authors (207, 208, 290, 306, 574). All studies agree that the maximal density increase in acoustic neurinomas is reached by 10 to 15 min after bolus injection. Therefore the CT examination has to be performed as soon as possible after contrast administration. If the examination time exceeds 20 min or if additional coronal views have to be performed, the high contrast level has to be maintained by a second bolus injection or by an additional drip infusion of contrast medium.

Tumor Shape

The overwhelming majority of acoustic neurinomas (80 to 92%) are round. If the intracanalicular tumor portion is taken into consideration they appear mushroom-shaped (Fig. 35) (360, 519, 574). This contrasts with cerebello-pontine angle

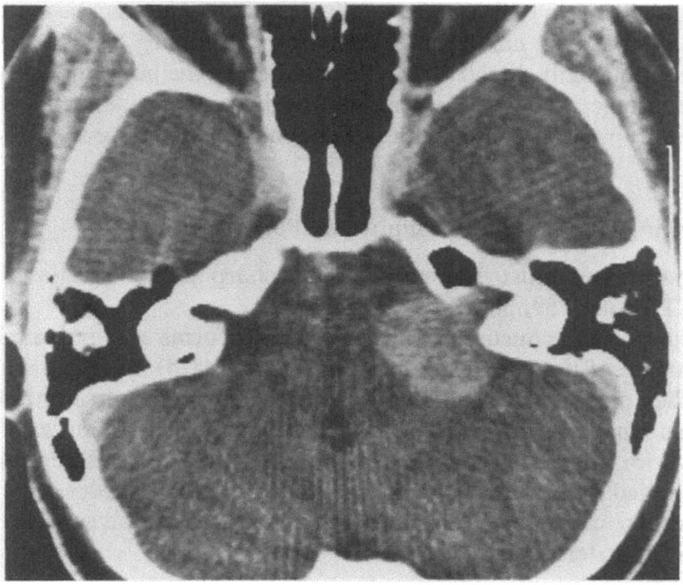

Fig. 35. Medium-sized acoustic neurinoma with typical mushroom appearance

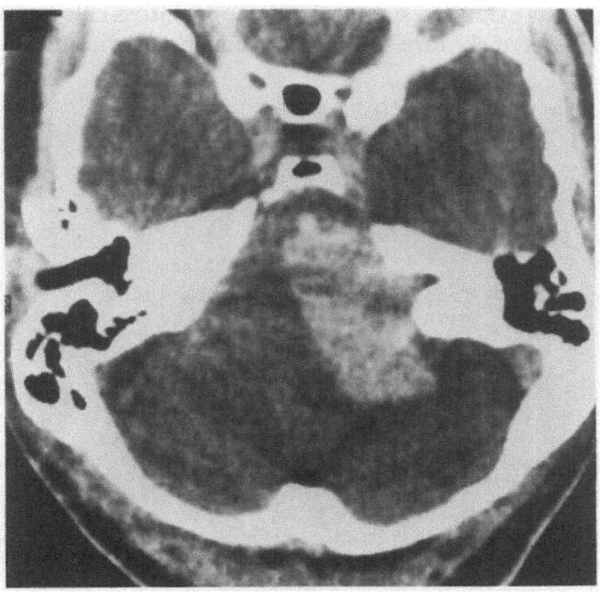

Fig. 36. Axial post contrast CT in a case of a large left-sided oval acoustic neurinoma

meningiomas which are typically oval (360, 519, 575). With increasing tumor size, the percentage of oval neurinomas increases. This may be explained by the hypothesis that medially directed growth is limited by the pons and cerebellum. At an advanced stage, acoustic neurinomas begin to grow antero-medially and postero-laterally in the direction of the least resistance, assuming an oval shape (Fig. 36).

Tumor Margin, Tumor Relationship to the Petrous Bone

Acoustic neurinomas most frequently exhibit sharp tumor margins on contrast enhanced CT scans (159, 387, 574).

The border of an acoustic neurinoma typically forms an acute angle with the posterior surface of the petrous bone (Fig. 37) (519, 574). Such an acute angle is found in 85% of medium-sized and large acoustic neurinomas. In contradistinction, meningiomas usually form an obtuse angle between the medial border of the tumor and the posterior surface of the petrous bone (519, 574). This differential angle sign cannot be applied to small acoustic neurinomas, since they start to grow within the internal auditory canal and only later begin to form tumor spheres within the pontocerebellar cistern (Fig. 38).

Calcifications

Calcifications are extremely rare in acoustic neurinomas. Only 2 of 400 cases of acoustic neurinomas exhibited small calcifications. Gross calcifications mimicking meningioma are extremely rare findings in acoustic neurinomas (562).

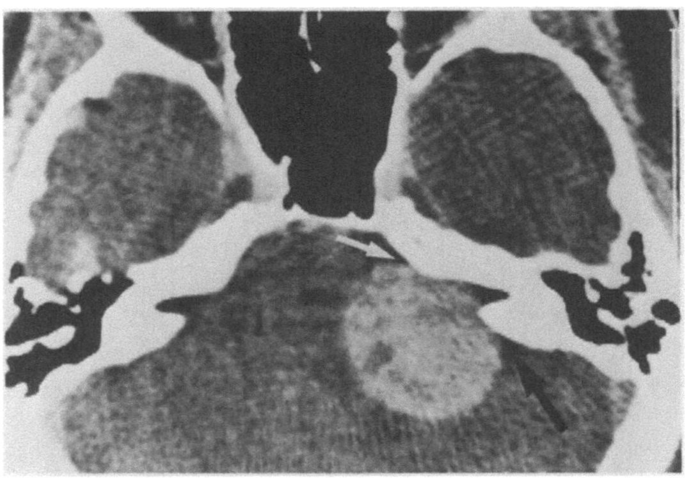

Fig. 37. Acoustic neurinoma with acute angle sign. Post contrast axial CT. The angle formed by the posterior surface of the petrous bone and the anterior and posterior margins of the tumor is acute (*arrows*)

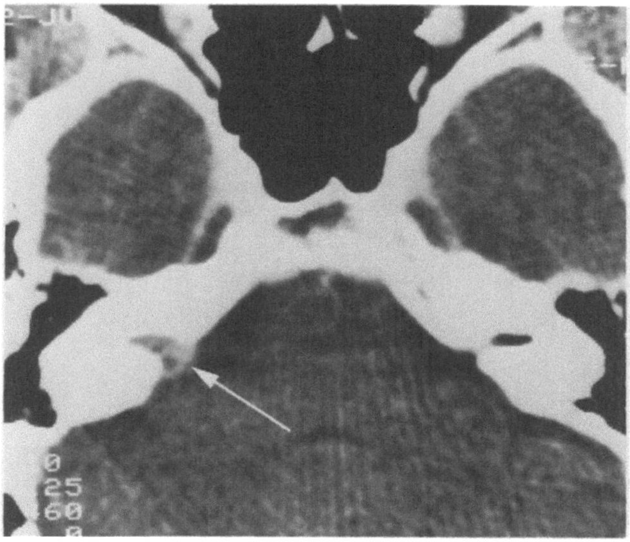

Fig. 38. Mainly intracanalicular right-sided acoustic neurinoma without acute angle sign. Axial post contrast CT section at the level of the internal auditory canal shows obliteration of the widened internal auditory canal by a small enhancing mass (*arrow*). Note the medially convex border of the tumor and absence of the acute angle sign. The medial contour of the tumor is surrounded by cerebro-spinal fluid

C. *The Internal Auditory Canal on High Resolution CT*

Second generation CT equipment demonstrates gross widening of the internal auditory canal as well as does conventional pluridirectional tomography (209, 515, 574, 620). Late-generation CT equipment with high resolution algorithms detects subtle abnormalities of the internal auditory canal as sensitively as does conventional pluridirectional tomography (559, 577, 590). High resolution CT successfully demonstrated dilatation of the internal auditory canal in 65 of 71 cases of acoustic neurinoma (92%). In 5 of the remaining 6 cases, there were medial acoustic neurinomas that did not extend into the internal auditory canal at surgery. In the 6th case, surgery disclosed a very small, purely intracanalicular neurinoma that did not enlarge the internal auditory canal.

The criteria developed for diagnosis of acoustic neurinomas with conventional pluridirectional tomography may be applied directly to diagnosis by high resolution CT (213). The different patterns of canalicular dilatation are extremely well shown on high resolution CT (Figs. 39 and 40). In addition, high resolution CT shows features that are poorly resolved on conventional tomograms, including shortening (Fig. 41), displacement and erosion of the falciform crest and fine erosions of the internal auditory canal.

Combined axial and direct coronal CT often demonstrate pressure erosion of the posterior surface of the petrous bone (Fig. 42), pressure erosion of the anterior border of the internal auditory canal, erosion of the inferior lip of the porus acusticus and, in large tumors, erosion of the dome of the jugular tubercle (556). In

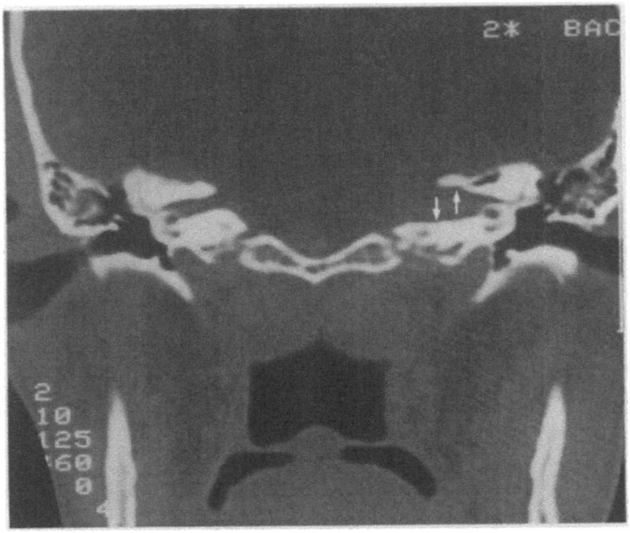

Fig. 39. Coronal high resolution CT in a case of left-sided acoustic neurinoma. The internal auditory canal shows funnel-shaped dilatation (*arrows*)

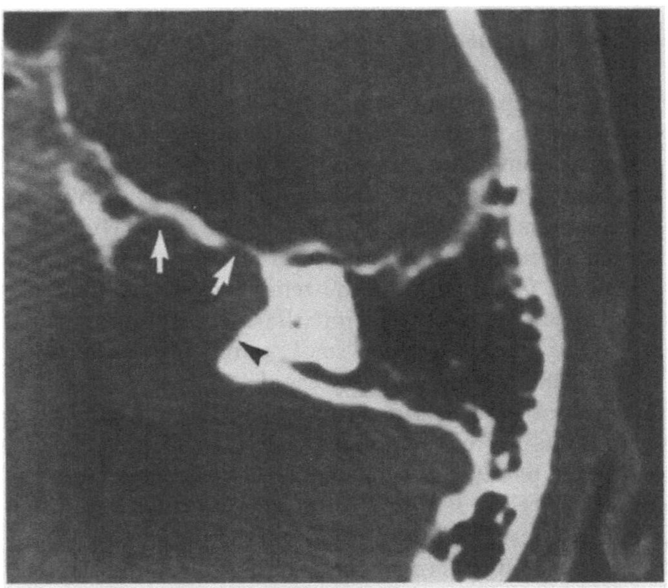

Fig. 40. Unusual, extensive erosion of the internal auditory canal in a case of left-sided acoustic neurinoma. High resolution axial CT. The posterior lip of the internal auditory canal (*arrowhead*) is eroded. Note the extensive bone erosion at the level of the antero-superior compartment of the internal auditory canal causing destruction of the petrous tip (*arrows*)

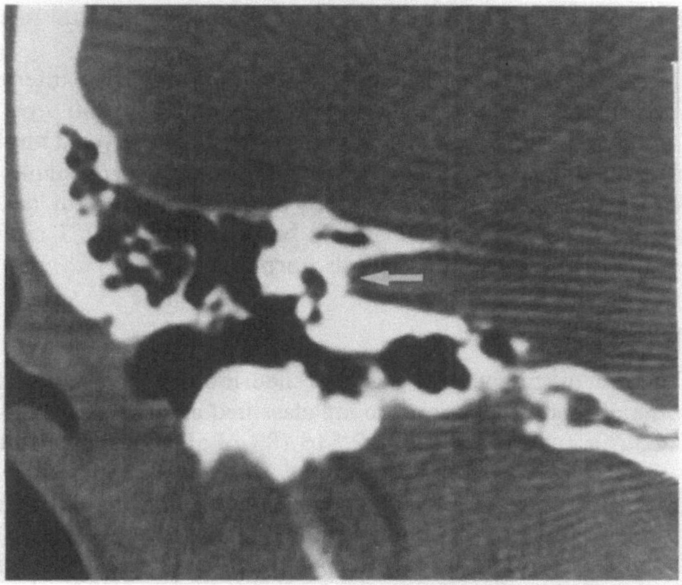

Fig. 41. High resolution coronal CT. Shortening of the falciform crest (*arrow*) by a right-sided acoustic neurinoma. The internal auditory canal shows ampullary dilatation

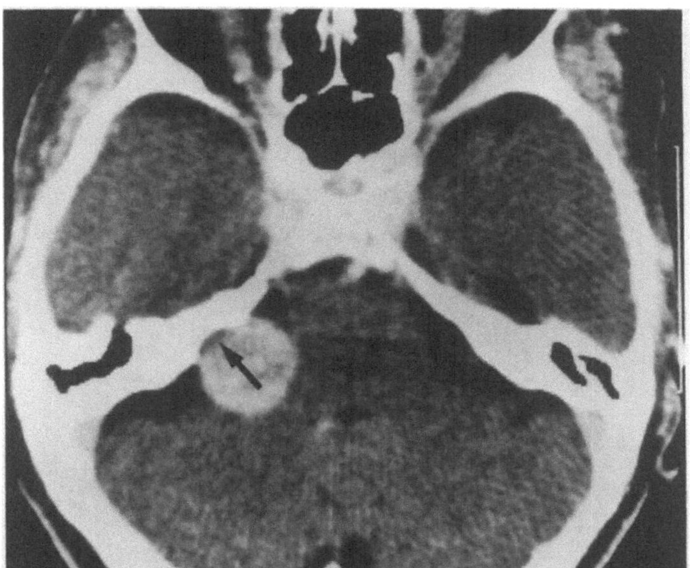

Fig. 42. Right-sided acoustic neurinoma. A post contrast axial CT section slightly above the level of the internal auditory canal shows focal pressure erosion of the posterior surface of the petrous bone (*arrow*)

exceptional cases a hyperostotic reaction may be observed lateral to the internal auditory canal (45).

It must be emphasized that CT demonstration of symmetrical internal auditory canals of normal size does not exclude the presence of a medial type of acoustic neurinoma. Conversely CT demonstration of significant (over 2 mm) unilateral enlargement of the internal auditory canal does not *necessarily* signify pathology (151, 177, 603). Rare normal individuals may have a "patulous" or "dilated empty internal auditory canal". This state should be proven by air CT cisternography before the patient is properly regarded as normal.

D. The Small Acoustic Neurinoma

Intracanalicular acoustic neurinomas and neurinomas protruding fewer than 10 mm into the pontocerebellar cistern are classified as small (138, 229, 449, 574). Such small acoustic tumors constitute 2.5 to 18% of all acoustic neurinomas (143, 229, 252).

With current CT equipment small acoustic neurinomas may be demonstrated directly on thin section, contrast enhanced CT scans (Figs. 38 and 43) (527, 528, 574, 577). Demonstrability is directly proportional to the size of the tumor and to the degree of canalicular enlargement. It varies from 20% for tumors that protrude 5 mm into the pontocerebellar cistern to 70% for tumors that protrude 10 mm into the cistern (111, 515, 573, 574, 576). Even when a small intracanalicular acoustic neurinoma is not demonstrated directly, enlargement of the internal auditory canal indicates the presence of the tumor in about 90% of cases. Additional indirect signs may be present and correlate with the tumor size.

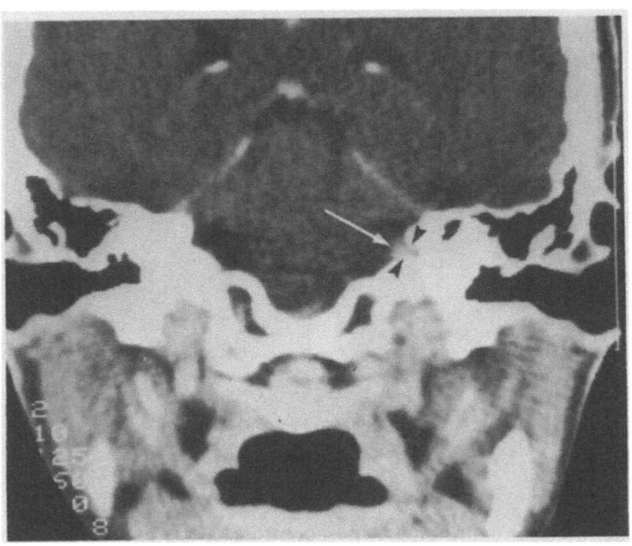

Fig. 43. Small mainly intracanalicular left-sided acoustic neurinoma. Direct coronal view. Dilatation of the internal auditory canal (*arrowheads*) is evidenced on this soft-tissue CT picture. The small acoustic neurinoma protrudes 2 mm into the pontocerebellar cistern (*arrow*). The neurinoma is completely surrounded by cerebro-spinal fluid

Histologically, small acoustic neurinomas are typically Antoni-A type tumors and present as homogeneously enhancing lesions (515, 574). This appearance of homogeneous enhancement may be mimicked by the hyperdense beam hardening artifact at the porus acusticus internus (Fig. 5). In most cases, the true tumor may be differentiated from the artifact by examining the non contrast scan. When the supposed blush is present prior to enhancement the "tumor" is probably a hyperdense artifact. If the tumor is isodense on non contrast CT, the blush probably does indicate true tumor. However, small hyperdense acoustic neurinomas and meningiomas may appear dense on both non contrast and contrast enhanced CT scans. In such cases, direct coronal CT may help to differentiate the hyperdense artifact from true tumor. The beam hardening artifact varies with precise beam path and is unlikely to be present at exactly the same site on the 2 right angle scans.

The most valuable method for evaluating possible small neurinomas is gas CT cisternography (7, 26, 65, 242, 253, 302, 336, 414, 430, 443, 444, 471, 536, 559, 577, 590, 612). This method combines high diagnostic accuracy with very low morbidity and is easy to perform rapidly in a busy CT suite (281, 559). Gas CT cisternography also demonstrates the seventh and eighth cranial nerves and the AICA loop, permitting assessment of the relationship of the tumor to the neurovascular bundle (Fig. 14). The use of intravenous enhancement in combination with gas CT cisternography provides even better demonstration of the AICA loop. The course of the eighth cranial nerve with respect to the tumor is of differential diagnostic value: In cases of acoustic neurinoma, the eighth nerve enters the tumor centrally and merges with the tumor (Figs. 44 and 45), whereas in cases of intracanalicular

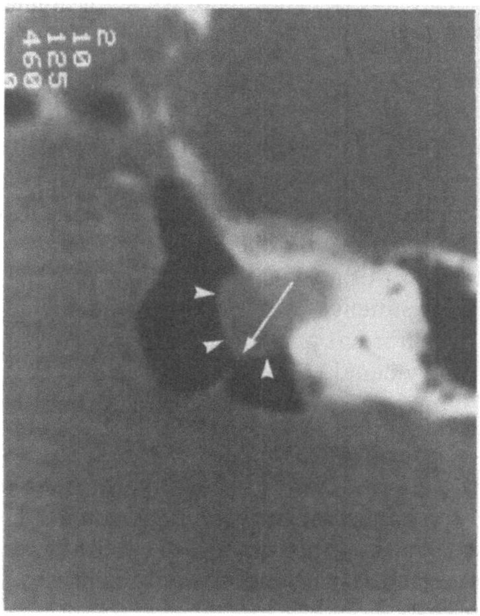

Fig. 44. Left-sided acoustic neurinoma. Gas CT cisternography. The neurinoma presents as a medially convex filling defect in the pontocerebellar cistern (*arrowheads*). The internal auditory canal contains a soft tissue tumor preventing entrance of gas into the canal. The vestibulocochlear nerve enters the tumor centrally (*arrow*)

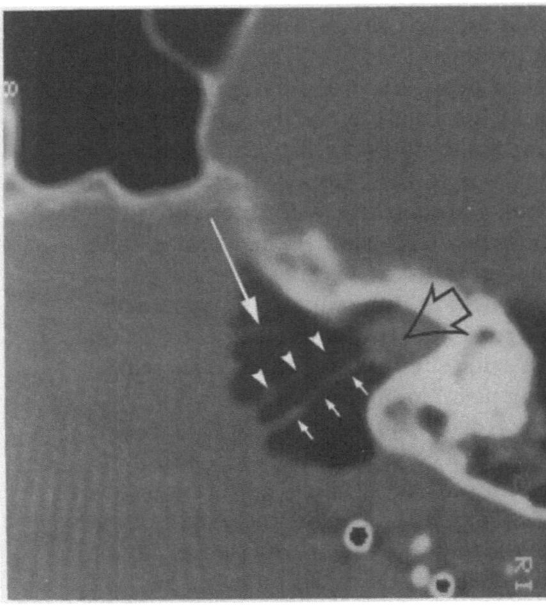

45

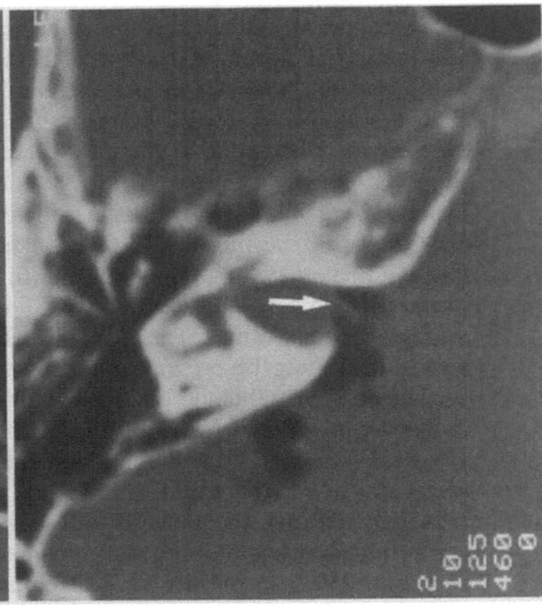

46

Fig. 45. Gas CT cisternography in a case of intracanalicular acoustic neurinoma (*open arrow*). Note the relation of the facial and vestibulocochlear nerves to the tumor: the facial nerve (*arrowheads*) bends anteriorly over the tumor, whereas the vestibulocochlear nerve (*short arrows*) enters into the tumor. The AICA loop (*arrow*) is located outside the internal auditory canal

Fig. 46. Gas CT cisternography in a case of right-sided acoustic neurinoma. Purely intracanalicular acoustic neurinoma with medially convex border. The neurovascular bundle enters the tumor centrally (*arrow*).

meningioma, the eighth nerve courses over the tumor surface and enters the internal auditory canal between the tumor and the osseous border of the internal auditory canal. In patients with predominantly intracanalicular neurinomas that protrude only a few millimeters into the pontocerebellar cistern, gas CT cisternography shows a medially convex soft tissue mass protruding from the porus acusticus into the gas-filled cistern. In patients with purely intracanalicular neurinomas, the pontocerebellar cistern is normal and filled with gas. However, the gas does not enter the internal auditory canal (Fig. 46).

Three different filling patterns may be distinguished in patients with small acoustic neurinomas (577):

1. Partial filling of the internal auditory canal with gas is indicative of a small, deeply situated, intracanalicular acoustic neurinoma.
2. Non filling of the internal auditory canal with gas in association with normal gas filling of the pontocerebellar cistern strongly suggests a diagnosis of intracanalicular neurinoma.
3. Non filling of the internal auditory canal with gas plus *partial* filling of the medial portion of the pontocerebellar cistern, is diagnostic of a small acoustic neurinoma that protrudes a few millimeters outside the internal auditory canal.

A gas-filled internal auditory canal, with well visualized neurovascular bundle and intracisternal portion of the seventh and eighth cranial nerves, safely excludes the presence of an acoustic neurinoma. In all cases, however, it must be remembered that non filling of the canal is *not diagnostic* of a mass within the canal. In exceptional cases, for example, a large AICA-loop may completely prevent entrance of gas into the internal auditory canal thus mimicking a tumor (263, 264, 319). In cases of artifactual non filling of the internal auditory canal, the air may be induced to enter the canal by shaking the head (479).

The incidence of false positive studies is lower with gas CT cisternography than with the previously performed Pantopaque meatocisternography (7, 108, 282, 471). Gas will enter narrow canals that would not fill with viscous Pantopaque. Gas will bypass a loop of the anterior inferior cerebellar artery that partially occludes the porus acusticus and will reach to and enter an internal auditory canal even if arachnoiditis partially loculates the cisterns (136, 310, 410, 587).

Pantopaque meatocisternography will often give false positive results. The incidence of false positive diagnoses with gas CT cisternography may be minimized by careful analysis of the shape of any filling defects observed. The filling defects caused by tumor regularly have a medially convex border, whereas the filling defects caused by arachnoiditis (Fig. 47) and by congenitally narrow canal are usually medially concave or straight. However, caution is urged in the case of very small

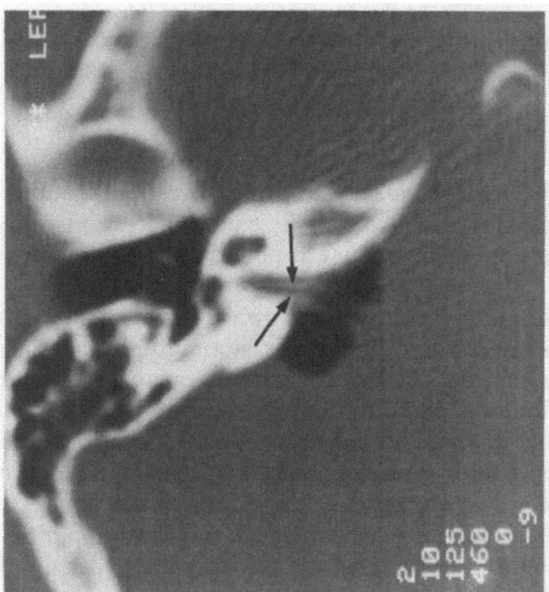

Fig. 47. Gas CT cisternography in a case of arachnoiditis. A soft tissue mass prevents entrance of gas into the internal auditory canal. The medial border of the mass is flat. Note that the intracanalicular course of the facial and vestibulocochlear nerves (*arrows*) is discernible despite the obliteration of the internal auditory canal by the soft tissue mass

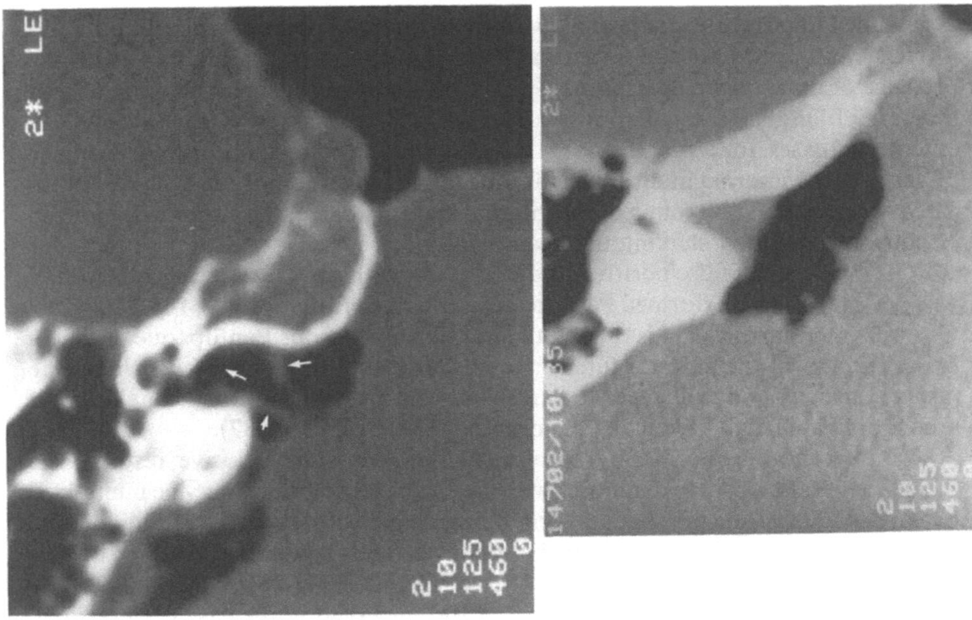

a b

Fig. 48. a Contrast enhanced gas CT cisternography showing intrameatal position of the AICA loop (*arrows*) in a case diagnosed clinically as acoustic neurinoma. **b** Intracanalicular cavernous hemangioma. Gas CT cisternography with intravenous contrast enhancement. The markedly dilated internal auditory canal is occupied by a soft tissue mass. Note intense and homogeneous enhancement of the mass as well as the flat contour of its medial border. These unusual features are atypical for acoustic neurinoma or meningioma

"tumors" measuring 3 mm or less. If the cochlear, vestibular and facial nerves are tightly applied to the posterior wall of the canal and are inseparable from one another, the apparent thickening may erroneously be diagnosed as a small tumor (242).

Whenever symptomatic patients are shown to have normal internal auditory canals and a normal eighth nerve on gas CT cisternography, special attention must be directed towards the loop of the anterior inferior cerebellar artery (Fig. 48). Auditory and vestibular symptoms may be caused by a complex interaction between the eighth cranial nerve and a prominent loop of the anterior inferior cerebellar artery that enters the internal auditory canal: the loop compresses the eighth nerve and the nerve compromises circulation to the inner ear. In contrast to patients with acoustic neurinomas, patients with this condition often have excellent speech discrimination and normal caloric test responses, despite the presence of sponataneous nystagmus (9).

Besides these non-neoplastic conditions, other neoplastic lesions simulating acoustic neurinoma may also be encountered on gas CT cisternography. These include meningioma (see p. 74), facial nerve neurinoma (see p. 130), cavernous hemangioma and metastastis.

Cavernous hemangioma is a rare lesion, which may be encountered in patients presenting clinically with symptoms of acoustic neurinoma. This rare tumor is believed to arise from the rich vascular network surrounding the intrameatal and geniculate portion of the facial nerve (142).

Cavernous hemangioma may mimic acoustic neurinoma or other intracanalicular tumors on gas CT cisternography. In the authors' experience intracanalicular cavernous hemangiomas may exhibit unusual features, which are not encountered with other lesions. These include intense and homogeneous enhancement as well as a rather flat medial tumor border (Fig. 48b).

Table 3 summarizes the intracanalicular neoplastic and non-neoplastic lesions, which may be detected by gas CT cisternography.

Table 3. Intracanalicular pathology

Neoplastic lesions
1. Acoustic neurinoma
2. Meningioma
3. Facial nerve neurinoma
4. Cavernous hemangioma
5. Metastasis
Non-neoplastic lesions
1. Arachnoiditis
2. Prominent AICA-loop

Meningioma of the Posterior Surface of the Petrous Bone

1 General Considerations

Meningioma is the second most frequent cerebello-pontine angle tumor, with an incidence of 6.7 to 9.5% (57, 575, 625, 630, 640, 641). Meningiomas of the cerebello-pontine angle constitute 5 to 8.4% of all meningiomas and 1 to 1.7% of all intracranial tumors (78, 365, 416, 418). Indeed, most infratentorial meningiomas (42 to 56.6%) originate from the posterior surface of the petrous bone and primarily involve the pontocerebellar cistern (57, 630).

Meningiomas of the pontocerebellar cistern were first described by Rokitansky in 1855 (214). A series of 3 cases and review of the literature was reported by Henschen in 1910 (214). Because of their clinical similarity to acoustic neurinomas, they were classified as "simulating acoustic neurinoma" by Cushing and Eisenhardt (78). Other terms have been used for this type of meningioma: "Meningioma of the cerebello-pontine angle" (54, 365, 464), "meningioma of the acoustic foramen" (78), "meningioma of the lateral recess" (433, 434) and "meningioma of the posterior surface of the petrous bone" (57). The term "meningioma of the posterior surface of the petrous bone" should be preferred, since it conforms to the general classification of intracranial meningiomas which is based upon the dural site of attachment and not upon the anatomical region involved by tumor growth (57).

Meningiomas of the posterior surface of the petrous bone originate from clusters of arachnoid cells that are distributed along the posterior surface of the petrous bone (8, 57). Such clusters of arachnoid cells are found around the porus acusticus internus, the superior and inferior petrosal sinuses, the jugular foramen and the trigeminal hiatus. Accordingly, meningiomas of the posterior surface of the petrous bone usually arise from these sites.

The dural implantation of meningiomas is commonly round in shape with a diameter of 1.5 to 2.5 cm (57). Vessels may enter the tumor through an exostosis at the tumor base (630). Meningiomas of the posterior surface of the petrous bone may infiltrate the petrous bone and invade the middle ear cavity in rare cases (145, 189, 381, 384, 497). Equally exceptional is primary origin of meningioma within the petrous bone (190). Sites of origin of intraosseous temporal bone meningiomas are, in order of decreasing frequency, the geniculate ganglion region, the internal auditory canal and the jugular foramen (142, 144, 146).

Clinically, meningiomas of the posterior surface of the petrous bone cause symptomatology similar to that of acoustic neurinomas. They occur more frequently in females than in males (57, 630). Small tumors usually present with signs of compression of cranial nerves eight and five. Facial nerve palsy is frequently present. Larger tumors cause additional cerebellar and pontine signs (54, 57, 99, 289, 300, 340, 433, 434, 630).

2 Conventional Radiology

Conventional radiologic studies demonstrate bone erosion and/or calcification in nearly 40% of meningiomas of the posterior surface of the petrous bone (57, 455, 630). The erosions are usually sharply delineated pressure erosions (455). Hyperostosis and small exostoses of the posterior surface of the petrous bone are observed infrequently (455). In the vast majority of cases the internal auditory canal is of normal size (55, 455). In unusual cases, it may be shortened by pressure erosion from adjacent large meningiomas or enlarged by rare primary intracanalicular meningiomas. The internal auditory canal may also be enlarged by impaired cerebrospinal fluid circulation.

The calcifications observed are commonly curvilinear capsular calcifications (55, 455, 599). Intratumoral psammomatous calcifications, commonly found on histological sections, are rarely observed by conventional radiologic techniques.

Angiography for meningiomas of the petrous bone is performed in the same way as is angiography for acoustic neurinoma. The arterial and venous displacements are essentially the same (259, 411, 498, 601, 630). The branches which most commonly supply a meningioma of the posterior surface of the petrous bone are the lateral clival branch of the internal carotid artery, the petrosal branch of the middle meningeal artery and the meningeal branches of the ascending pharyngeal and occipital arteries (102, 103, 259, 630). Characteristically, the feeding dural arteries of meningiomas are dilated and tortuous. Meningiomas show a tumor blush in 40 to 80% of the cases (259, 411), which is more often than in acoustic neurinoma. The tumor blush appears in the capillary phase, is homogeneous and is more intense than with acoustic neurinomas (259, 411).

3 Computed Tomography

Density and Contrast Enhancement

Meningiomas typically present as hyperdense masses on non contrast CT (Fig. 49) (73.3–77.4%) (257, 594). The hyperdensity of the meningioma is related to the presence of psammoma bodies within the meningioma. Such psammoma bodies are often found in the syncytial, transitional and fibroblastic meningiomas that are commonly encountered in the cerebello-pontine angle. Uncommon meningiomas may be isodense with cerebellum (Fig. 50); only 1% are primarily hypodense (257).

Contrast enhancement is observed in up to 97.3% of cases and is typically homogeneous (257, 259, 361, 387, 575). Total hypodensity is an extremely rare finding in meningiomas and may be caused by fatty degeneration (106, 257, 492, 493, 555). Focal intratumoral hypodensities from organized hemorrhage or intratumoral necrosis are found in only 1 to 2% of meningiomas of the posterior surface of the petrous bone (493, 575). The detection of such defects in an enhancing pontocerebellar mass favors a diagnosis of acoustic neurinoma rather than meningioma. Since focal non enhancing hypodensities are commonly encountered with large acoustic neurinomas the homogeneous contrast enhancement regularly observed with meningiomas is a very reliable differential diagnostic criterion (361, 575, 596).

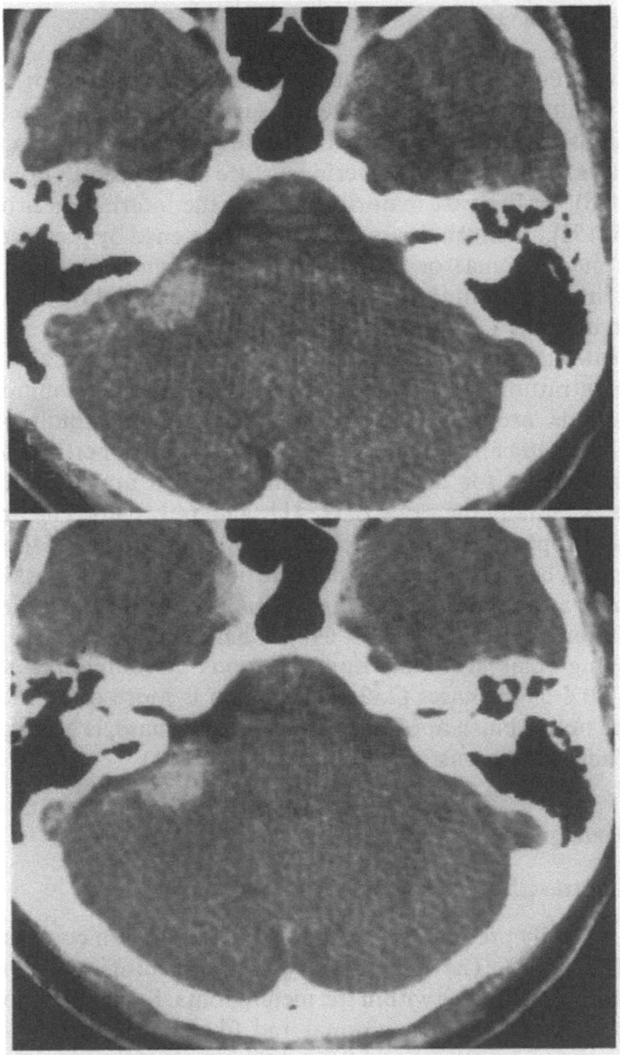

a

b

Fig. 49a, b. Meningioma of the right cerebello-pontine angle. **a** Non contrast scan. The meningioma is hyperdense. It lies in the retromeatal portion of the cerebello-pontine angle. **b** Post contrast scan. The meningioma exhibits a homogeneous, but not very intense enhancement. Note the broad contact of the meningioma with the posterior surface of the petrous bone

Dynamic CT studies show that the maximal density peak of meningiomas is reached 2 to 3 min after a bolus injection of contrast. Thereafter the time-density curve nearly parallels the density measured over a vessel (27, 207, 306, 540). From this time-density curve, it can be concluded that the contrast enhancement in meningiomas is primarily due to the vascular compartment. In contradistinction, the time-density curves of acoustic neurinomas support the concept that their enhancement results from leakage of contrast into the extracapillary space.

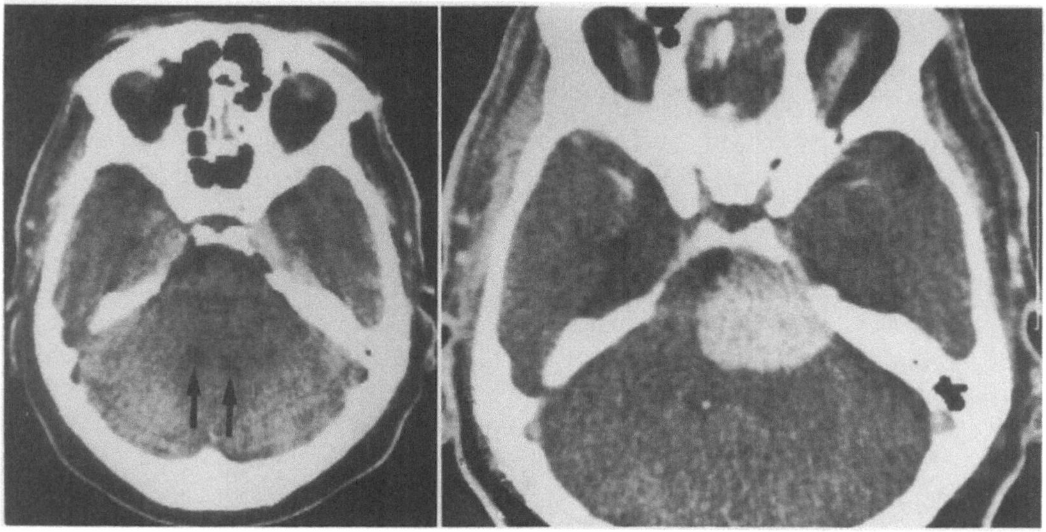

a b

Fig. 50 a, b. Primary isodense cerebello-pontine angle meningioma. **a** Non contrast scan. The left-sided meningioma is isodense and therefore invisible on a non contrast scan. Note however the posteriorly displaced, compressed fourth ventricle (*arrows*). **b** Post contrast CT. On the post contrast scan, the meningioma shows very intense, homogeneous contrast enhancement

Tumor Margin

Meningiomas of the posterior surface of the petrous bone nearly always have sharp margins. Occasionally, the tumor capsule may be visible as an enhancing rim (Figs. 51 and 54). Meningiomas without capsule and malignant meningiomas may present with irregular margins (459, 630).

Tumor Shape

Approximately 71 to 81% of meningiomas of the posterior surface of the petrous bone are ovoid and are oriented with their long axis parallel to the petrous bone (Fig. 52) (361, 575). This is a helpful differential diagnostic criterion especially with medium-sized tumors, since medium-sized acoustic neurinomas almost never are oval. Tumor shape is of less differential diagnostic value in large tumors, since large acoustic neurinomas and neurinomas of the medial type more often assume an oval shape.

The lateral, petrous border of the meningioma is usually rather straight. The angle formed between the bony surface and the medial free tumor border is obtuse (Fig. 52). This "obtuse angle sign" is present in 80% of meningiomas, and is almost never observed with medium- and large-sized neurinomas (519, 575).

Some difficulties arise in applying these criteria to small lesions. Small acoustic neurinomas that extend minimally into the cerebello-pontine angle initially assume a hemispherical shape. Therefore an obtuse angle is formed between the round medial tumor margin and the petrous bone. Rarely, meningiomas may be connected to the dura by a stalk (630). In such cases, the meningioma assumes a spherical

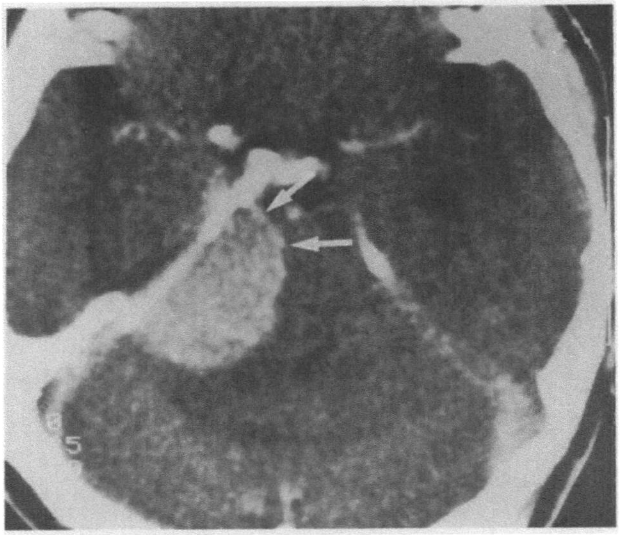

Fig. 51. Cerebello-pontine angle meningioma. Post contrast CT. A very faint peripheral blush, representing the tumor capsule (*arrows*) can be seen

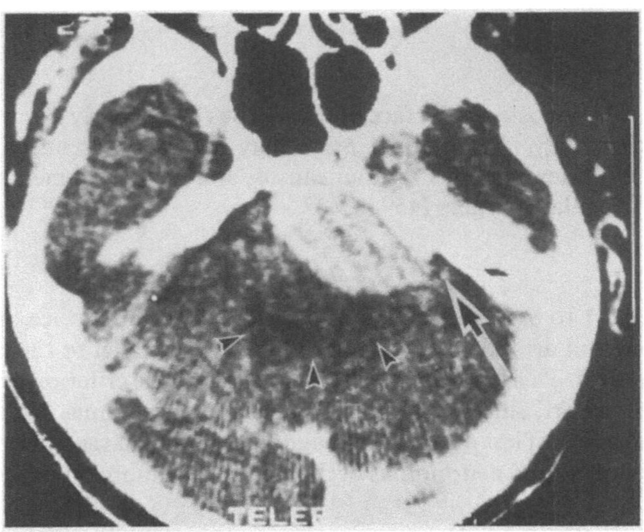

Fig. 52. Cerebello-pontine angle meningioma. Post contrast axial scan. The meningioma is located in the premeatal portion of the cerebello-pontine angle. It is oval in shape and presents with intense, homogeneous contrast enhancement. Note the broad contact of the tumor with the posterior surface of the petrous bone and the open angle formed between the posterior tumor margin and the posterior surface of the petrous bone (*arrow*). Peritumoral hypodensity (*arrowheads*)

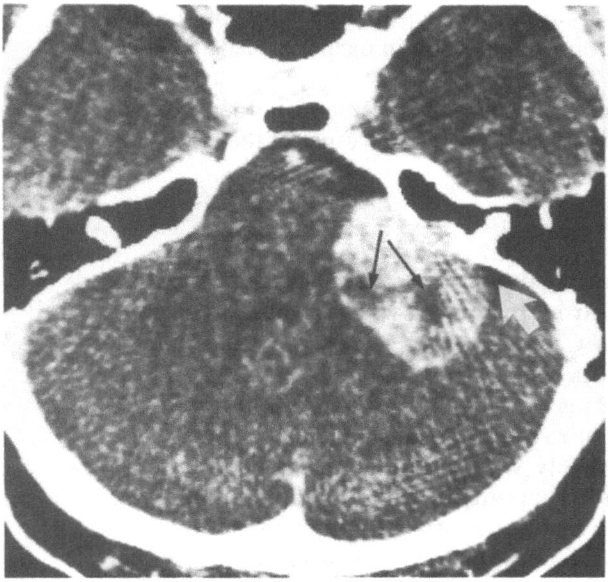

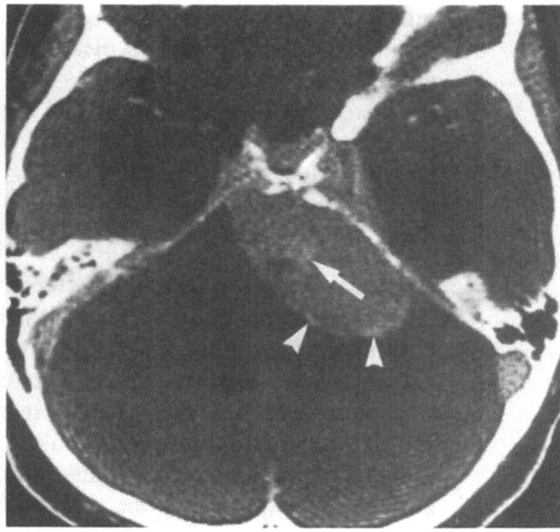

◄ Fig. 53 ▲ Fig. 54

Fig. 53. Atypical CT features of a cerebello-pontine angle meningioma. Post contrast CT. This meningioma presents with focal intratumoral hypodensity (*black arrows*). Another atypical feature is its short contact with the posterior surface of the petrous bone, causing an acute angle between the tumor borders and the posterior surface of the petrous bone (*white arrow*). Operation in this case showed a meningioma connected to the dura of the posterior surface of the petrous bone by a small stalk

Fig. 54. Cerebello-pontine angle meningioma. High resolution post contrast CT. A central calcification (*arrow*) is seen in this large meningioma. Note also a peripheral linear blush, representing the tumor capsule (*arrowheads*)

configuration so the "obtuse angle sign" is not formed (Fig. 53). Such meningiomas must be differentiated from a medial type of acoustic neurinoma by use of other diagnostic criteria.

Peritumoral Hypodensity

Peritumoral hypodensity is an inconstant finding, observed in approximately 50% of cases (Fig. 52) (575). Such hypodensity is more common with large tumors. It is not known whether peritumoral hypodensity represents edema, atrophy, or a combination of the two. However, persistence of peritumoral hypodensity in the cerebellar white matter after surgical removal of the meningioma suggests that atrophy is a factor in at least some cases (Valavanis, unpublished data).

Calcifications

Tumor calcification is found in 40 to 50% of meningiomas of the posterior surface of the petrous bone (361, 575). The calcification may be central (Fig. 54), peripheral or mixed. Totally calcified meningiomas may appear homogeneously white on routine brain window images but typically exhibit irregular, inhomogeneous density when viewed with bone windows.

Detection of calcification has special significance since acoustic neurinomas calcify only exceptionally (208, 575). Chordomas and chondromas of the cerebello-pontine angle often calcify.

Osseous Changes

Pressure exerted on the bone by the growing tumor may cause sharply demarcated erosion of the posterior surface of the petrous pyramid. Typically, the cortical bone is thinned, but intact. High resolution CT demonstrates focal or diffuse hyperostosis of the petrous pyramid in up to 22% of cases (Figs. 55 and 56). Focal hyperostosis at the porus acusticus internus may narrow the internal auditory canal. Diffuse hyperostosis may thicken the entire posterior surface of the petrous bone. Diffuse hyperostosis occurs less commonly with meningiomas of the posterior surface of the petrous bone than with the supratentorial meningiomas, however.

A special form of hyperostosis is a small exostosis located at the base of the tumor (Figs. 57–62) (257, 519, 575, 630). These exostoses represent the hilum of the tumor where feeding vessels penetrate the tumor (630).

Meningiomas may infiltrate the bone at the site of dural attachment (Fig. 63). Large meningiomas with caudal extension may erode the jugular foramen, the jugular tubercle and the basal parts of the occipital squama.

The internal auditory canal is usually normal in size (57, 330, 455, 575). Rare primarily intracanalicular meningiomas widen the canal. Secondary extension of a petrous tumor into the canal may also widen the canal. However, tumor extension into the canal is not necessarily accompanied by canalicular dilatation (630). In exceptional cases, entrapment of cerebro-spinal fluid within the canal may create an internal auditory canal cerebro-spinal fluid cyst deep to the obstructing meningioma.

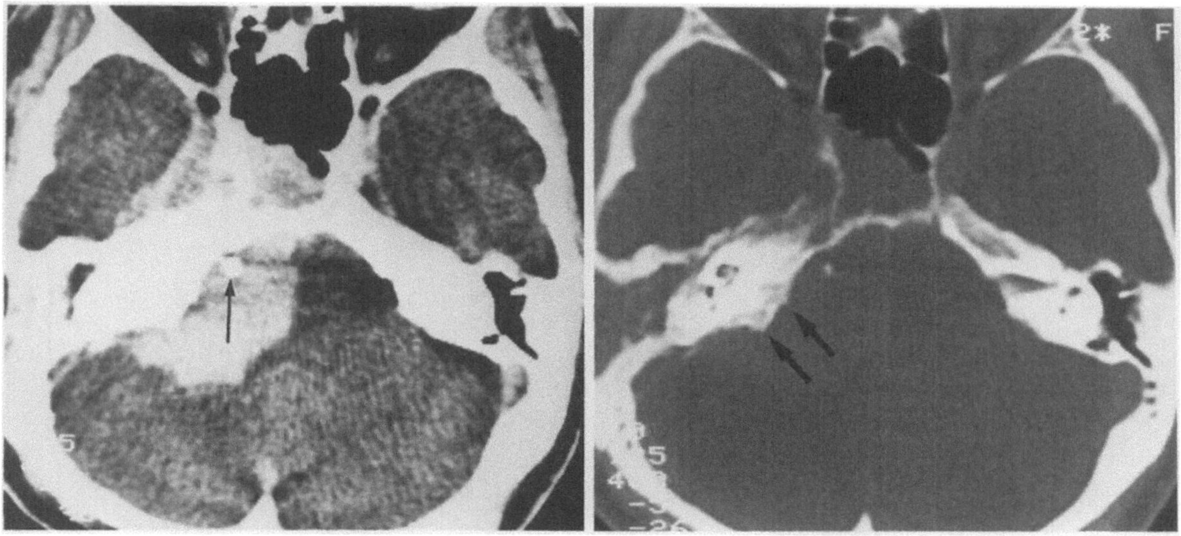

a b

Fig. 55 a, b. Spheno-petro-clival meningioma. **a** Post contrast axial CT. The tumor shows intense and homogeneous enhancement, is broadly attached to the posterior surface of the petrous bone and contains small, eccentric calcification (*arrow*). **b** High resolution CT at the same level shows diffuse hyperostosis of the posterior surface of the petrous bone (*arrows*)

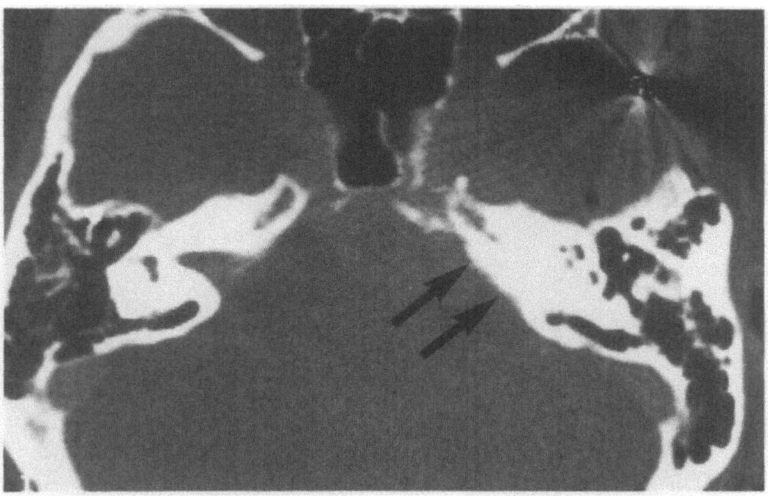

Fig. 56. Cerebello-pontine angle meningioma. High resolution axial CT. Hyperostosis (*arrows*) is present at the posterior surface of the petrous bone

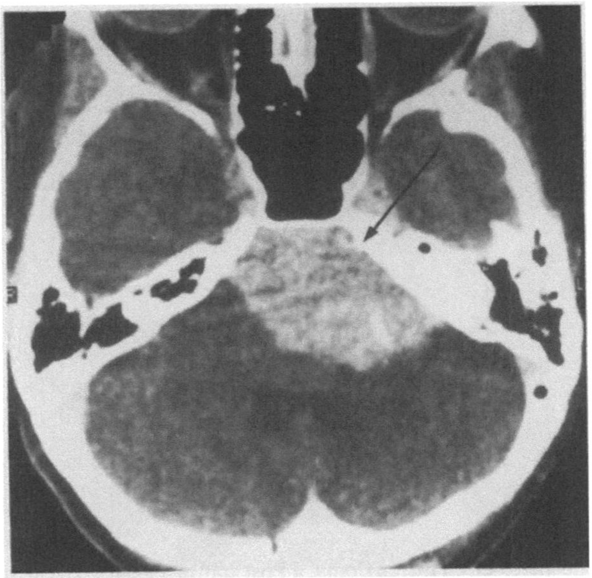

Fig. 57. Large spheno-petro-clival meningioma. Post contrast axial CT. A very small exostosis, representing the hilum of the tumor is seen (*arrow*) even without high resolution algorithm. The exostosis was only visible on this single 1.5 mm thin slice. Higher and lower sections did not show the exostosis

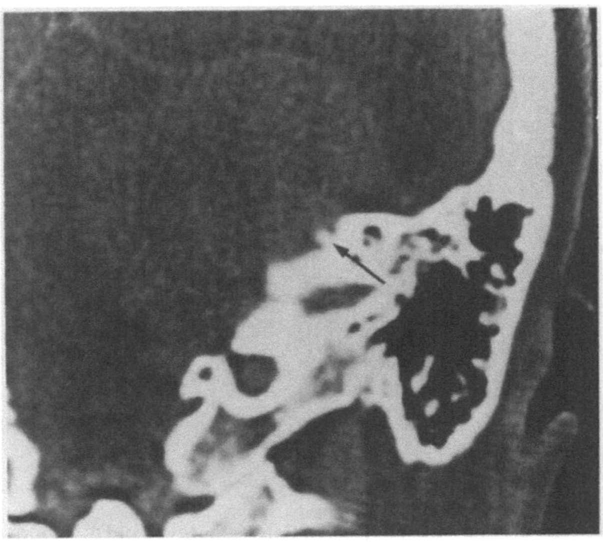

Fig. 58. Superomeatal exostosis in a case of large cerebello-pontine angle meningioma. High resolution CT. The exostosis (*arrow*) is located between the internal auditory canal and the tentorium

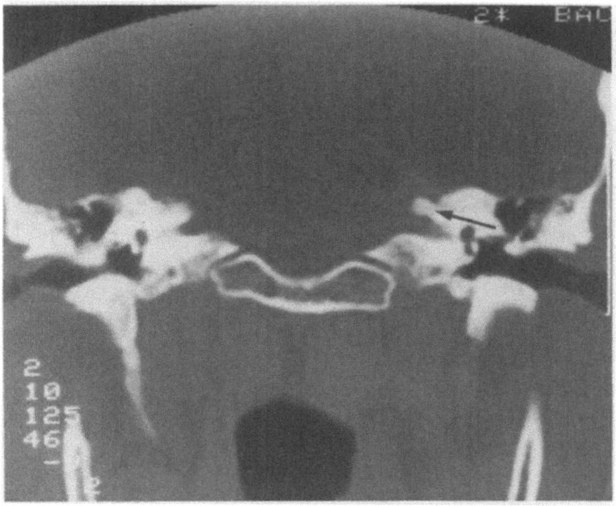

Fig. 59. Cerebello-pontine angle meningioma with superomeatal origin. High resolution coronal CT. The roof of the internal auditory canal ends in a thick exostosis (*arrow*)

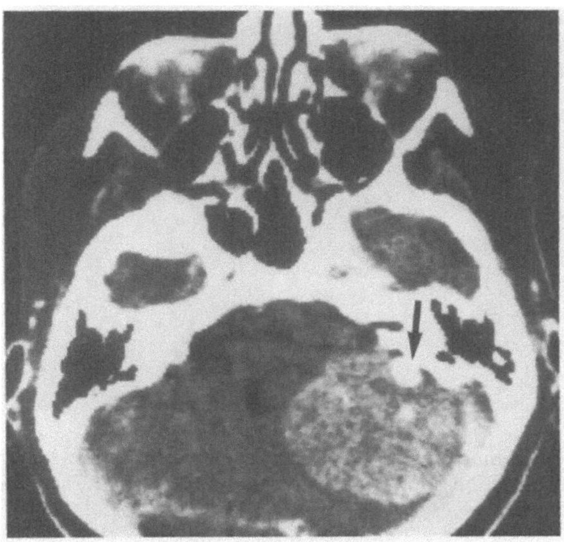

Fig. 60. Retromeatal cerebello-pontine angle meningioma. Post contrast CT. A spherical exostosis (*arrow*) is seen at the point of tumor contact with the posterior surface of the petrous bone

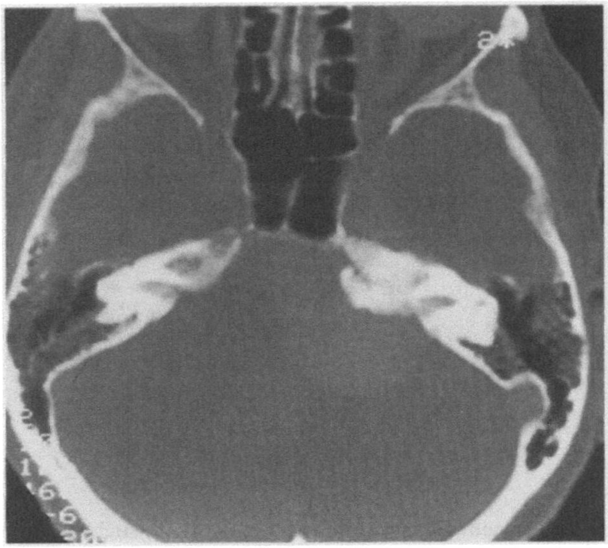

Fig. 61. Spheno-petro-clival meningioma. High resolution axial CT. A thick, elongated exostosis, indicating the origin of the tumor, is seen at the medial end of the anterior lip of the internal auditory canal

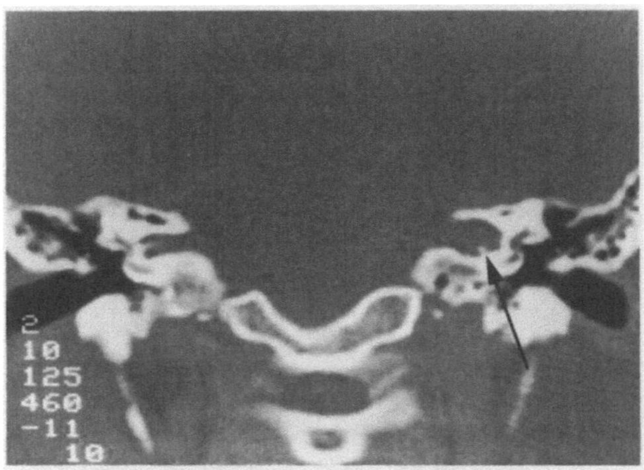

Fig. 62. Purely intrameatal meningioma. Coronal high resolution CT shows a small exostosis (*arrow*) at the medial portion of the floor of the internal auditory canal. The internal auditory canal is significantly enlarged

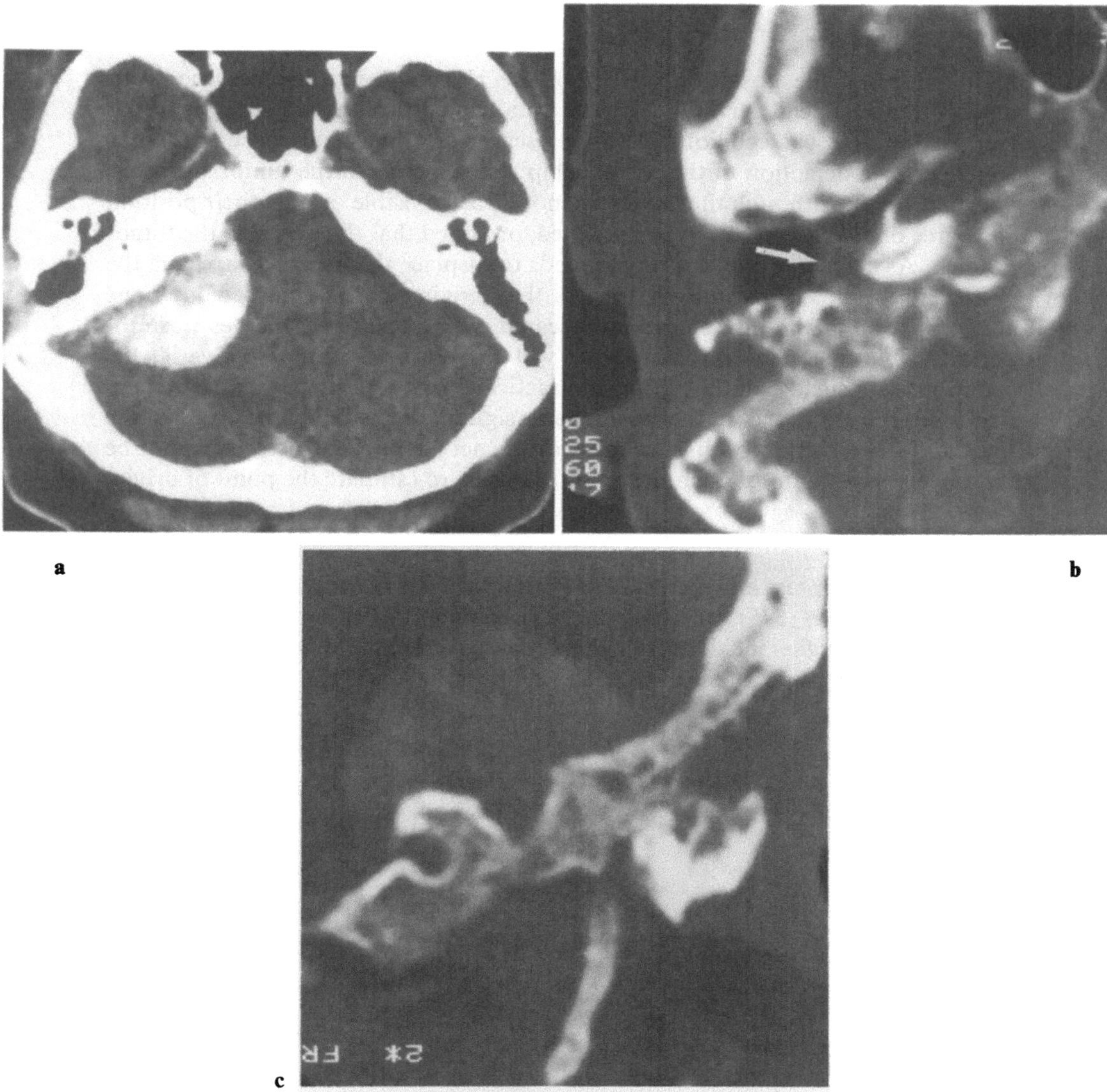

a b c

Fig. 63a–c. Cerebello-pontine angle meningioma. **a** Post contrast CT shows intense, homogeneous enhancement of the tumor and broad attachment to the posterior surface of the petrous bone. Axial **b** and coronal **c** high resolution CT in the same case show extensive invasion of the medial aspect of the petrous bone and tumor extension into the middle ear (*arrow*)

Relation to Cranial Nerves

Meningiomas of the posterior surface of the petrous bone displace the vestibulocochlear and facial nerves, but do not usually incorporate them into the tumor mass. Current surgical techniques permit preservation of the neurovascular bundle, so preoperative depiction of the relationship of the nerves to the tumor surface is important (630). Although the nerves are not directly visible on CT, their position and degree of displacement can be predicted, provided that the origin of the tumor is known. As a general rule, the tumor tends to displace the nerves away from the point of its origin. For example, tumors that originate from the petrous bone antero-superior to the internal auditory canal, will displace the nerves postero-inferiorly. During operation the nerves will therefore be found to overlie the postero-inferior surface of the tumor. In practical terms, identification of the small exostosis at the tumor base is the most reliable sign for determining the origin of the tumor and the direction of displacement of the nerves. If the exostosis cannot be seen, one uses the point of greatest tumor thickness to estimate the point of origin.

Fourth Ventricle

Meningiomas compress and displace the fourth ventricle about as commonly as do acoustic neurinomas (575). Obstructive hydrocephalus is found in more than 60% of cases. This much higher incidence of hydrocephalus in meningiomas as compared to acoustic neurinomas is explained by the greater tumor size at the time of detection (95).

Supratentorial Growth

Meningiomas may extend into the supratentorial compartment either transcisternally or transtentorially. In approximately 75% of cases supratentorial growth occurs by transcisternal, transincisural extension (390, 575). In these cases, the ipsilateral ambient cistern is dilated, the quadrigeminal plate cistern is deformed or obliterated, and the pons and mesencephalon are rotated. Depending upon the size of the supratentorial portion of the tumor, the posterior third ventricle may be compressed and displaced to the contralateral side and the ipsilateral temporal horn may be displaced antero-laterally.

The supero-lateral border of the meningioma abuts upon the tentorium. The supero-lateral tumor margin is therefore straight. If the tumor grows through the incisura, the supratentorial portion of the tumor will not be constrained by the tentorium and will grow into a spherical shape instead. The free margin of the tentorium will appear to "notch" the lateral border of the tumor deeply. If the flat infratentorial portion of the tumor "tail", the round supratentorial portion of the tumor "head" and the lateral "notch" are included in the same slice simultaneously, the tumor will appear to have a comma shape (Fig. 64). This "comma-sign" (390) is characteristic and nearly specific for meningiomas. It is found with other tumors only exceptionally (575).

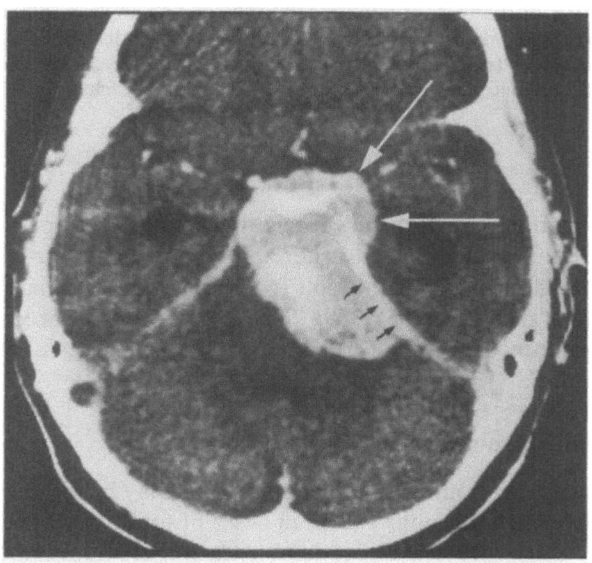

Fig. 64. Comma sign with cerebello-pontine angle meningioma. The infratentorial lateral border of the tumor lies on the tentorium and is straight (*short black arrows*). The supratentorial portion of the tumor assumes a round shape (*white arrows*). Together, the infra- and supratentorial portions of the tumor form a comma

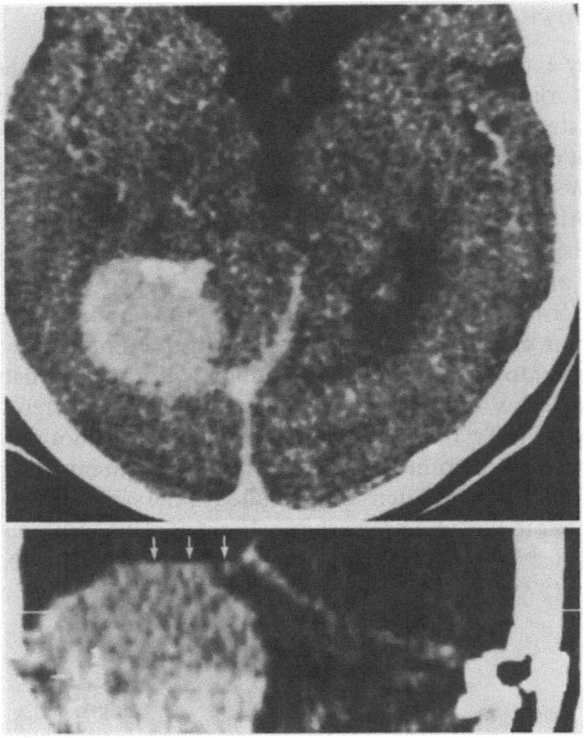

a

b

Fig. 65a, b. Elevation of the tentorium with cerebello-pontine angle meningioma, mimicking transtentorial growth. **a** Axial post contrast CT. The tumor bulk seems to be located lateral to the tentorium, which suggests true transtentorial growth. **b** Coronal reformation shows, that the tentorium is elevated (*arrows*) and overlies the tumor. The tentorium can be separated from the tumor

True transtentorial growth occurs rarely and is most commonly encountered with tumors exhibiting histological criteria of malignancy. True transtentorial extension of meningioma may be difficult to demonstrate on axial CT, and is best seen on thin coronal slices (Fig. 65) (389, 390, 575). In rare instances, supratentorial extension may occur by direct bone erosion through the petrous apex or by growth into Meckel's cave.

Diagnosis of Small Meningiomas

Like small acoustic neurinomas, small meningiomas may be difficult to detect and to differentiate from other lesions except in cases of totally calcified meningiomas (Fig. 66). Artifacts may prevent direct demonstration of small tumors. Therefore, gas CT cisternography is indicated whenever high resolution CT demonstrates bone changes suggestive of meningioma and whenever there is strong clinical suspicion of tumor (Figs. 67 and 68) (430, 471, 575). Cisternographic demonstration of displaced vestibulocochlear and facial nerves may then aid in diagnosis (Fig. 69).

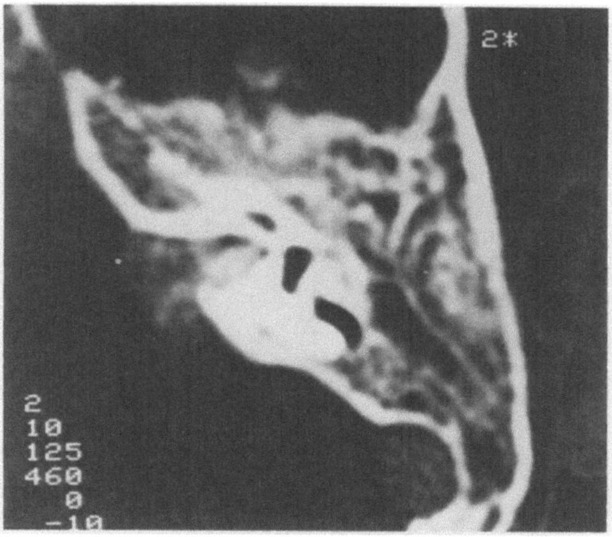

Fig. 66. Small mainly intracanalicular meningioma. The internal auditory canal is enlarged. It is filled out by an inhomogeneously calcified mass, which extends into the cerebello-pontine angle

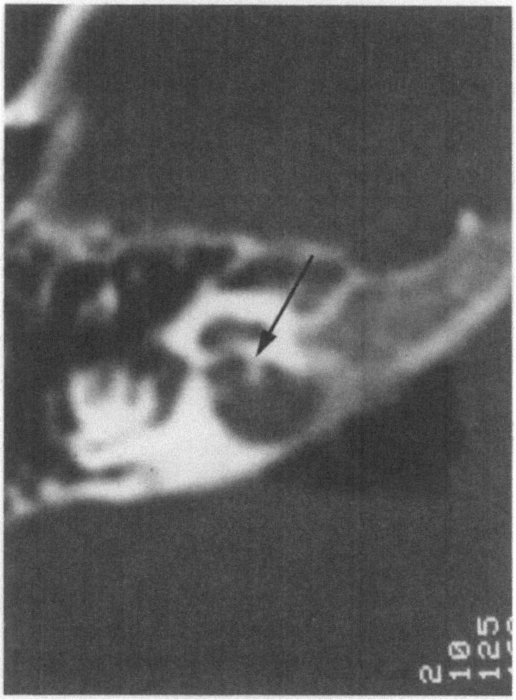

Fig. 67. Purely intrameatal meningioma. Gas CT cisternography shows the enlarged internal auditory canal to be filled with a mass. Air does not enter the internal auditory canal. Note the small exostosis at the medial aspect of the anterior border of the internal auditory canal (*arrow*) (same case as Fig. 62)

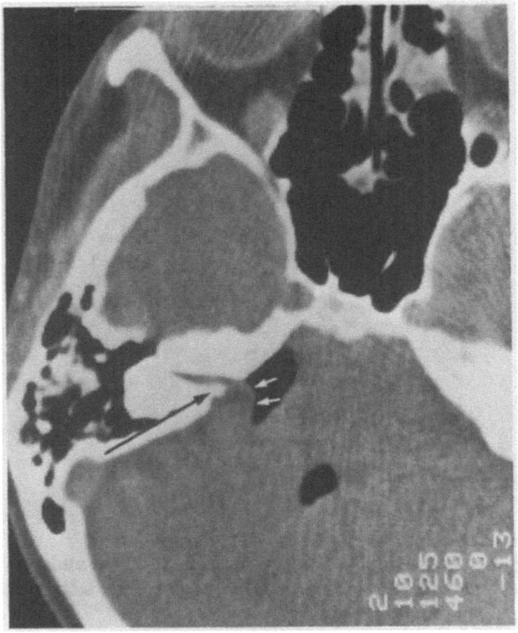

Fig. 68. Small cerebello-pontine angle meningioma. Gas CT cisternography. The anterior border of the small meningioma is delineated by gas (*short arrows*). Note the exostosis at the posterior lip of the internal auditory canal indicating the origin of the tumor (*arrow*)

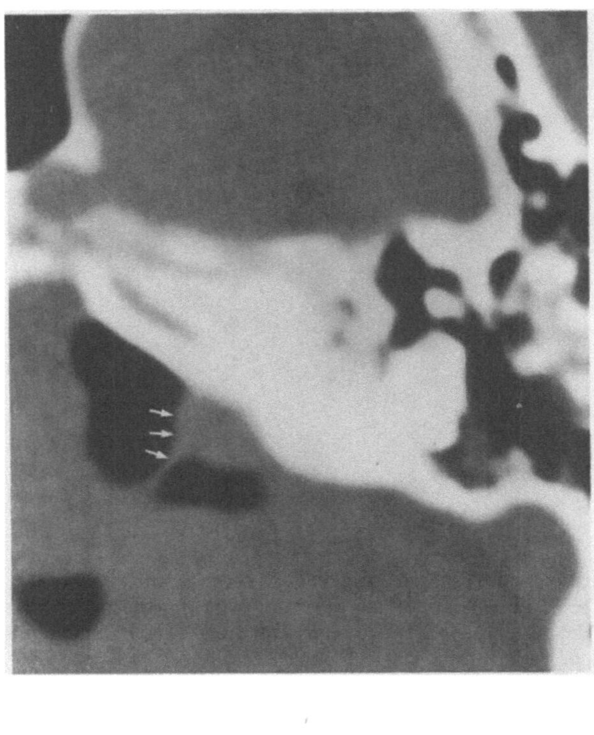

Epidermoid Tumors

1 General Considerations

Intracranial epidermoid tumors are rare tumors constituting 0.75 to 0.85% of all primary intracranial neoplasms (57, 77, 461) and 2% of all infratentorial tumors (166). The most frequent site of posterior fossa epidermoids is the cerebello-pontine angle. Epidermoids are the third most common tumor of the cerebello-pontine angle with a frequency of 2.8 to 6.3% of all cerebello-pontine angle masses (218, 473, 629, 640).

Clinical Findings

Although epidermoids are congenital tumors, most of them first become symptomatic in middle age after they have reached considerable size (304, 412, 473, 569, 570). Mean patient age at the time of diagnosis is about 35 years. Clinical misinterpretation of their symptoms as multiple sclerosis or trigeminal neuralgia is common (412, 569, 629). The most common initial symptoms are hypoacusis and tinnitus, related to the eighth cranial nerve. Facial and trigeminal palsy may also occur. Large tumors cause additional cerebellar symptoms (412, 569). Rupture of the tumor capsule permits cholesterin to escape into the cerebro-spinal fluid causing aseptic meningitis (176, 569). Extremely rarely, a primary intracranial squamous cell carcinoma may originate from a preexisting benign epidermoid (158).

2 Conventional Radiology

X-ray studies including pluridirectional tomography may show sharply demarcated erosion of the medial aspect of the posterior surface of the petrous bone (55, 325). Calcification may rarely be found at the periphery of the tumor (55, 331).

Angiography shows an avascular mass of the cerebello-pontine angle. In some cases narrowing and irregularities of the arteries indicate tumor encasement of the vessels (355). The most reliable and specific conventional diagnostic study is pneumoencephalography. Air entering into the interstitium of the tumor produces a characteristic "cauliflower" or "cottage cheese" appearance (325).

←

Fig. 69. Small cerebello-pontine angle meningioma. Gas CT cisternography. The whole circumference of the tumor is delineated by gas. The vestibulocochlear nerve overlies the tumor anteriorly (*short arrows*)

3 Computed Tomography

Density and Contrast Enhancement

Epidermoids usually appear on CT as homogeneously hypodense masses (Fig. 70) (128). The majority of epidermoids present with density values near that of cerebro-spinal fluid. In rare cases the density may vary between −20 and +30 HU (93, 355, 387, 401). Since the density of the tumor is nearly the same as cerebro-spinal fluid, these lesions may be misinterpreted as arachnoid cysts or hygromas. Quantitative analysis of the scan permits correct differential diagnosis, however, because the standard deviation in density of epidermoids is higher than that measured in cerebro-spinal fluid (257). Tumor hypodensity is caused by desquamated epithelial cells containing keratin and cholesterin. The more cholesterin the tumor contains, the lower its overall density will be (62, 93, 257, 355). Uniformly hyperdense epidermoid cysts are described as extremely rare variants (38, 379, 518). Such hyperdensity is thought to be the result of formation of calcified soaps (38). Punctate and curvilinear calcifications are extremely rare in epidermoids and appear to be confined to the tumor capsule (378, 437, 492).

Epidermoids are nearly avascular tumors (93, 128, 166, 629) and do not enhance after contrast administration (Figs. 70–73). They are surrounded by a thin capsule, which is not usually visible on CT. However, a few epidermoids with total or partial ring enhancement have been reported (355, 401, 499). The ring enhancement in these cases has been interpreted as thickened tumor capsule, possibly related to

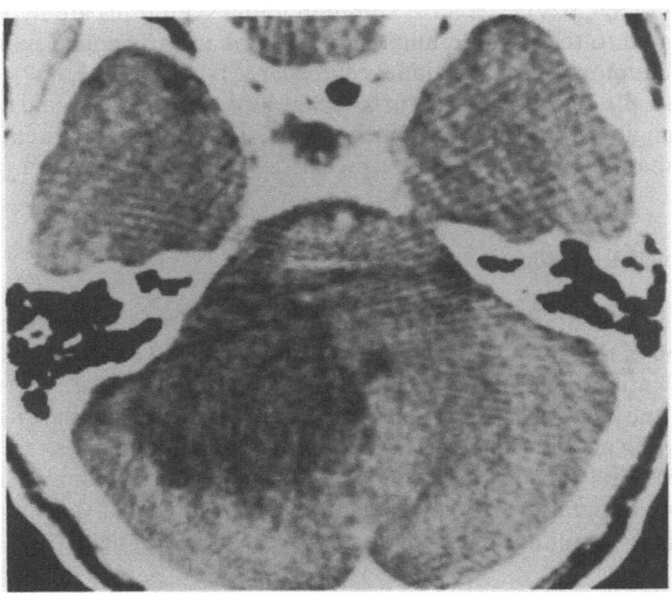

Fig. 70. Epidermoid tumor of the right cerebello-pontine angle. Post contrast axial CT. The tumor is homogeneously hypodense and shows no enhancement. Pons and cerebellum are displaced medially. Note the dentate, irregular appearance of the tumor border, especially at its posterior surface

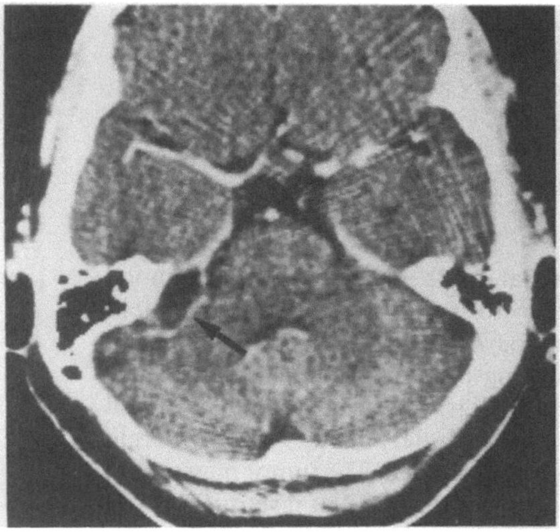

▲ Fig. 71

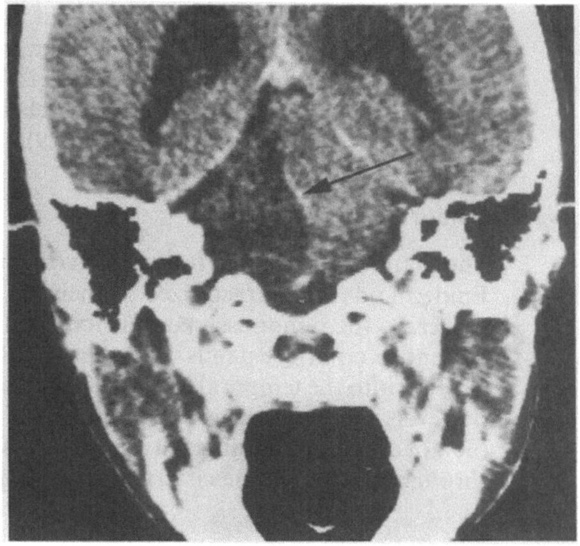

Fig. 72 ▶

Fig. 71. Small epidermoid tumor of the cerebello-pontine angle with thick tumor capsule. Post contrast axial CT. Note the thick enhancing rim surrounding the epidermoid (*arrow*). At operation, a thick capsule was found

Fig. 72. Epidermoid tumor of the cerebello-pontine angle. Post contrast coronal CT. The capsule of the epidermoid is visible as an enhancing rim (*arrow*)

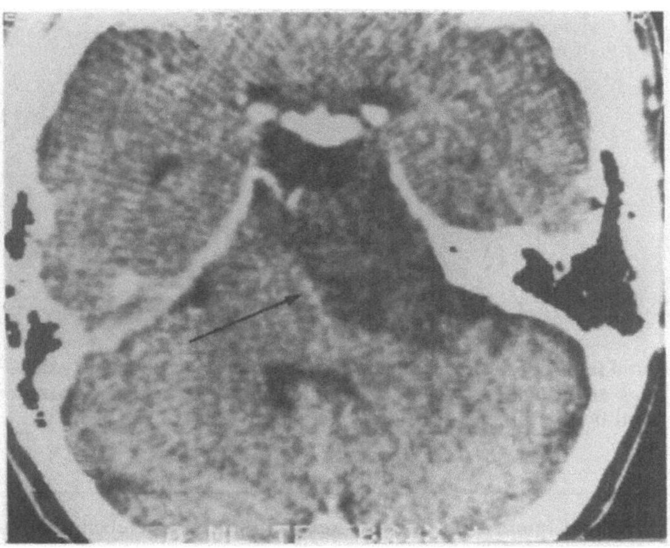

Fig. 73. Thin tumor capsule in a large epidermoid tumor of the cerebello-pontine angle. Post contrast axial CT. Only a very small linear enhancement is seen partially outlining the tumor (*arrow*)

leakage of cyst content and perilesional inflammation (Figs. 71–73). Peritumoral gliosis, known to occur in rare instances, may also explain the ring enhancement (262). Since the capsule of epidermoids is frequently adherent to adjacent vessels, nerves, pia mater, brainstem and cerebellum, CT demonstration of a capsule suggests the presence of adhesions (629).

Tumor Shape

The shape of epidermoid tumors differs from that of other pontocerebellar tumors. Epidermoids are characterized by their tendency to spread along the subarachnoid spaces, so the tumor assumes an elongated shape, fills out the edges and curves of the entire cistern, extends into the neighbouring cisterns, and even crosses the incisura into the temporal cisterns (70% of cases) (Figs. 74–78). This tendency to fill out every free space gives the appearance of an irregular, dentate tumor margin (60% of cases). All the affected cisterns are slightly expanded. The tumor may extend through the prepontine cistern into the opposite pontocerebellar cistern (Fig. 76).

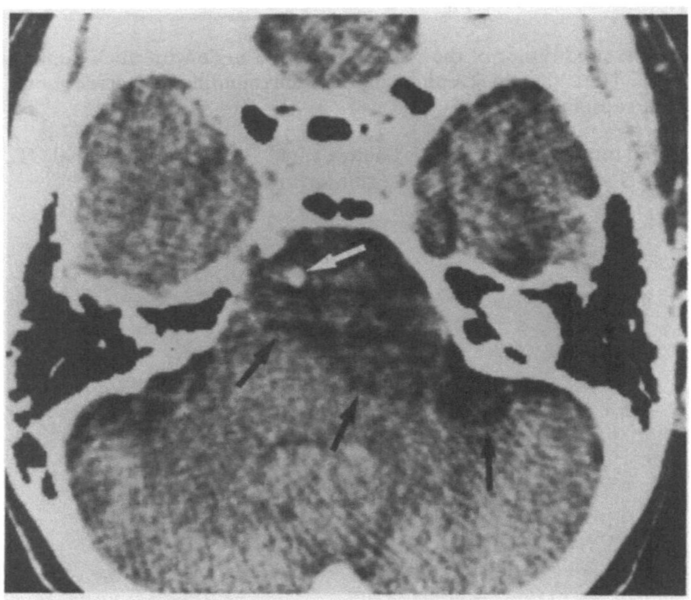

Fig. 74. Epidermoid tumor of the left cerebello-pontine angle. Post contrast axial CT. The tumor (*black arrows*) has an elongated, oval shape. Note the basilar artery (*white arrow*) which is completely encased by the tumor

Fig. 76a, b. Epidermoid tumor with diffuse extension into both cerebello-pontine angles and supratentorial cisterns. **a** Axial post contrast CT section shows bilateral widening of the prepontine and cerebello-pontine angle cisterns by a hypodense tumor mass (*arrows*). The basilar artery (*short white arrows*) courses through the tumor. **b** Coronal reformation shows tumor extension in front of the pons (*arrowhead*) and additional supratentorial tumor extension (*arrow*)

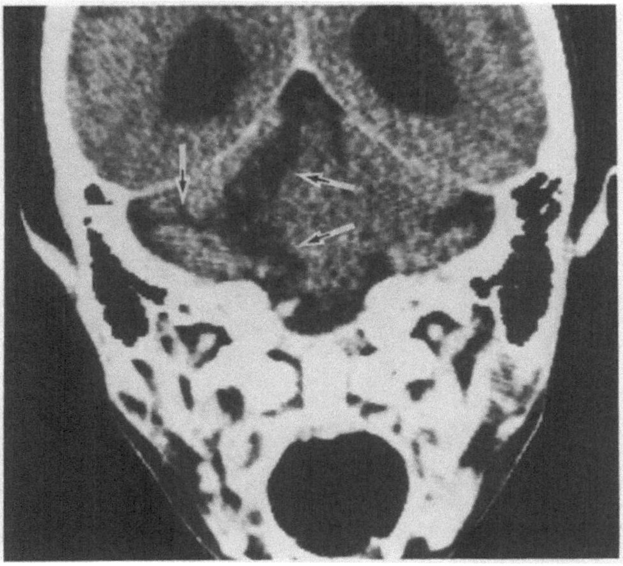

Fig. 75. Epidermoid tumor of the cerebello-pontine angle. Post contrast coronal CT. The tumor originates from the right cerebello-pontine angle and shows finger-like extensions within the cerebro-spinal fluid spaces and along a cerebellar sulcus (*arrows*)

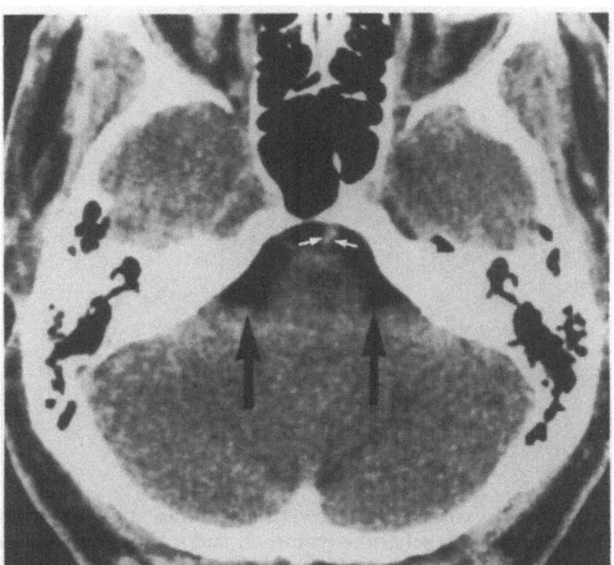

a

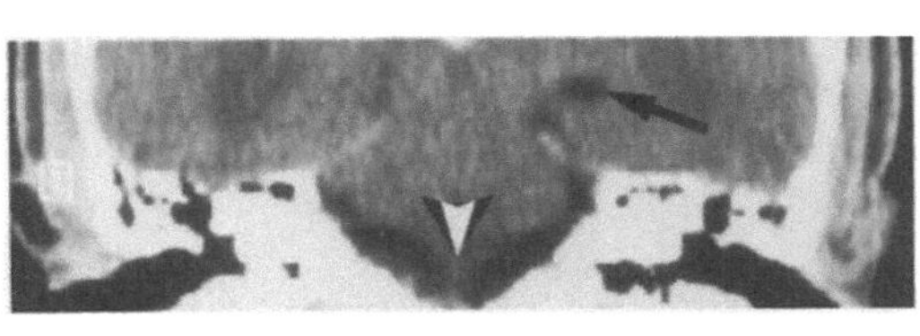

b

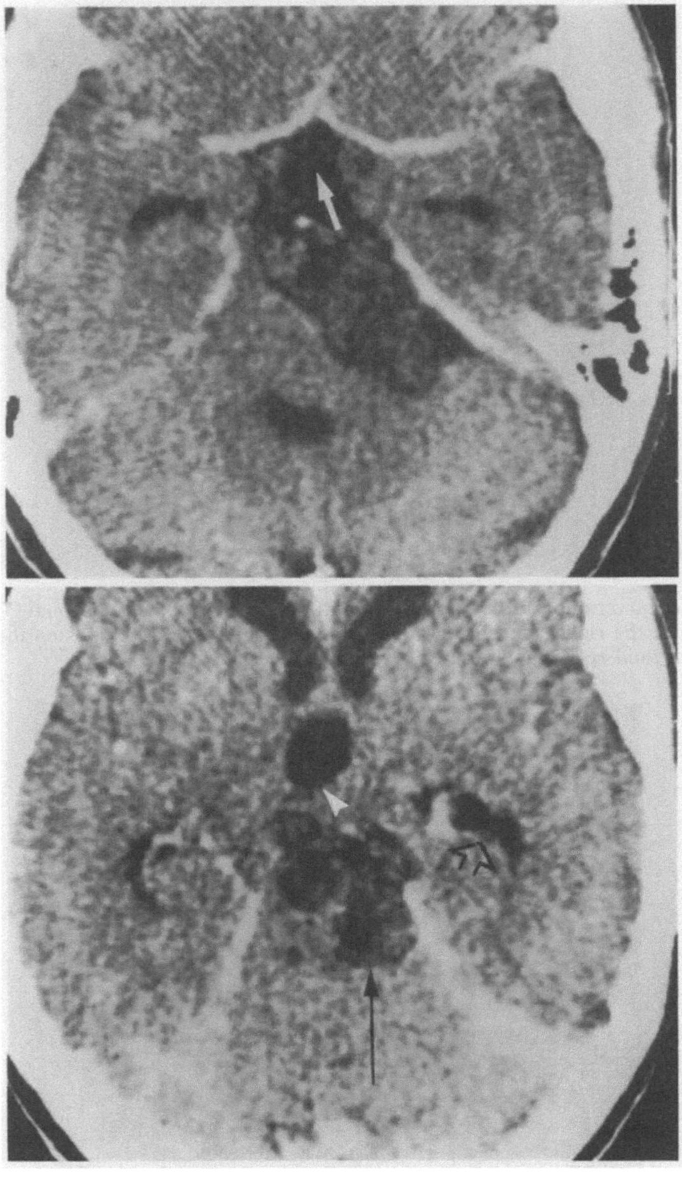

a

b

Fig. 77a, b. Supratentorial extension of a cerebello-pontine angle epidermoid tumor. Post contrast CT. **a** The epidermoid reaches the tentorium and extends into the suprasellar cistern (*arrow*). **b** At a slightly higher level, transincisural growth is seen with tumor masses in the posterior wing of the ambient cistern and in the quadrigeminal plate cistern (*arrow*). Note the angular cutoff of the posterior third ventricle (*arrowhead*) and slight antero-lateral displacement of the temporal horn (*open arrow*)

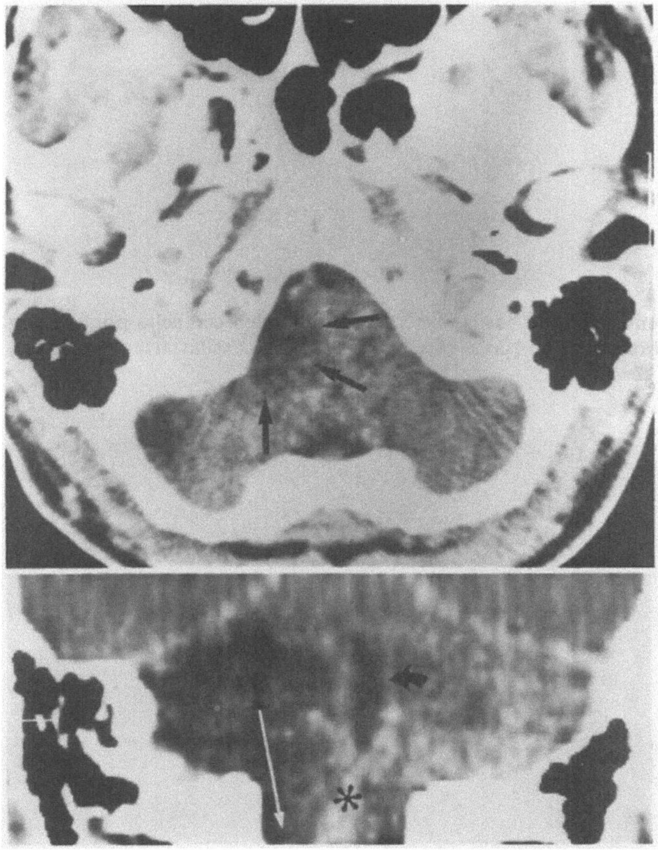

a

b

Fig. 78a, b. Epidermoid tumor of the right cerebello-pontine angle. Post contrast CT. **a** The axial section at the level of the lateral cerebellomedullary cistern shows cisternal obliteration and expansion by the epidermoid (*arrows*). **b** Coronal reformation shows tumor extension into the upper cervical subarachnoid space (*arrow*). The medulla (*asterisk*) and the fourth ventricle (*short curved arrow*) are displaced to the left side

Less commonly, the tumor extends downward to the lateral cerebello-medullary cistern (30% of cases). Very large tumors may reach the foramen magnum or even the cervical subarachnoid space (Fig. 78).

Vessel Encasement

Contrast enhanced CT regularly demonstrates displacement of the large vessels surrounding the tumor. Thin section contrast enhanced CT often permits demonstration of encasement of the cisternal vessels by the epidermoid. Depending on the direction of the vessel course in respect to the scanning plane, encasement appears as linear, curvilinear or punctate vascular enhancement, completely surrounded by the hypodense tumor tissue (Figs. 74, 79 and 80).

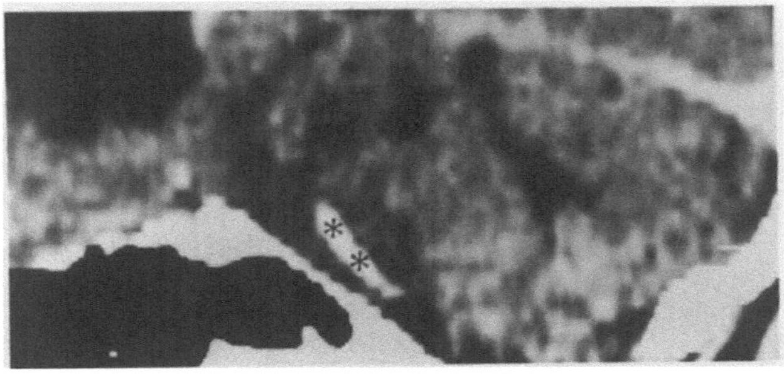

Fig. 79. Encasement of the basilar artery with left-sided cerebello-pontine angle epidermoid tumor. Sagittal reformation (same case as Fig. 74). The basilar artery (*asterisks*) is completely surrounded by the tumor

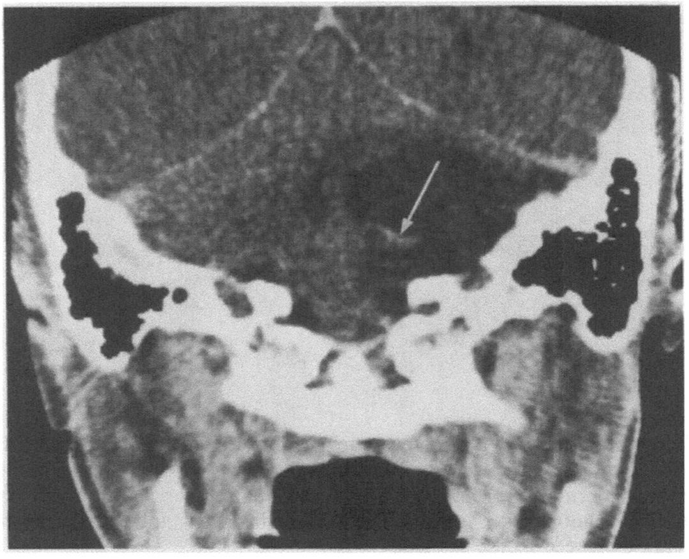

Fig. 80. Encasement of the choroid plexus with left-sided cerebello-pontine angle epidermoid tumor. Post contrast coronal CT. The choroid plexus of the fourth ventricle (*arrow*) is completely embedded in the epidermoid

Perifocal Hypodensity

Perifocal hypodensity is usually not observed with epidermoids, although it is a common finding with other cerebello-pontine angle tumors. Pressure exerted on the surrounding cerebellar parenchyma may be too low to cause edema. Obstructive hydrocephalus also occurs more rarely with epidermoids than with other cerebello-pontine angle tumors, perhaps because cerebro-spinal fluid may percolate through the interstices of the tumor to pass the obstruction. However, normal pressure hydrocephalus may occur by impaired cerebro-spinal fluid circulation at the level of the tentorial incisura or as a sequel of aseptic meningitis, caused by escaping cholesterin.

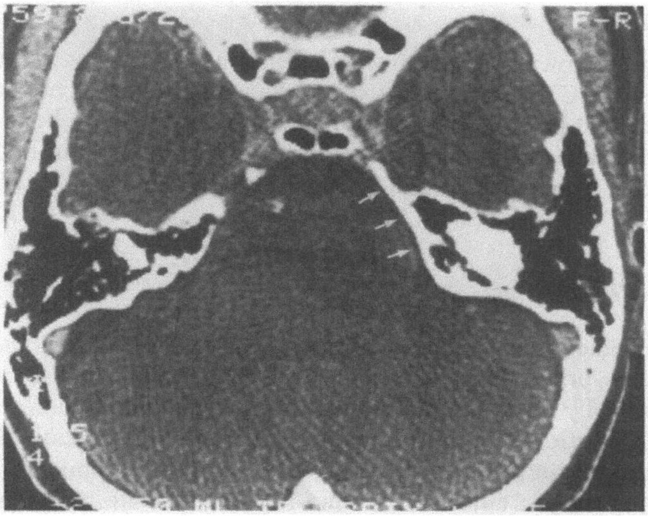

Fig. 81. Pressure erosion of the petrous pyramid in a case of epidermoid tumor of the left cerebello-pontine angle. Axial high resolution CT (same case as Fig. 74). A sharply marginated pressure erosion of the petrous pyramid (*small arrows*) is seen

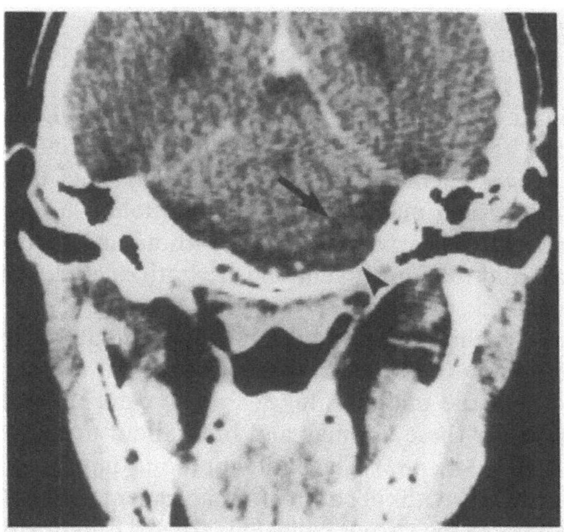

Fig. 82. Pressure erosion of the left basiocciput in a case of cerebello-pontine angle epidermoid tumor. Post contrast coronal CT. The tumor (*arrow*) assumes an oval shape and fills out the expanded pontocerebellar cistern. Pressure erosion at the basiocciput (*arrowhead*) is seen even without bone imaging parameters

Osseous Changes

Osseous changes, known to occur from conventional X-ray studies, have found little attention in the CT literature. In 40% of the authors' material, pressure erosion of the antero-medial part of the posterior surface of the petrous bone assumes a laterally-convex shape and the cortical surface may be thinned but not destroyed (Figs. 81 and 82). The internal auditory canal usually remains intact.

4 Differential Diagnosis

The differential diagnosis of epidermoid tumors includes the other hypodense non enhancing lesions, primarily the arachnoid cyst. Epidermoids and arachnoid cysts are characterized by hypodensity, elongated shape, bone erosion and lack of enhancement. Detection of irregular, dentate tumor margins indicates the presence of epidermoid and excludes an arachnoid cyst. Similarly pseudopodic extensions to adjacent cisterns suggest epidermoid tumor, not arachnoid cyst. Water soluble positive-contrast CT cisternography may also help to differentiate the lesions, since the epidermoid will often show the "cauliflower" appearance previously described for pneumoencephalography, whereas arachnoid cysts will appear as smooth filling defects within the contrast or as opacifying collections in delayed CT scans. Penetration of water soluble positive-contrast agent into a cystic acoustic neurinoma has been described as a very rare finding. The differential diagnostic value of entrance of positive-contrast into a tumor is therefore rather limited (266). Vessel encasement is not observed with arachnoid cysts.

Chronic subdural hygroma may mimic an epidermoid. Like arachnoid cysts, subdural hygromas are confined to the pontocerebellar cistern. The subdural membrane often shows enhancement on contrast enhanced CT.

Cerebellar atrophy also may mimic an epidermoid (93). Cerebellar atrophy presents as symmetrical cisternal dilatation without mass effect. Since the infratentorial cisterns and the fourth ventricle are both dilated, differentiation from an epidermoid should be possible.

Lipoma of the cerebello-pontine angle may also simulate an epidermoid on CT. Lipomas are rare tumors (0.1 to 0.4% of all intracranial tumors) and are usually located within or near the midline (46, 598). The cerebello-pontine angle is an uncommon location for these lipomas and only about a dozen cases have been reported (155, 174, 273, 345, 482). The pathognomonic pattern is hypodensity with values as low as -100 HU without contrast enhancement (124, 257). Calcifications, common with lipomas of the corpus callosum, are not found with pontocerebellar lipomas.

The rare hyperdense variant of an epidermoid has to be differentiated from meningioma and choroid plexus papilloma (38). Since the hyperdense epidermoid shows no contrast enhancement, it is readily differentiated from enhancing meningiomas and papillomas. It may usually be distinguished from the completely calcified, non enhancing meningiomas by its far lower density measurements.

Finally, primary, intradural epidermoid of the pontocerebellar cistern must be distinguished from the primary cholesteatoma of the petrous pyramid (431, 438).

The main clinical symptom of primary cholesteatoma is facial palsy, caused in most cases by involvement of the geniculate ganglion. These cholesteatomas may erode through the posterior surface of the petrous bone into the epidural intracranial space. In that location the cholesteatoma is nearly indistinguishable from primary epidermoid tumor. The non contrast density varies from a few HU below zero to cerebro-spinal fluid density in the same way as in intradural epidermoids (333, 438, 550). On contrast enhanced CT, however, the position of the enhancing dura distinguishes the two lesions: The dura is displaced medially by epidural extension of the petrous cholesteatoma and is not detectable when it is pushed laterally against the petrous bone by the expanding intracisternal epidermoid (Figs. 83 and 84).

The extremely rare expanding intrapetrous granuloma may be nearly impossible to differentiate from primary cholesteatoma by clinical or radiological criteria (322).

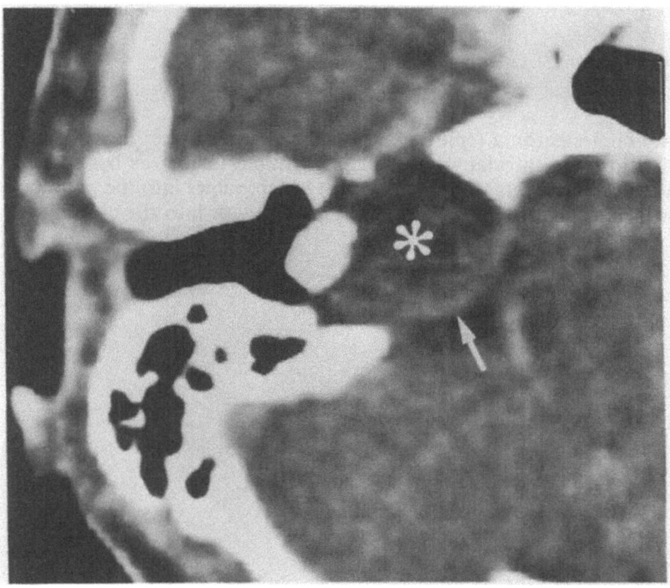

Fig. 83. Primary cholesteatoma (epidermoid) of the right petrous bone. Post contrast axial CT. The petrous pyramid is destroyed by a hypodense epidermoid (*asterisk*). Intrapetrous origin of the epidermoid is evidenced by the medially-convex dura (*arrow*) which separates the tumor from the pontocerebellar cistern

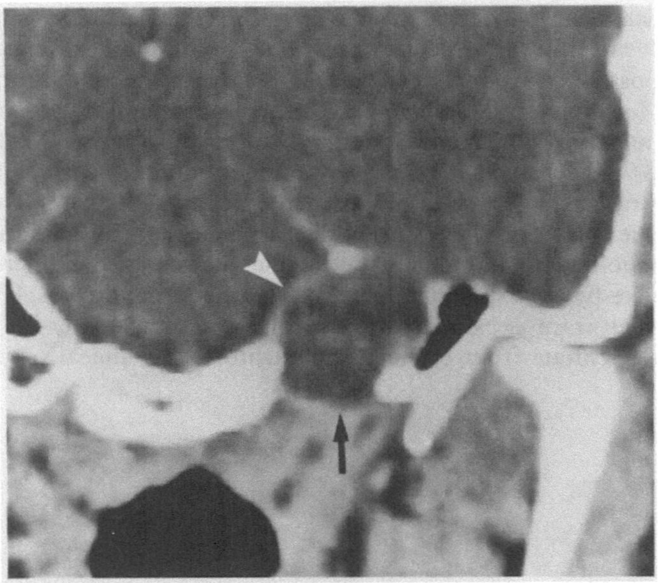

Fig. 84. Primary cholesteatoma (epidermoid) of the petrous bone. Post contrast coronal CT. Tumor extension into the infralabyrinthine compartment (*arrow*) is best assessed on coronal views. Note the thick enhancing dura (*arrowhead*) which bulges into the pontocerebellar cistern and obliterates it partially. There is no direct tumor growth into the cistern

Arachnoid Cysts of the Cerebello-Pontine Angle

1 General Considerations

Arachnoid cysts constitute 0.4 to 0.8% (629, 640) of all lesions of the cerebello-pontine angle. The first description of an arachnoid cyst of the posterior fossa was given by Mannsell in 1889 (339). The true etiology remains obscure. Congenital (28), inflammatory (6) and traumatic factors (557) have been postulated. Histologic (538) and electron-microscopic studies (469) show that arachnoid cysts are intra-arachnoid lesions originating from clefting of the arachnoid membrane. Gardner et al. (161) have postulated that arachnoid cysts of the posterior fossa originate from a primary impermeability of the primitive membranes covering the roof of the fourth ventricle. Impermeability of the membrane covering the foramen of Magendie leads to formation of a retrocerebellar midline Dandy-Walker cyst. Impermeability of the membrane covering the foramen of Luschka leads to arachnoid cysts of the cerebello-pontine angle. The developing cyst then extends from the lateral recess of the fourth ventricle into the pontocerebellar cistern. At best, such explanation would account for only a fraction of the cysts observed. Secondary loculation of the subarachnoid space by arachnoiditis may cause a superficially similar lesion, but such lesion may be differentiated from true arachnoid cysts pathologically.

Clinically, arachnoid cysts of the cerebello-pontine angle cause pressure-related pontine and cerebellar symptoms. Obstructive hydrocephalus may occur with large arachnoid cysts.

2 Conventional Radiology

Conventional X-ray studies including pluridirectional tomography show thinning and pressure erosion of the posterior surface of the petrous bone (90). Pneumoencephalography usually discloses a non communicating mass lesion. In some cases, air does enter the cyst, permitting correct diagnosis (558). Vertebral angiography gives evidence of an avascular cerebello-pontine angle mass (558, 622).

3 Computed Tomography

Arachnoid cysts present as hypodense, sharply demarcated extraaxial lesions with smooth margins and without contrast enhancement (Figs. 85 and 86) (6, 21, 257, 301, 303, 460, 593). Quantitative density analysis characteristically discloses homogeneous fluid very similar to cerebro-spinal fluid (257). Arachnoid cysts of the cerebello-pontine angle commonly are biconvex, lentiform lesions (21). Rarely they

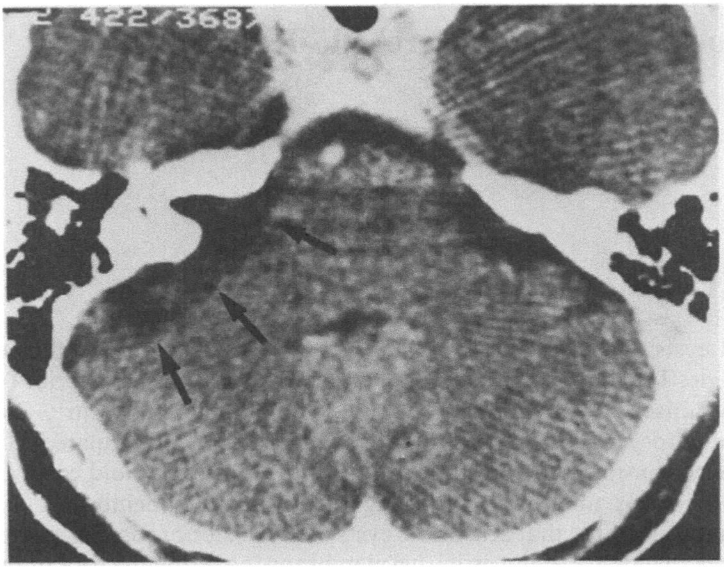

Fig. 85. Arachnoid cyst of the cerebello-pontine angle. Post contrast axial CT. The arachnoid cyst presents as an oval, sharply delineated hypodense mass without contrast enhancement (*arrows*). The pontocerebellar cistern is dilated. The fourth ventricle is distorted and slightly displaced posteriorly

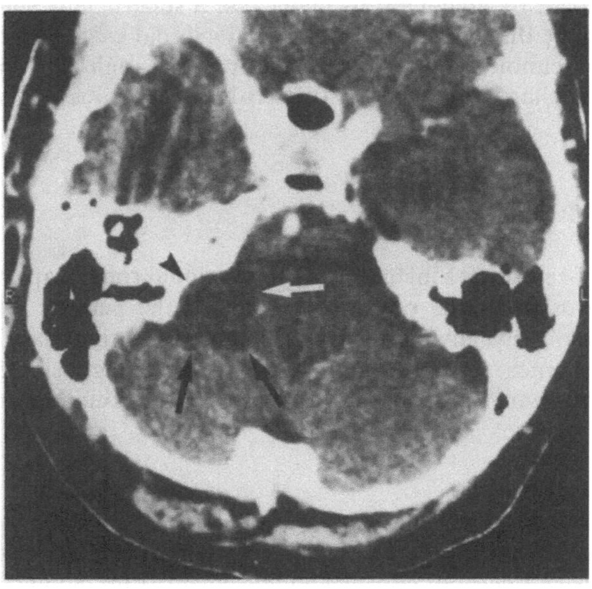

Fig. 86. Arachnoid cyst of the cerebello-pontine angle. Post contrast axial CT. The hypodense cyst has slightly irregular borders (*arrows*). Typical pressure erosion of the posterior surface of the petrous bone (*arrowhead*) is seen

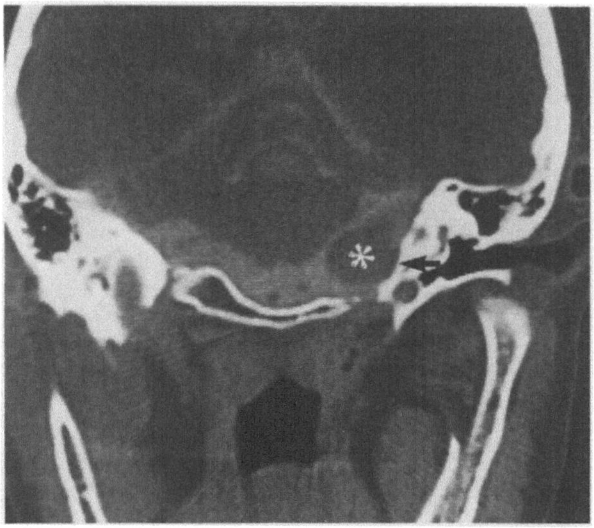

Fig. 87. Arachnoid cyst of the cerebello-pontine angle. Coronal metrizamide CT cisternography. The arachnoid cyst presents as a round filling defect in the cerebello-pontine angle (*asterisk*). Pressure erosion (*arrow*) of the inferior portion of the posterior surface of the petrous bone and of the lateral clivus is well seen

may be round. Depending upon their size and mass effect, the fourth ventricle may be compressed or displaced. Osseous changes are common and consist mainly in a sharply demarcated pressure erosion of the posterior surface of the petrous bone (Figs. 86 and 87). The cortical bone is thinned but remains intact. With large cysts, the bone erosion may encroach upon the neighbouring structures such as the jugular tubercle, the occipital condyle or the clivus.

Three types of arachnoid cysts are distinguished on the basis of their appearance on water soluble positive-contrast CT cisternograms including late scans performed after 6, 12, and 24 h in order to prove or exclude communication (110, 181, 196, 303, 491, 623). Considerable evidence suggests that these 3 types are directly related to cyst size (or perhaps vice versa).

1. Rapidly communicating arachnoid cysts. Non contrast CT scans show a wide "cistern" that appears to displace or indent the adjacent brain. CT scans performed immediately following instillation of positive-contrast show opacification of the cistern and partial opacification of a separate space within the cistern. This space usually contains less contrast and is somewhat lower in density than the adjacent cistern. It frequently exhibits a layering or sedimentation gradient of density within the cyst. A membrane usually demarcates the cyst border from the adjacent cistern.
2. Slowly communicating arachnoid cysts usually appear as non opacified filling defects on the immediate post contrast CT scan, but increase in density and "fill in" during the subsequent 6 to 24 h (Fig. 88). Late filling may be explained either by intermittent communication or by active or passive transmembraneous diffusion (110, 196, 623).

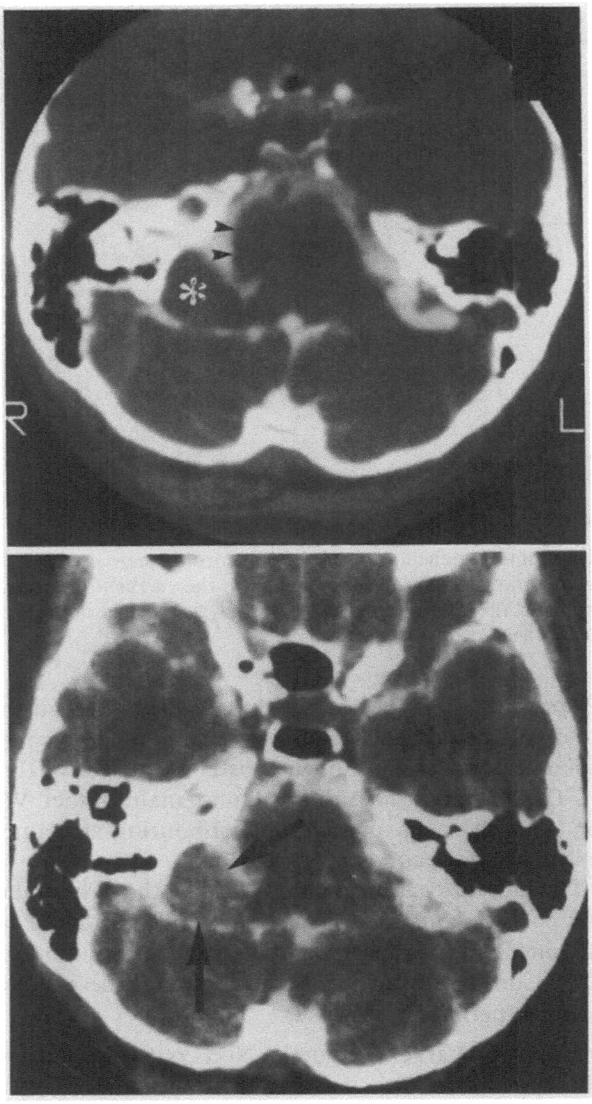

a

b

Fig. 88a, b. Slowly communicating arachnoid cyst of the cerebello-pontine angle. Axial metrizamide CT cisternography (same case as in Fig. 86). **a** Scan immediately after intrathecal contrast instillation. The arachnoid cyst (*asterisk*) presents as a sharply marginated filling defect in the contrast filled pontocerebellar cistern. The slight distortion and rotation of the pons (*small arrowheads*) is much better seen on the metrizamide CT cisternography than on the routine CT (Fig. 86). **b** Scan 5 h after contrast instillation. Absorption of the contrast medium has begun and the density in the pontocerebellar cistern has diminished when compared with the density immediately after contrast instillation. The arachnoid cyst (*arrows*) is now partially filled with contrast medium. The density of the cyst-content is less elevated than that of the cerebero-spinal fluid. The scan 24 h after contrast instillation (not shown) showed the same slightly elevated density in the cyst as in the cerebello-pontine angle

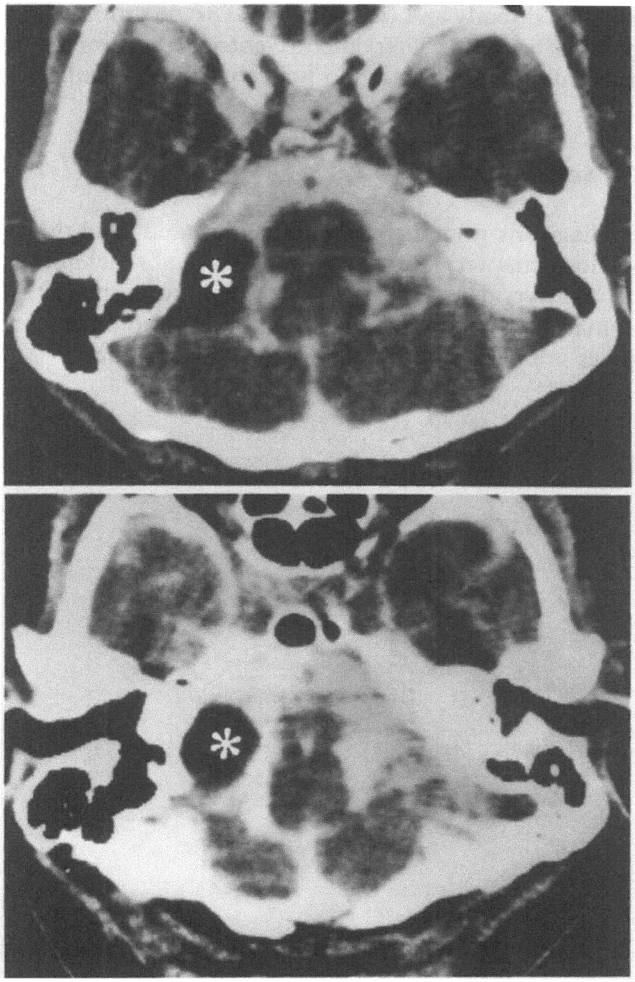

a

b

Fig. 89a, b. Non communicating arachnoid cyst of the cerebello-pontine angle. Metrizamide CT cisternography. **a** The scan immediately after intrathecal contrast instillation shows the arachnoid cyst as a filling defect in the pontocerebellar cistern (*asterisk*). **b** The scan 4 h later still shows the arachnoid cyst as a hypodense filling defect (*asterisk*) in the pontocerebellar cistern. The scan 24 h after contrast instillation (not shown) showed no entrance of contrast into the arachnoid cyst

3. Non communicating arachnoid cysts remain as low density filling defects within the opacified subarachnoid space for the duration of the study (Fig. 89). Depending on their size and location they may prevent filling of the fourth ventricle or not.

Treatment regimens for arachnoid cysts vary widely. Non communicating cysts are shunted directly into the cyst (623). In some cases the cyst wall is resected and a shunt is then placed into the cyst bed, or the lateral ventricle. Slowly communicating cysts are also shunted directly and followed by CT to determine the success of the therapy and possible need for later lateral ventricular shunt or cyst resection. Rapidly communicating cysts usually do not require treatment.

4 Differential Diagnosis

The differential diagnosis primarily includes epidermoids and the extremely rare lipomas (cf. previous chapter). Rarely, a round or oval arachnoid cyst has to be differentiated from a hypodense intraaxial cerebellar tumor such as astrocytoma or hemangioblastoma (257). The extraaxial origin of arachnoid cysts and lack of any enhancing nodules are helpful differential diagnostic criteria.

Trigeminal Neurinoma

1 General Considerations

Trigeminal neurinomas are not primarily cerebello-pontine angle tumors. However, they frequently extend secondarily into the pontocerebellar cistern, and constitute 1.5 to 2% of all cerebello-pontine angle lesions (473, 629).

Clinically and radiologically, trigeminal neurinomas can be classified as middle fossa, posterior fossa and dumbbell middle-posterior fossa lesions (4, 276, 278, 311, 507). Those neurinomas originating from the Gasserian ganglion are usually confined to the middle fossa, until they grow large. The petroclinoid ligament prevents early extension into the posterior fossa. Only later may limited infratentorial extension occur.

Trigeminal neurinomas that originate from the trigeminal root are characterized by their tendency to spread along the fifth nerve through the porus trigeminus. These tumors grow in dumbbell fashion with both supra- and infratentorial nodules. The two nodules are separated by the petroclinoid ligament which forms the rigid roof of the porus trigeminus. Less commonly a trigeminal neurinoma may originate directly from the cisternal segment of the trigeminal root and, thus, may first present as a cerebello-pontine angle tumor (249, 276, 278, 311).

The clinical presentation of trigeminal neurinomas correlates with the direction of their growth. Tumors confined to the middle fossa present with symptoms related to the trigeminal and the intracavernous nerves, whereas tumors extending into the pontocerebellar cistern manifest additional cerebello-pontine angle symptoms.

2 Conventional Radiology

Conventional radiologic studies frequently demonstrate characteristic changes of the middle fossa and the petrous apex (15, 311, 324, 465, 599). Neurinomas confined to the middle fossa cause enlargement of the foramen ovale. Large tumors may also erode the sphenoid wing and widen the superior orbital fissure. Infratentorial extension of trigeminal neurinomas is associated with erosion of the posterior clinoid process and the petrous apex. Pressure erosion of the petrous apex typically manifests as excavation of the impressio trigemini (311, 323, 425).

In cases with infratentorial extension, vertebral angiography shows evidence of a high pontocerebellar mass with elevation of the posterior cerebral and superior cerebellar arteries and caudal displacement of the anterior inferior cerebellar artery. The basilar artery is displaced contralaterally (486, 553, 554, 614, 622). The tumor is vascularized mainly from the tentorial artery or from the clival branches of the internal carotid artery. Less commonly, the middle meningeal artery, the ascending pharyngeal artery or the superior cerebellar artery may be involved in the arterial supply of the tumor (259).

3 Computed Tomography

Only a few reports deal with the CT morphology of trigeminal neurinomas (159, 167, 249, 259, 387, 535, 574, 577). However, analysis of the tumor morphology, osseous changes and tumor location usually permits correct diagnosis.

Density and Contrast Enhancement

Trigeminal neurinomas exhibit variable CT appearance on non contrast CT scans. Approximately 50% present as hypodense lesions. Approximately 17% each present as isodense, hypodense, and mixed density tumors. More than half the cases show homogeneous contrast enhancement (Fig. 90). About 20% exhibit ring enhancement (Fig. 91), and about 20% show inhomogeneous enhancement (Fig. 92). Correlation of the enhancement pattern with tumor appearance on non contrast CT shows that many iso- or hypodense tumors enhance homogeneously; some exhibit ring blush. Tumors with mixed density on non contrast CT usually show irregular enhancement. Correlation of CT images with operative findings indicates that many of the hypodense lesions are cystic (167). Indeed cystic transformation is much more frequent with trigeminal neurinomas than with acoustic neurinomas. Peripheral calcification is present in more than 10% of the reported trigeminal neurinomas. Perifocal hypodensity is encountered only rarely.

Tumor Localization and Osseous Changes

Trigeminal neurinomas that originate from the postganglionic trigeminal root lie within the ventro-medial compartment of the pontocerebellar cistern. Large tumors may grow to reach or cover the internal auditory canal, but the center of the tumor clearly remains ventro-medial to the canal. This ventro-medial location helps to identify a tumor as a possible trigeminal neurinoma. With careful study, the tumor can usually be shown to extend into the porus trigeminus (Fig. 90) and to erode the incisura trigemini of the petrous apex. The antero-medial aspect of the posterior surface of the petrous bone may exhibit sharply demarcated pressure erosion (Figs. 90 and 93). Large tumors may erode the lips of the internal auditory canal, and shorten the canal, but they do not enlarge the canal itself (311, 599).

Trigeminal neurinomas that originate from the Gasserian ganglion and grow primarily within the middle fossa show bone erosion of the foramen ovale and, if large, of the sphenoid wing and dorsum sellae.

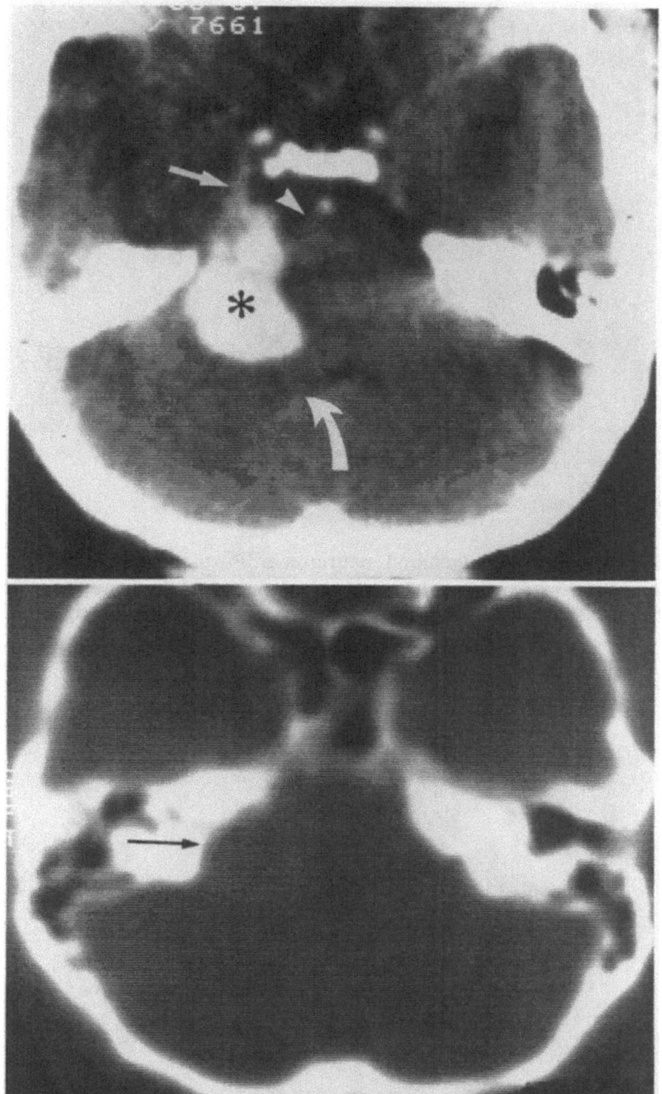

a

b

Fig. 90 a, b. Mainly infratentorial trigeminal neuroma. **a** Post contrast axial CT. The tumor (*asterisk*) shows intense and homogeneous contrast enhancement. The main tumor mass is located infratentorially filling out the supero-medial portion of the pontocerebellar cistern. A linear tumor extension through the porus trigeminus into Meckel's cave is seen (*arrow*). Note the cisternal dilatation (*arrowhead*) and distortion of the fourth ventricle (*curved arrow*). **b** Lower axial section viewed with bone window settings shows sharply demarcated pressure erosion of the posterior surface of the petrous bone (*arrow*)

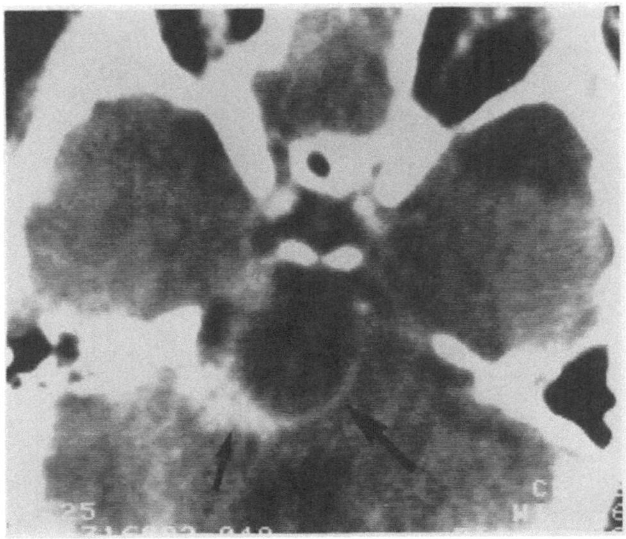

Fig. 91. Purely infratentorial trigeminal neurinoma. Post contrast axial CT. A centrally hypodense lesion with irregular ring enhancement (*arrows*) occupies the supero-medial portion of the pontocerebellar cistern. Operation proved the cystic nature of this trigeminal neurinoma

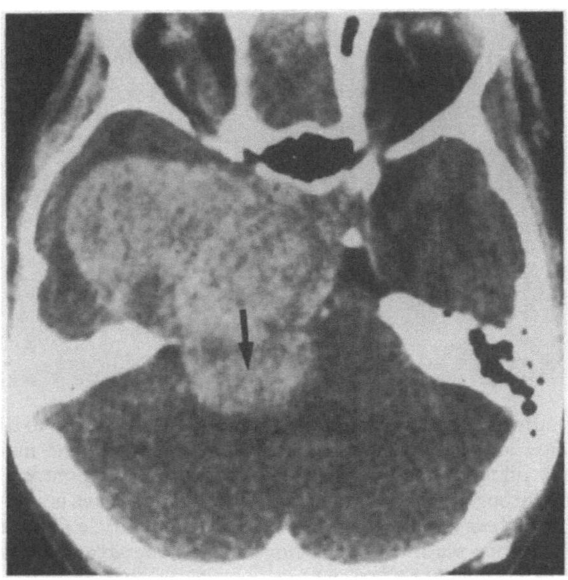

Fig. 92. Infra- and supratentorial (dumbbell) trigeminal neurinoma. Post contrast axial CT. The tumor shows slightly inhomogeneous contrast enhancement. The mainly supratentorial tumor shows a spherical extension underneath the petroclinoid ligament into the supero-medial portion of the pontocerebellar cistern (*arrow*)

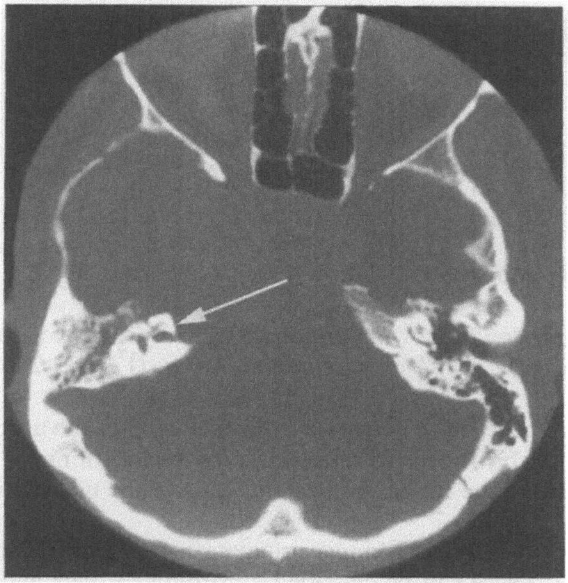

Fig. 93. Bone erosion of the petrous apex in a case of large dumbbell trigeminal neurinoma (same case as in Fig. 92). The petrous tip is completely eroded. The pressure erosion reaches the anterior lip of the internal auditory canal (*arrow*), but the internal auditory canal itself is not enlarged

4 Differential Diagnosis

Infratentorial extensions of trigeminal neurinomas are readily identified by their characteristic dumbbell shape and location. They are differentiated from dumbbell temporal fossa – pontocerebellar epidermoid tumors by their greater density (solid tumors) and more frequent ring enhancement (cystic tumors). Cystic trigeminal tumors are usually round or oval, well defined masses, whereas epidermoids are more irregular and pseudopodic. Greater difficulty may be encountered with purely infratentorial trigeminal neurinomas. As compared with trigeminal neurinomas, even medially situated acoustic neurinomas lie more laterally, near to the internal auditory canal and cause fewer, more subtle bone erosions. Spheno-petro-clival meningiomas typically exhibit homogeneous contrast enhancement, specific bone changes and the obtuse angle sign, which has proved to be a helpful differential criterion. Giant intracranial aneurysms may be differentiated from trigeminal neurinoma by their specific morphology (516).

Unusual lesions may be mistaken for trigeminal neurinoma. Thus a primary intracranial melanoma that presented as a round, hyperdense, homogeneously enhancing mass in the antero-medial compartment of the pontocerebellar cistern, that extended slightly into the middle fossa and that eroded the petrous apex was misinterpreted as a trigeminal neurinoma. Another tumor, histologically classified as desmoid fibroma, presented with the characteristic appearance of a middle fossa trigeminal neurinoma with secondary extension into the posterior fossa. In a third case, hypernephroma metastatic to the Gasserian ganglion mimicked the appearance of a trigeminal neurinoma completely.

Chordoma of the Cerebello-Pontine Angle

1 General Considerations

Chordoma is a rare, slowly growing tumor with locally invasive growth characteristics. It constitutes 0.1 to 0.2% of intracranial tumors (17, 269, 280, 435, 450, 468, 508).

Chordomas are believed to originate from remnants of the notochord (chorda dorsalis) (378). Probably for that reason, the common locations for chordomas are the clivus and sacrum, the rostral and caudal ends of the notochord, respectively (280).

Approximately 40% of chordomas originate in the skull base as extradural tumors (565, 572). These can be classified according to their main location and direction of growth as sellar, parasellar and clival (125, 173, 508). Clival chordomas may be subclassified as medial, lateral and occipital (280).

Of these, the lateral clival chordoma most commonly affects the cerebello-pontine angle causing palsies of cranial nerves three to five and/or five to eight. Large chordomas may also cause cerebellar and pontine signs.

2 Conventional Radiology

Chordoma of the cerebello-pontine angle presents with destruction of the petrous apex and of the lateral clivus (55, 260, 505, 572). The internal auditory canal is usually not involved. In rare instances, the eroded bone may show reactive sclerosis (112, 309). With conventional techniques, calcifications are found in more than 30% of cases (260, 314, 508).

Prior to introduction of CT, pneumoencephalography was the most reliable method for documenting the intracranial extent of the tumor (260, 505). Angiography remains useful for demonstrating or excluding encasement of the internal carotid artery at the horizontal segment of the carotid canal or the cavernous sinus (89, 132, 260, 450, 505, 615). Since chordomas are predominantly avascular masses, tumor blush is rarely observed. When seen, tumor blush derives from the meningeal branches of the internal carotid, external carotid and vertebral arteries (260, 404).

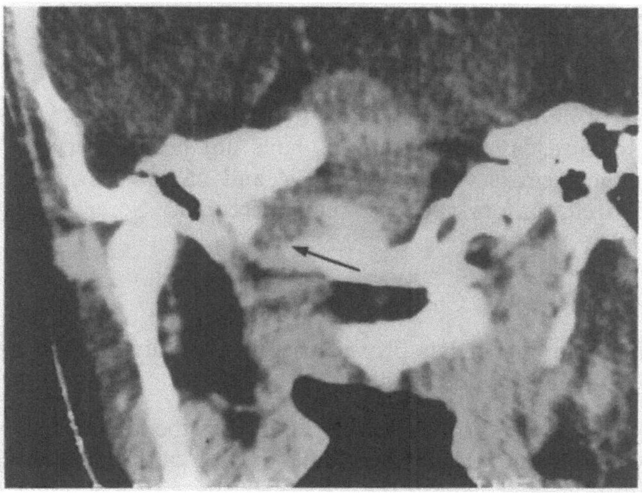

Fig. 94. Chordoma of the right cerebello-pontine angle. Coronal post contrast CT. The tumor is sharply marginated and presents with homogeneous, intense contrast enhancement. The tumor infiltrates the inframeatal compartment of the petrous bone (*arrow*)

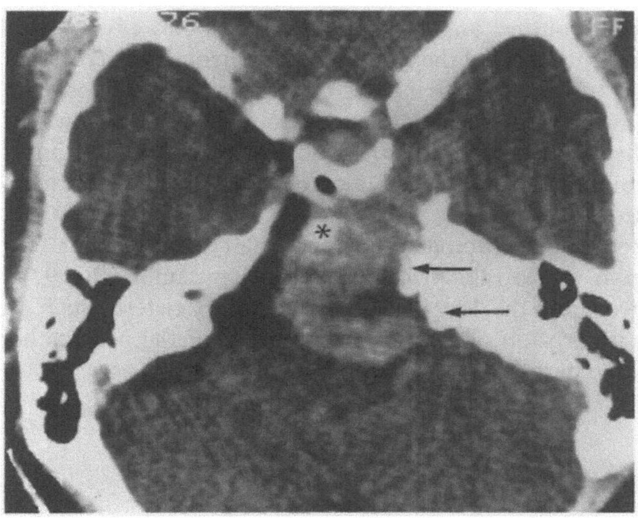

Fig. 95. Left spheno-petro-clival chordoma. Axial post contrast scan. The chordoma invades the parasellar region and destroys the lateral part of the sphenoid. The tumor exhibits less intense contrast enhancement than that shown in Fig. 94. Note the nodular calcification within the tumor (*asterisk*) and at the periphery of the tumor (*arrows*) where it contacts the petrous bone

3 Computed Tomography

Density and Contrast Enhancement

The majority of chordomas present as hyperdense lesions (257, 260, 284, 378). Fewer are isodense. Hypodense lesions have not been observed. The degree of contrast enhancement is variable (Figs. 94 and 95), but is never as great as in hypervascularized tumors such as chemodectomas. Some chordomas do not enhance at all.

Localization and Osseous Changes

For operative planning, it has proved useful to subdivide the cerebello-pontine angle chordomas into two groups:

1. Spheno-petro-clival chordomas originate from the lateral border of the clivus and grow mainly into the antero-medial portion of the cerebello-pontine angle. These chordomas grow into the parasellar space (Fig. 95).
2. Jugulo-petrosal chordomas originate caudo-laterally in the region of the jugular foramen and extend primarily into the lateral cerebellomedullary cistern. With further growth, the tumor may encroach upon the infero-lateral part of the pontocerebellar cistern. These chordomas resemble chemodectomas with intracranial extension (Type-D) (Figs. 96 and 97) (147, 679).

Chordomas usually cause far more extensive bone erosion and destruction than do other cerebello-pontine angle lesions. Spheno-petro-clival chordomas usually destroy the lateral aspect of the clivus and the petrous apex (Figs. 98 and 99). Some 75% of these tumors extend into the parasellar middle fossa and from there, commonly invade the cavernous sinus. Rarely, the tumor grows through foramen ovale into the infratemporal fossa. Tumor extension into the infratemporal fossa and erosion of the horizontal segment of the carotid canal are best assessed on direct coronal sections.

Jugulo-petrosal chordomas erode and enlarge the jugular foramen and may encroach upon the infralabyrinthine petrous pyramid (Fig. 97). These tumors commonly grow into the lateral cerebellomedullary cistern. Such growth is usually associated with erosion of the posterior surface of the petrous bone. Exocranial growth into the paravertebral space is possible.

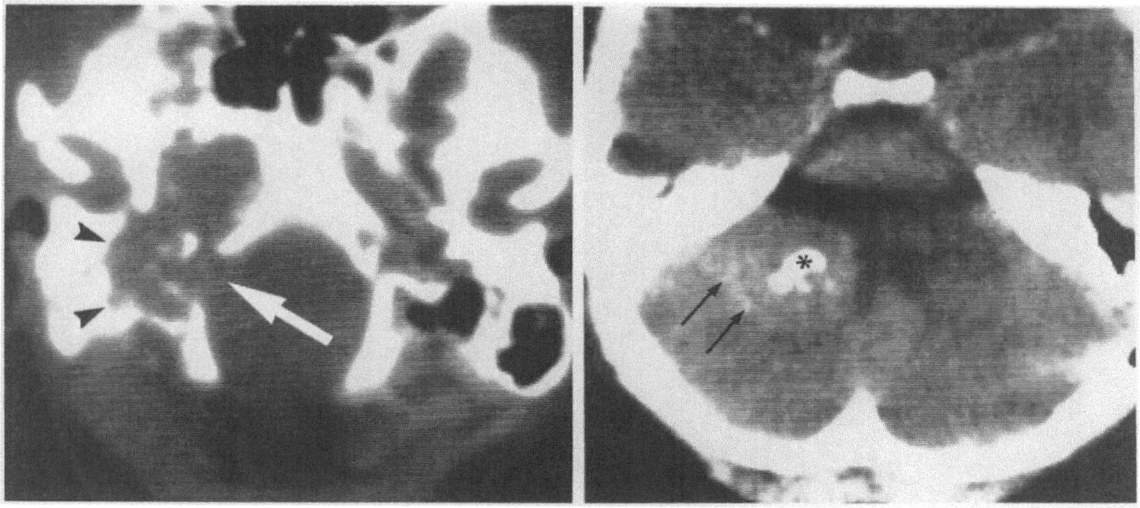

a b

Fig. 96a, b. Jugulo-petrosal chordoma. **a** Axial section through the jugular foramen viewed with bone window settings. The tumor enlarges and erodes the right jugular foramen (*arrowheads*). It invades the infralabyrinthine compartment of the temporal bone. The tumor destroys the hypoglossal canal and extends into the posterior fossa (*arrow*). **b** Post contrast axial CT. The chordoma fills out the posterior part of the pontocerebellar cistern. It enhances moderately. The posterior margin of the tumor can be delineated by fine reticular calcifications (*arrows*). Another nodular calcification is seen within the tumor (*asterisk*)

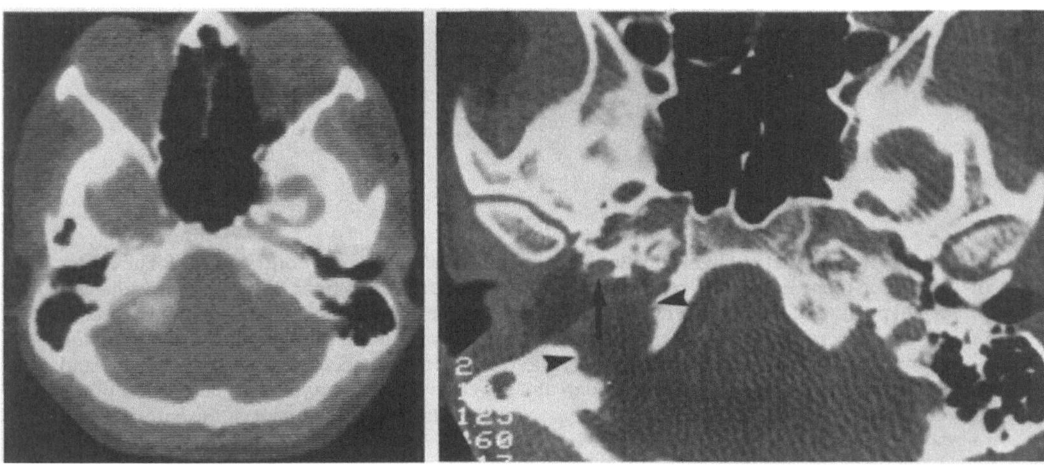

a b

Fig. 97a, b. Calcified jugulo-petrosal chordoma. **a** The retro- and inferomeatal compartment of the pontocerebellar cistern and the lateral cerebellomedullary cistern are filled with a calcified chordoma. **b** High resolution CT at the level of the lateral cerebellomedullary cistern shows erosion of the jugular foramen (*arrowheads*), of the vertical segment of the carotid canal (*arrow*) and of the infralabyrinthine compartment of the petrous bone. The pattern of bone erosion in this case is identical to that seen with chemodectomas. The only distinguishing feature is the calcification of the intracranial tumor portion

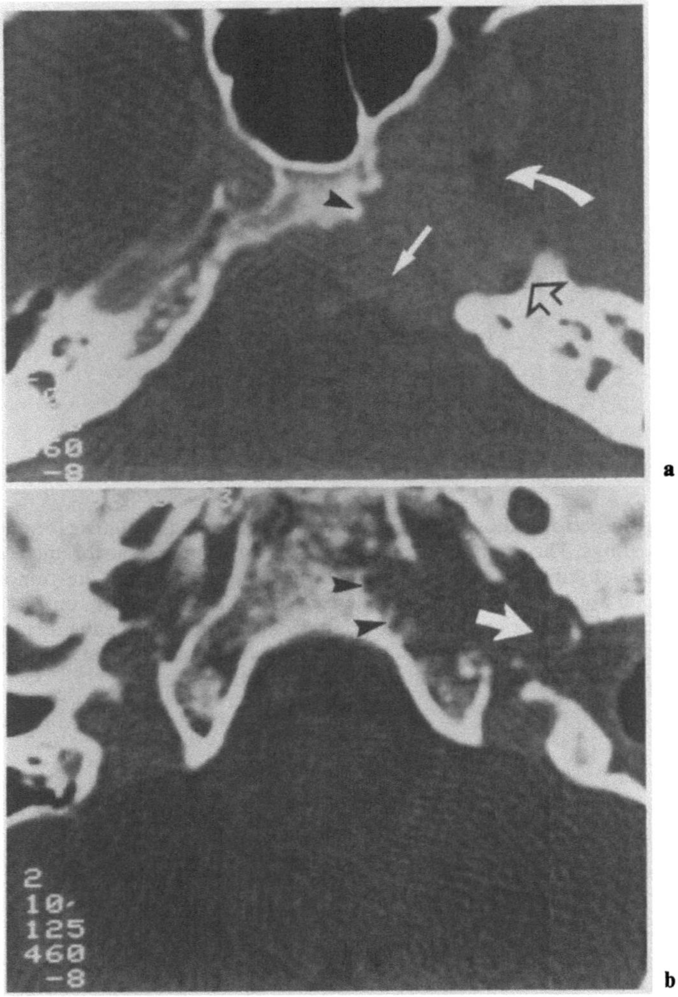

Fig. 98 a, b. Spheno-petro-clival chordoma. Axial high resolution post contrast CT. **a** The center of the tumor mass lies in the region of the petrous apex. From here, the tumor invades the premeatal portion of the pontocerebellar cistern (*arrow*), the prepontine cistern and the parasellar region. The cavernous sinus can not be distinguished from the tumor. The Gasserian ganglion however (*curved arrow*) is displaced laterally. Bone erosion of the petrous apex (*open arrow*) and the lateral clivus (*arrowhead*) is seen. **b** Scan at a lower level shows a typical bone erosion of the lateral clivus (*arrowheads*). Laterally, the tumor reaches the vertical segment of the carotid canal (*arrow*)

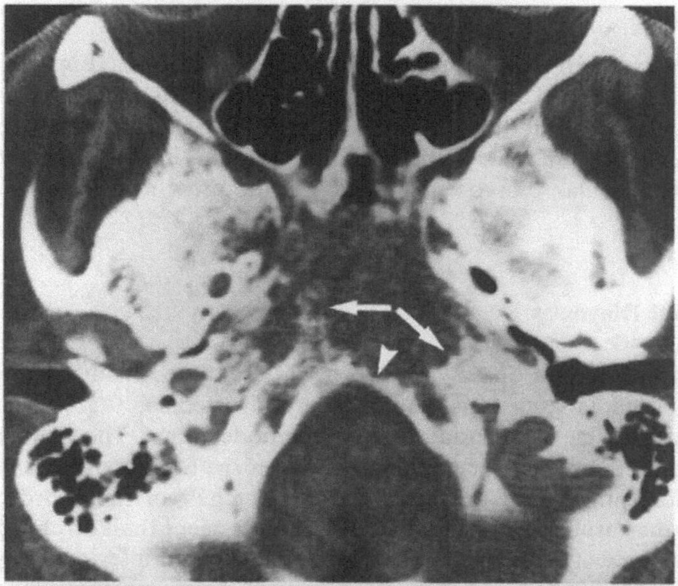

a

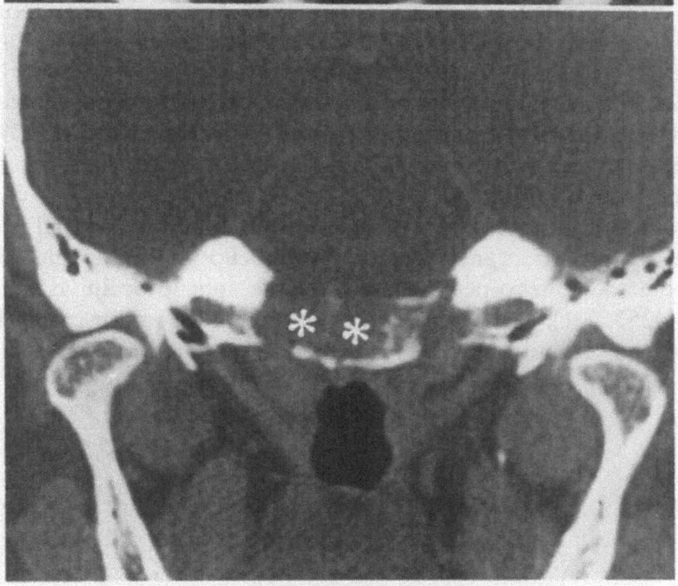

b

Fig. 99a, b. Spheno-petro-clival chordoma. Post contrast high resolution CT. **a** The axial scan demonstrates the bone infiltration of the inferior petrous apex and of the clivus (*arrows*). The tumor crosses the midline. Note the preservation of the cortical outline of the clivus (*arrowhead*). **b** Coronal CT demonstrates the mainly intraosseous location of this chordoma which destroys the petrous apex and invades the clivus (*asterisks*)

Calcifications

Chordomas characteristically form intratumoral calcifications (Figs. 95–97). These are demonstrable by CT in about 40% of cases (260). The pattern of calcification may be reticular, solid-nodular, cystic or mixed (314). Unfortunately the different patterns of calcification are not specific for chordoma. In the authors' experience, however, the reticular type of calcification is the most nearly characteristic for chordoma.

4 Differential Diagnosis

Spheno-petro-clival chordomas need to be differentiated from meningioma and rare tumors such as metastasis, chondroma and osteoma. Jugulo-petrosal chordomas must also be differentiated from chemodectoma. The main differential diagnostic criteria are the very intense enhancement found with chemodectomas and the calcifications that are present in almost half of the chordomas. Since chemodectomas usually show more intense enhancement than do chordomas, and usually do not calcify, intensely enhancing non calcified inferior pontocerebellar tumors are more probably chemodectomas than jugulo-petrosal chordomas. In some cases however, the lesions appear identical and cannot be differentiated successfully.

Osteomas are bone tumors that may be connected to the posterior surface of the petrous bone but which do not produce erosion of the petrous bone (257). They are not calcified, per se, and show no enhancement. These lesions are readily differentiated from chordomas.

Chondromas constitute 0.09% (484) of intracranial tumors and are therefore one of the rarest intracranial tumors. Cerebello-pontine angle chondromas originate from the spheno-petrosal or from the spheno-occipital synchondrosis (about 66%) (257, 501). The non calcified portions of the tumor regularly enhance. For these reasons chondromas may not be differentiated from chordomas.

Chemodectomas of the Petrous Bone

1 General Considerations

Chemodectomas of the petrous bone are also known as glomus tumors or nonchromaffin paragangliomas. These lesions originate from microscopically small, nonchromaffin paraganglia (or "glomera"). Histologically, glomus structures are composed of capillary and precapillary blood vessels and epitheloid cells. Their size varies from 1 to 1.5 mm in diameter (186, 187). Glomus structures are found along the tympanic branch of the glossopharyngeal nerve (Jacobson's nerve) and along the auricular branch of the vagal nerve (Arnold's nerve). In order of decreasing frequency, the main locations of glomus structures are the dome of the jugular bulb, the canaliculus tympanicus in which Jacobson's nerve courses, and the promontory of the cochlea, where the ramifications of Jacobson's nerve are located. The least frequent location of glomus structures is along Arnold's nerve (187).

Chemodectomas may originate from glomus structures in any of these locations and may grow sufficiently to cause clinical symptoms. Differences in the clinical signs with which the glomus tumors present are probably explained by different tumor origins (173).

The first author to recognize the nonchromaffin paraganglia was Valentin in 1840 (581) who termed them "Gangliolum tympanicum". Guild in 1941 (186) studied nonchromaffin paraganglia extensively and introduced the term "glomus jugulare". In 1937, Lübbers (326) noted histologic similarity between an operated ear tumor and glomus caroticum tumors. In 1945, Rosenwasser (483) first described a case of histologically proven chemodectoma of the middle ear.

Chemodectomas are 5 times more frequent in middle aged females than in males. Multicentric tumors and familial occurrence are well known (173). In rare cases, chemodectomas may metastasize to distant sites (173). The first clinical symptoms of chemodectomas depend on tumor origin. Chemodectomas that originate within the middle ear cavity first cause tinnitus and conductive hearing loss. Chemodectomas that originate from the jugular bulb first cause palsies of the cranial nerves nine to eleven. With increasing tumor size and tumor extension into the infratemporal compartment and the middle ear respectively, symptoms from the middle ear and from the caudal cranial nerves become superimposed (3, 173). Eventually, the tumor reaches the cerebello-pontine angle and causes additional cerebello-pontine angle symptoms (150, 173, 537).

Chemodectomas form one part of the so-called APUD system (*A*mine-*P*re-cursor-*U*ptake-*D*ecarboxylation) (177, 428). Histochemical examinations indicate that chemodectomas may have a secretory activity, producing Vanillyl-mandelic-acid and 5-hydroxy-indol-acetic-acid (177). However, clinical evidence of secretory activity seems to be uncommon and was found in only 3 of 19 cases reported by Lasjaunias et al. (296).

2 Conventional Radiology

Conventional X-ray studies permit diagnosis of large chemodectomas that erode the petrous bone (123, 201, 210, 475, 476, 488). Complex motion tomography can demonstrate erosion of the jugular foramen and tumor invasion into the middle ear cavity (43, 113, 126, 152, 153, 168, 591).

Superselective external carotid angiography is now the most reliable modality for the diagnosis of chemodectomas (102, 367). Superselective angiography is a prerequisite for preoperative or palliative embolization (102, 440).

Chemodectomas are supplied by vessels normally supplying the area involved by the tumor. The tympanic and jugular portions of the tumor are supplied by the inferior tympanic and jugular branches of the ascending pharyngeal artery (292). Mastoid extension of the tumor is supplied by the stylomastoid artery (294). The anterior (pericarotid) intratemporal tumor extension is supplied by the tympanic branch of the internal carotid artery (246), as well as by the anterior tympanic branch of the internal maxillary artery (296). The superior intratemporal extension of the tumor is supplied by the superior tympanic branch of the middle meningeal artery (293, 295). Intracranial extradural tumor extension is supplied posteriorly by the mastoid branch of the occipital artery, centrally by the jugular branch of the ascending pharyngeal artery and anteriorly by the clival branches of the internal carotid artery (294, 295). Intracranial intradural tumor extension is constantly supplied by the posterior inferior and anterior inferior cerebellar arteries (367).

The jugular vein is well shown in the venous phase of superselective angiograms. Therefore, venous obstruction or tumor infiltration of the jugular vein can be assessed without need for jugular phlebography (162).

3 Computed Tomography

On CT scans, chemodectomas present as iso- or slightly hyperdense mass lesions with intense, homogeneous enhancement (59, 341). Before the introduction of high resolution reconstruction algorithms, the main indication for CT was demonstration of the intracranial extent of the tumor (59, 92, 171, 237, 341, 458, 504). Since the introduction of high resolution algorithms, CT has completely replaced conventional tomography.

Micro-oto-neurosurgical techniques (141, 148) now allow radical removal of large chemodectomas with minimal morbidity and no mortality (147). Selection of the appropriate surgical approach depends upon the location, size and extension of the tumor as well as upon the degree of involvement of surgically important intratemporal structures. According to Fisch and Valavanis chemodectomas are classified into four main Types (147, 579, 580).

Classification of Jugulo-Tympanic Chemodectomas

Type-A tumors represent *tympanic* chemodectomas located solely within the tympanic cavity. These tumors are removed by conventional tympanoplastic techniques. On high resolution CT, Type-A tumors appear as homogeneous, intensely-enhancing soft tissue masses in the tympanic cavity. They are usually broadly attached to the promontory of the cochlea and may have secondary attachment to the lateral surface of the carotid canal. They do not cause bone erosion.

Tumors Type-B, C, and D represent forms of jugular chemodectomas (glomus jugulare).

Type-B tumors are located in the tympanomastoid area and are also removed by conventional tympanoplastic techniques. Type-B tumors infiltrate the hypotympanic bone plate and extend from the bone plate into the hypotympanum. Type-B tumors do *not* form a mass within the jugular fossa. Therefore, for a tumor to be classified as Type-B, the cortical outline of the jugular fossa must be intact. CT evidence of erosion of the cortical outline of the jugular fossa indicates that the tumor has extended from the hypotympanic bone plate into the jugular fossa and precludes classification of the tumor as Type-B. Since removal of the intrajugular part of the tumor is not possible with conventional tympanoplastic technique, such a tumor is classified as Type-C instead.

Type-C tumors involve the jugular foramen and bulb and show variable degrees of extension into the infralabyrinthine compartment of the temporal bone. Since the size and shape of the two jugular foramina are frequently asymmetrical, erosion of the cortical outline of the jugular fossa is more reliable evidence of extension into the temporal bone than is enlargement of the fossa itself. Type-C tumors are subclassified into four subtypes by the degree to which they involve the carotid canal. Each subtype is resected by a specifically modified infratemporal fossa approach (147).

In *C-1 tumors*, the carotid canal is intact or exhibits only minimal erosion of the posterior aspect of the vertical segment of the carotid canal. The extent of such erosion is best evaluated on axial sections (Fig. 100) and on reformatted sagittal sections (for evaluation of the posterior wall of the vertical segment of the carotid canal). Coronal views through the jugular foramen show the extent of tumor infiltration of the jugular vein and bulb.

In *C-2 tumors*, the vertical segment of the carotid canal is eroded significantly, usually circumferentially. Axial and direct coronal sections are necessary for precise assessment of the tumor size and the degree of bone erosion. Axial sections show the true extent of invasion of the infralabyrinthine compartment. Coronal sections are more sensitive for demonstrating minimal bone erosion.

The involved bone shows a mottled appearance. Type-C-2 tumors often extend medially to involve the inframeatal compartment (i.e. the bone plate below the floor of the internal auditory canal). Such extension is best seen on coronal CT sections. Medial extension of C-2 tumors may also cause erosion of the hypoglossal canal. Coronal CT sections demonstrate best the enlargement and erosion of the cortical outline of the hypoglossal canal. When the tumor extends into the hypoglossal canal, either axial or coronal CT sections through the tongue may demonstrate ipsilateral hypodensity, which is attributed to denervation hemiatrophy of the tongue (392).

C-3 tumors are similar to C-2 tumors except that they also extend into the apical compartment (i.e. the bone space ventral to the infralabyrinthine compartment and around the horizontal segment of the carotid canal). Therefore, C-3 tumors are

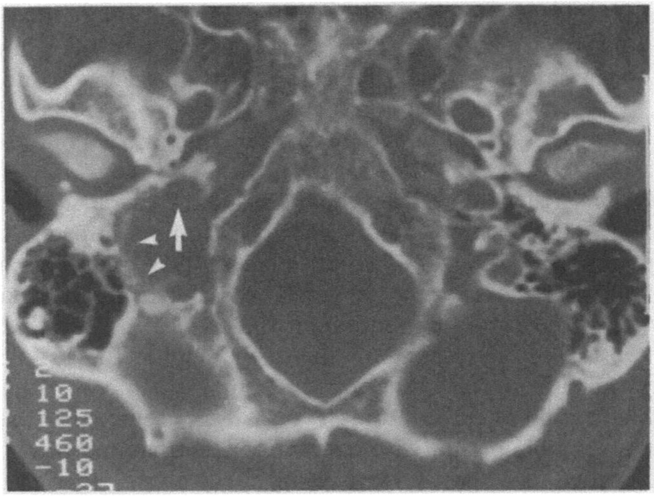

Fig. 100. Type-C-1 chemodectoma. Axial high resolution CT section at the level of the skull base shows significant enlargement of the right jugular foramen compared to the normal left side. There is circumferential erosion of the right jugular foramen with unsharp margins (*arrowheads*). The vertical segment of the carotid canal is eroded in its posterior aspect (*arrow*), compatible with Type-C-1 tumor

characterized by additional erosion of the horizontal segment of the carotid canal (Fig. 101). Erosion first occurs at the proximal part of the horizontal segment of the carotid canal and usually involves the lateral wall.

C-4 tumors cause erosion of the foramen lacerum. C-4 tumors may also extend along the internal carotid artery into the ipsilateral cavernous sinus.

Type-D tumors extend into the intracranial space. Depending on their *e*xtradural or *i*ntradural intracranial extension, Type-D tumors are further classified into types De and Di respectively. Depending on the size of the intracranial component of the tumor, tumors Type-De and Di are subclassified into subtypes De-1 to De-3 and Di-1 to Di-3 respectively. Intracranial tumor extension of less than 1.5 cm is defined as Type-D-1. Intracranial extension of 1.5 to 2.5 cm is defined as Type-D-2. Intracranial tumor extension greater than 2.5 cm is defined as Type-D-3. Tumors Type-De-1 to De-3 and Di-1 can be radically removed by the infratemporal fossa approach. Tumors Type Di-2 usually require a combined oto-neurosurgical approach. Tumors Type-Di-3 are regarded as inoperable.

Intracranial Tumor Extension

Different patterns of intracranial extension are found. Most commonly, glomus jugulare tumors Type-D extend superomedially from the jugular foramen and come to occupy the lateral cerebellomedullary cistern. With further cranially directed growth, the tumor may occupy the cerebello-pontine angle (Fig. 102). Further increase in tumor size causes compression of the cerebellum and of the pons.

Infrequently, the tumor first involves the infralabyrinthine, then the inframeatal compartment, grows through the floor of the internal auditory canal intrameatally

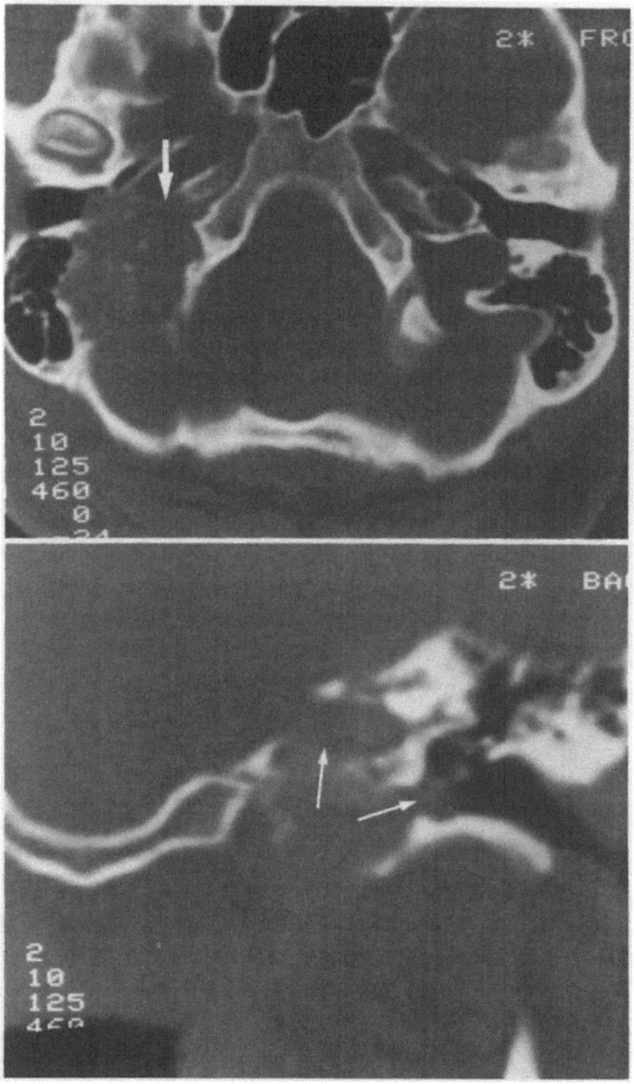

a

b

Fig. 101 a, b. Type-C-3 chemodectoma. **a** Axial high resolution CT section through the skull base shows enlargement and circumferential erosion of the right jugular foramen. In addition, the horizontal segment of the carotid canal has been eroded by the tumor in its postero-medial aspect (*arrow*). **b** Coronal high resolution CT section at the level of the internal auditory canal. There is infiltration of the inframeatal compartment of the temporal bone and tumor extension into both, the middle ear and the internal auditory canal (*arrows*)

and finally extends from there into the cerebello-pontine angle. Such a tumor may be misinterpreted as an acoustic neurinoma (Fig. 103). However, infiltrative bone erosion of the floor of the internal auditory canal and of the inframeatal compartment of the petrous bone plus presence of tumor in the jugular foramen

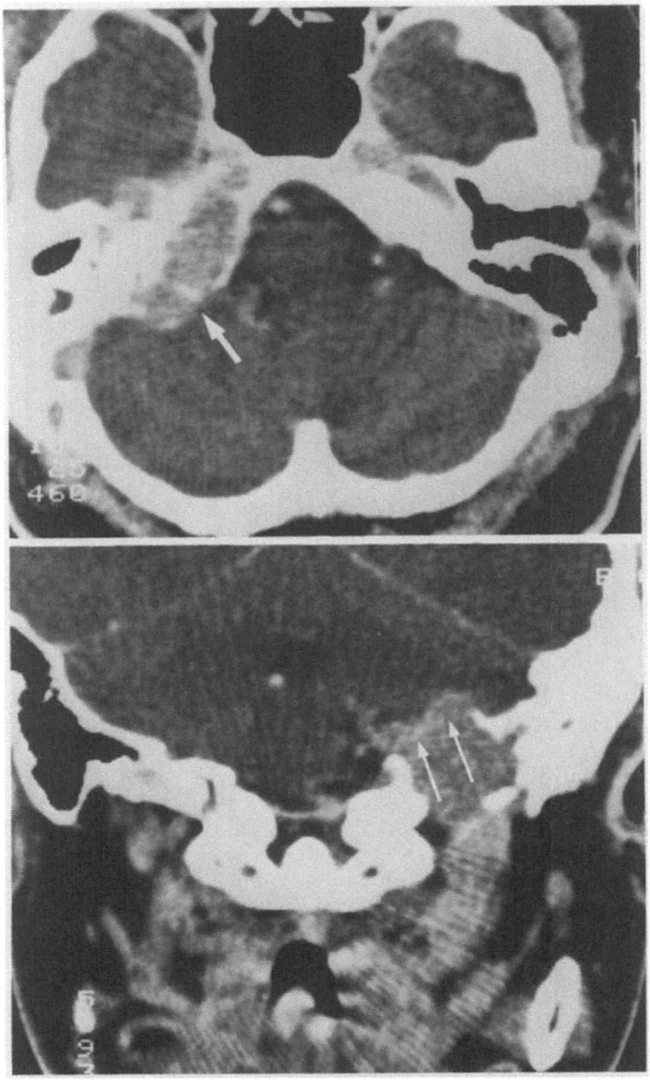

a

b

Fig. 102a, b. Type-D-2 chemodectoma. **a** Axial contrast enhanced CT section shows homogeneously enhancing tumor mass in the right cerebello-pontine angle. There is extensive erosion of the posterior surface of the petrous bone (*arrow*). **b** Coronal contrast enhanced section at the level of the mastoid tip shows tumor extension in a cranial direction from the jugular fossa towards the cerebello-pontine angle (*arrows*)

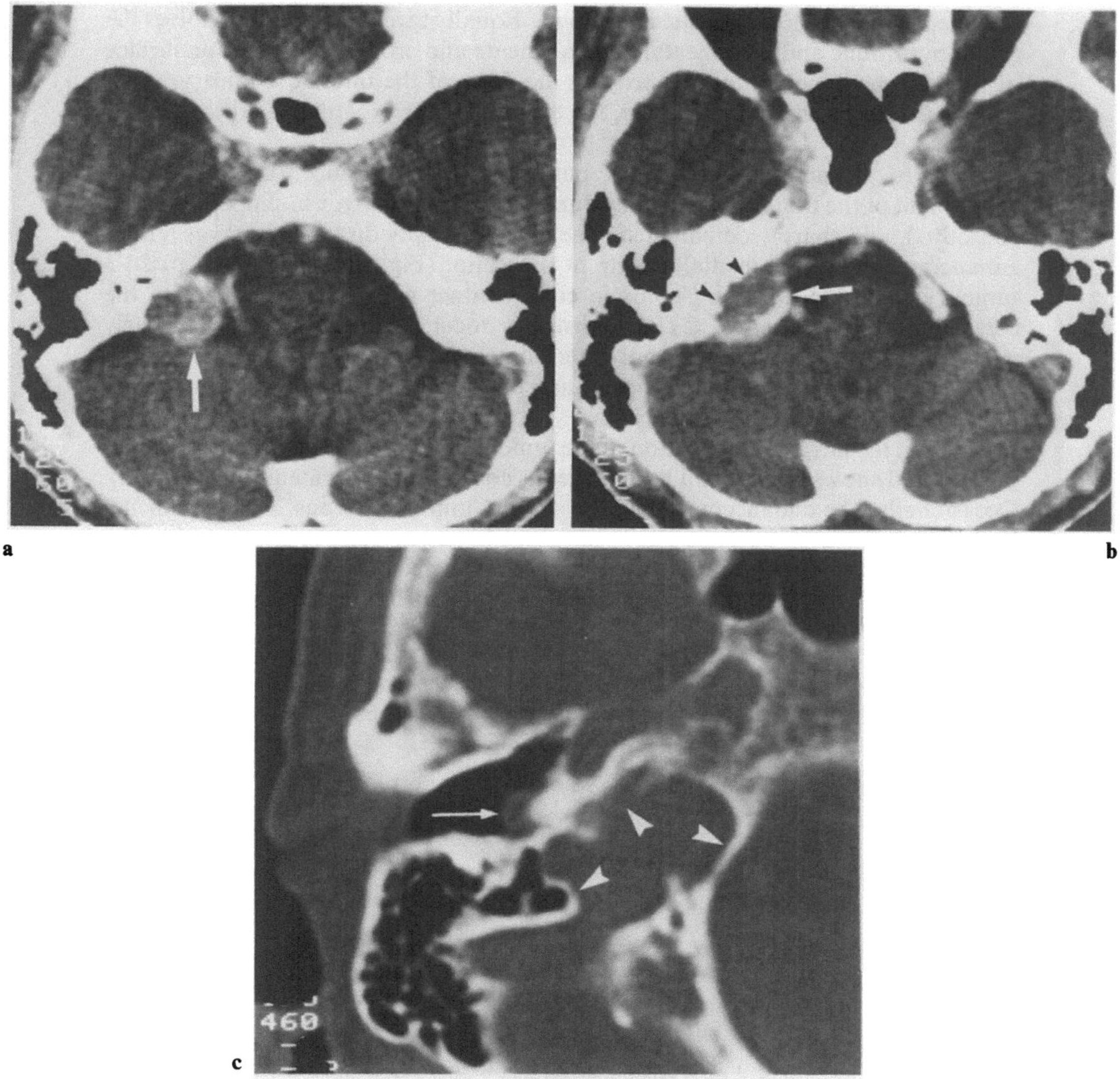

a b c

Fig. 103a–c. Type-De-1 chemodectoma. **a** Axial contrast enhanced CT section. An enhancing tumor nodule is seen within the cerebello-pontine angle, slightly posterior to the internal auditory canal (*arrow*). **b** A lower section shows the chemodectoma lying inbetween the eroded posterior surface of the petrous bone (*arrowheads*) and the jugular tubercle (*arrow*). **c** High resolution CT through the jugular foramen shows the enlarged, eroded jugular foramen (*arrowheads*). Note tumor extension into the middle ear (*arrow*) exclude the diagnosis of acoustic neurinoma. Equally rarely, the tumor involves the infralabyrinthine and inframeatal compartments and erodes the posterior surface of the petrous bone without destroying the floor of the internal auditory canal. From the inframeatal compartment, the tumor extends broadly into the posterior fossa.

Initially, intracranial growth is purely extradural. Since the intracranial component of the tumor is covered by dura it is typically convex in shape, smoothly contoured, and sharply demarcated. The dura is usually directly visible as a thin, enhancing band at the medial margin of the tumor (Fig. 104). Type-Di-1 to Di-3 tumors invade the dura and come in close contact with or even adhere to the cerebellum. In such cases, CT demonstrates focal interruption of the linearly enhancing dura plus nodular tumor extension into the intradural space (Figs. 105 and 106). Therefore, nodular appearance of the medial tumor border usually indicates intradural tumor extension.

On CT, the intracranial portion of the tumor behaves similar to the extracranial portion and shows intense and homogeneous contrast enhancement (59, 341, 579). Occasionally, the enhancement may be slightly inhomogeneous. Non enhancing hypodense, cystic or necrotic zones have not been reported to occur within the tumor. Calcification of glomus tumors has been reported in one case in the literature (363). Multiple tiny intratumoral calcifications have also been seen in one personal case.

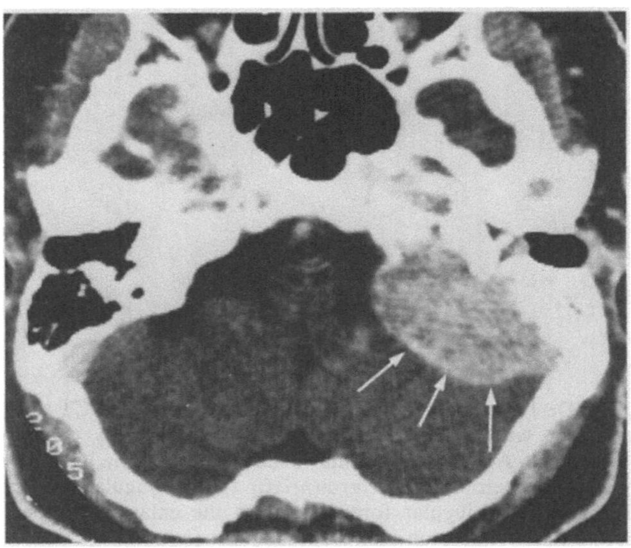

Fig. 104. Type-De-2 chemodectoma. Axial contrast enhanced CT section at the level of the jugular foramen. The homogeneously enhancing tumor occupies the left jugular foramen and extends intracranially. The medial tumor border is covered by the linearly enhancing dura (*arrows*), indicating its extradural location

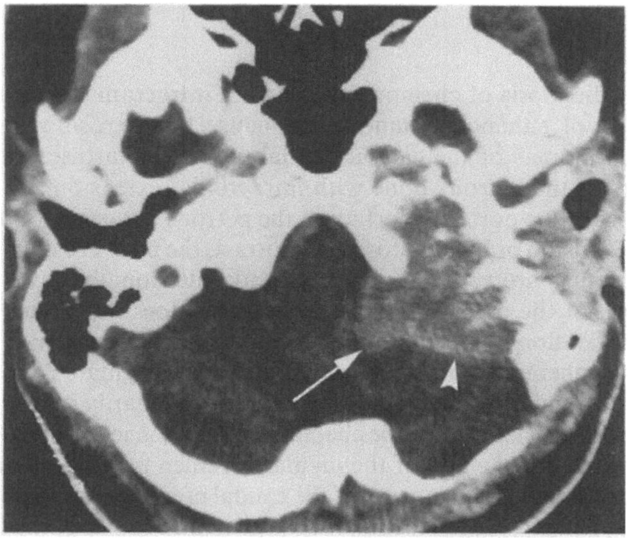

Fig. 105. Type-De-2, Di-1 chemodectoma. Axial contrast enhanced CT section at the level of the jugular foramen. The left jugular foramen is occupied by a homogeneously enhancing tumor. The tumor extends in a medial direction towards the intracranial space. The postero-medial border of the tumor is covered by the linearly enhancing dura (*arrowhead*). In its antero-medial portion, there is focal interruption of the dura and nodular tumor extension (*arrow*) into the intradural space

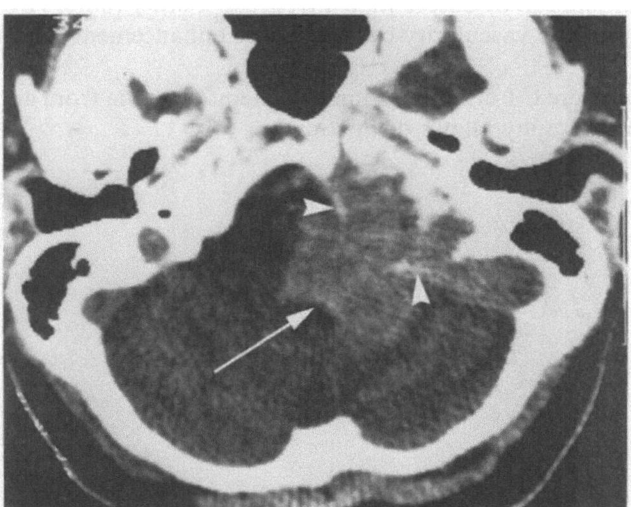

Fig. 106. Type-De-1, Di-2 chemodectoma. Axial contrast enhanced CT section at the level of the jugular foramen. The tumor mass occupies and destroys the right jugular foramen. It extends in a medial direction towards the intracranial space. There is focal interruption of the linearly enhancing dura (*arrowheads*) and significant tumor extension into the intradural space (*arrow*)

4 Differential Diagnosis

The differential diagnosis of chemodectomas with intracranial extension includes the whole group of enhancing tumors that cause bone erosion: meningiomas, chordomas, neurinomas of the caudal cranial nerves, metastases and malignant primary tumors of the petrous bone with intracranial extension.

Meningiomas of the posterior surface of the petrous bone may produce sharply delineated bone erosion or hyperostosis. In contrast, the bone erosions encountered with chemodectomas are typically irregular and, additionally, involve the infralabyrinthine part of the petrous bone. Hyperostosis does not occur with chemodectomas. Calcifications are commonly found with meningiomas, but are extremely rare with chemodectomas. Meningiomas that originate from the sigmoid sinus or from the jugular foramen and that extend secondarily into the pontocerebellar cistern may occasionally mimic chemodectomas, since erosion of the inferior surface of the petrous bone and of the jugular foramen may be encountered with this type of meningioma. Neurinomas of the caudal cranial nerves may originate in the jugular foramen and cause foraminal enlargement. However, the bone erosion seen with neurinomas is pressure-related and therefore is sharply delineated. The infiltration of bone typically seen with chemodectomas is not encountered with neurinomas.

Metastases within the jugular foramen may behave like chemodectomas; CT-differentiation may be impossible, especially in patients without a known primary tumor.

Glomus tumors can be differentiated from most other tumors by dynamic CT, because their profuse vascularity causes intense enhancement during the arterial phase (333).

In all cases where CT differentiation of a chemodectoma from another lesion is impossible, angiography allows distinction.

Neurinomas of the Caudal Cranial Nerves

Classification

Neurinomas of the caudal cranial nerves may originate from the glossopharyngeal, vagal, spinal accessory and hypoglossal nerves. At first, the tumors occupy the lateral cerebellomedullary cistern. With further growth they extend into the cerebello-pontine angle. Neurinomas of the caudal cranial nerves are extremely rare intracranial tumors, constituting 1.2 to 3% of all cerebello-pontine angle tumors (445, 473, 629).

Anatomical differences in the cisternal courses of the lower cranial nerves justify classification of these neurinomas into two main groups (70). The hypoglossal nerve assumes a latero-medullary course and then enters the hypoglossal canal. Neurinomas originating from the hypoglossal nerve constitute one distinct group (70, 255, 445). The glossopharyngeal, vagal and spinal accessory nerves course laterally in the lateral cerebellomedullary cistern and reach the neck through the jugular foramen. Because of their relation to the jugular foramen, neurinomas originating from cranial nerves nine to eleven are classified together as jugular foramen neurinomas. Classification of caudal neurinomas into hypoglossal neurinomas and neurinomas of the jugular foramen is also justified from the clinical point of view. Hypoglossal neurinomas grow in the narrow subarachnoid space between the bulb of the medulla oblongata and the occipital foramen (70). Therefore they cause signs of medullary compression earlier than do jugular foramen neurinomas.

A. Neurinomas of the Hypoglossal Nerve

1 General Considerations

Neurinomas of the hypoglossal nerve are very rare tumors. Only 22 cases were reported between 1933 and 1982 (11, 18, 24, 97, 105, 154, 206, 238, 350, 364, 407, 462, 480, 522, 545, 571, 577, 584, 616). These tumors originate from a motor nerve, although most other intracranial neurinomas originate from sensory nerves.

Hypoglossal neurinomas most commonly remain completely within the intracranial space. Infrequently, hypoglossal neurinomas present as dumbbell neurinomas with combined intra- and extracranial extension (24) or as purely extracranial tumor masses. 70% of cases occur in middle aged females. The most frequent clinical presentations are suboccipital or generalized headache, difficulties in swallowing and speaking and palsies of the other caudal cranial nerves (31).

Increasing tumor size results in cerebellar symptoms and, later, in signs of raised intracranial pressure (238, 571).

The most common and most reliable clinical sign of hypoglossal neurinoma is ipsilateral hemiatrophy of the tongue. Unilateral atrophy of the tongue should be an indication for CT examination of the cerebello-pontine angle, including the craniocervical junction.

2 Conventional Radiology

Hypoglossal neurinomas characteristically cause widening of the hypoglossal canal. This widening may be detected on standard radiographs or on multidirectional tomograms (268). Large hypoglossal neurinomas may also erode the jugular foramen (268).

Routine angiography demonstrates an avascular or poorly vascularized mass in the caudal cerebello-pontine angle (24, 480). Superselective angiography of the external carotid branches, the internal carotid artery and the vertebral artery may show neovascularity and tumor blush (370). Depending on tumor size, vertebral angiography may display displacement of the vertebral and the posterior inferior cerebellar arteries with elevation of the anterior inferior cerebellar artery over the upper border of the mass (154). Extracranial extension of tumor causes anterior displacement of the extracranial internal carotid and the ascending pharyngeal arteries (24).

3 Computed Tomography

Density and Contrast Enhancement

Hypoglossal neurinomas exhibit variable CT morphology. They may be iso- or slightly hypodense on non contrast CT and may exhibit homogeneous (Fig. 107) or inhomogeneous (Fig. 108) enhancement. The pattern of enhancement depends upon the regressive changes of the tumor. Antoni-B type tumors present as inhomogeneously enhancing tumors, and may have intratumoral cysts.

Extracranial Growth, Osseous Changes

High resolution CT is required to evaluate the skull base, since diagnosis and differential diagnosis of hypoglossal neurinomas depends in part on detection of specific bone changes. Hypoglossal neurinomas usually originate within the hypoglossal canal. Therefore, widening of the hypoglossal canal is the first radiological evidence of the presence of tumor (Fig. 107). As the tumor grows laterally, it reaches, erodes and enlarges the jugular foramen (Fig. 108). With further growth the tumor then resembles a chemodectoma that grows ventrally along the undersurface of the petrous bone into the infralabyrinthine and inframeatal compartments of the petrous bone. As the tumor grows it extends into the para- and retropharyngeal spaces (Fig. 107).

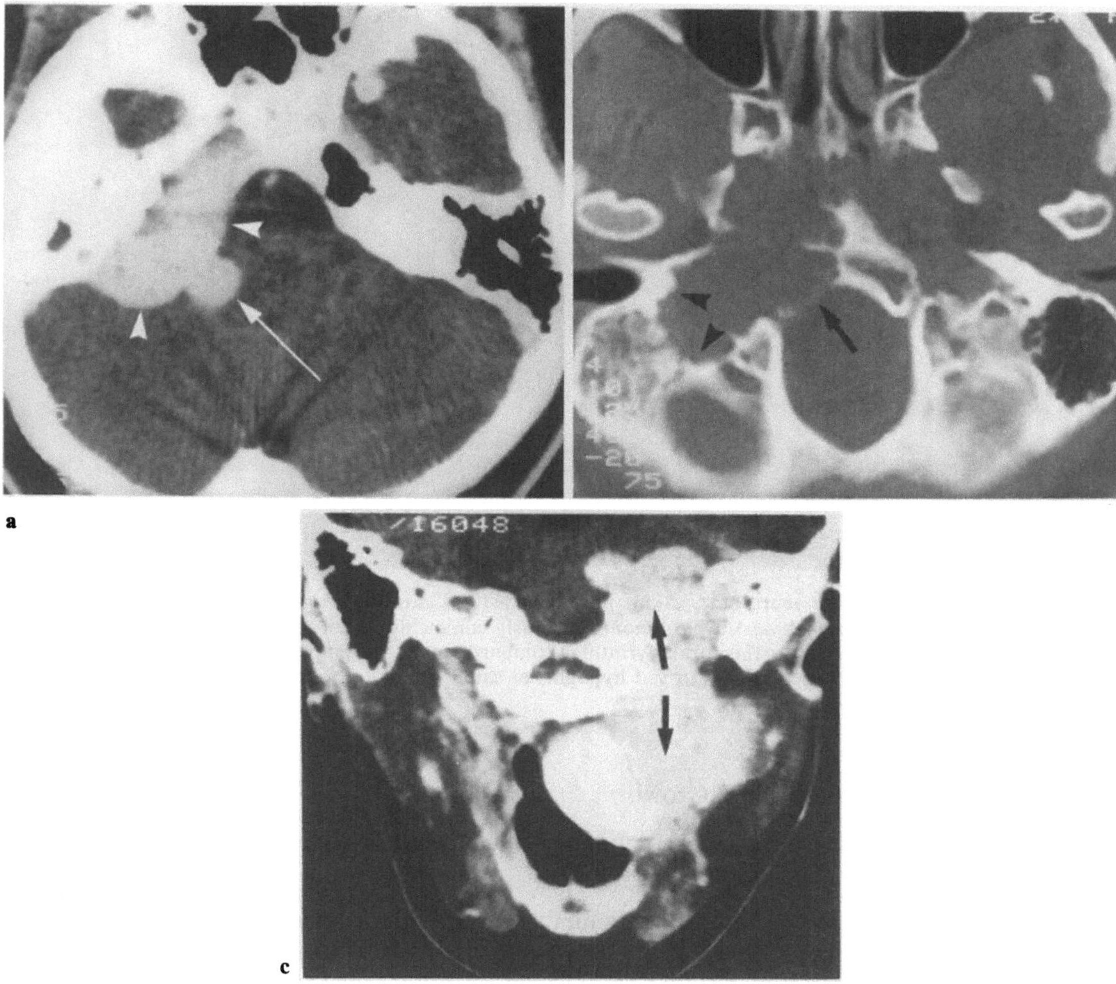

a b c

Fig. 107a–c. Hypoglossal neurinoma. **a** Axial post contrast CT. The tumor shows intense and homogeneous enhancement. The tumor extends into the extradural compartment of the cerebello-pontine angle. It is covered by linearly enhancing dura (*arrowheads*). There is focal interruption of the dura with nodular intradural tumor extension (*arrow*). **b** Axial high resolution section at a lower level shows destruction of the right hypoglossal canal (*arrow*) and sharply demarcated enlargement of the jugular foramen (*arrowheads*). **c** Coronal CT section shows typical dumbbell growth pattern (*arrows*) of this neurinoma with the extracranial, parapharyngeal component being larger than the intracranial component

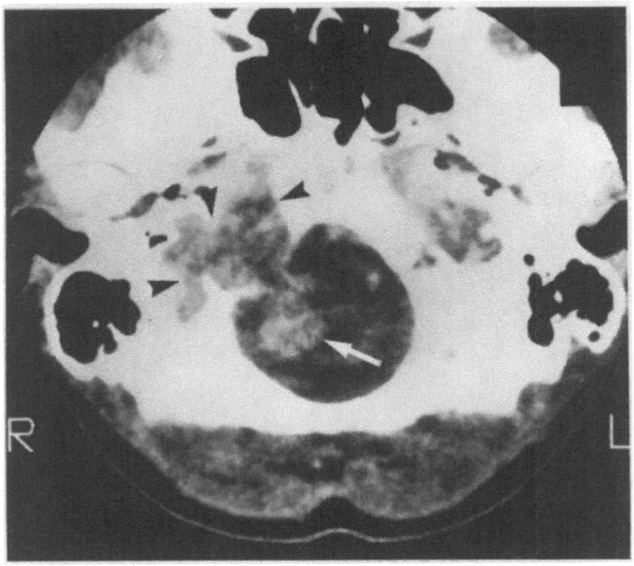

Fig. 108. Hypoglossal neurinoma. Axial post contrast CT shows destruction of the right hypoglossal canal (*arrowheads*) by an inhomogeneously enhancing tumor. The tumor occupies the jugular foramen, invades the infralabyrinthine compartment of the temporal bone and shows nodular extension through the destroyed hypoglossal canal into the inferior lateral cerebello-medullary cistern (*arrow*)

Intracranial and Intraspinal Growth

The intracranial and intraspinal components of a hypoglossal neurinoma typically form a trilobular mass as the tumor grows:

- caudally through the foramen magnum to form a tumor nodule lateral to the cervical spinal cord,
- medially to form a tumor nodule between the cerebellar tonsil and the bulb of the medulla (Fig. 108), and
- cranially to form a large tumor nodule within the cerebello-pontine angle (Fig. 107) (70).

This unique growth pattern with caudally, medially and rostrally directed tumor extensions probably arises because the narrow subarachnoid spaces prevent spherical growth of the tumor.

The relationship of the tumor to the dura is of special importance in planning the appropriate surgical approach. Medially directed components of the tumor may break through the dura and become adherent to the bulb of the medulla. Such intradural extension should be suspected whenever the medial border of the tumor appears indistinct and nodular (Fig. 107).

4 Differential Diagnosis

The differential diagnosis of hypoglossal neurinomas includes Type-D chemodectomas with intracranial extension. As compared with hypoglossal neurinomas, chemodectomas manifest more homogeneous and intense contrast enhancement and lack the trilobular finger-like intracranial extensions common with hypoglossal neurinomas. In doubtful cases, angiography allows differentiation of neurinoma from chemodectoma. Meningiomas originating in this region often show specific bone changes and usually do not cause dilatation of the hypoglossal canal. Metastases may usually be identified by their characteristic infiltration of bone.

B. Jugular Foramen Neurinomas

1 General Considerations

Neurinomas of the glossopharyngeal, vagal and spinal accessory nerves are grouped together as jugular foramen neurinomas, because clinical and even operative identification of the exact nerve of origin is often impossible. When precise identification is possible, glossopharyngeal neurinomas are more common than the other types. Vagal and spinal accessory neurinomas are found predominantly in patients with neurofibromatosis (70, 131).

Jugular foramen neurinomas are as rare as hypoglossal neurinomas. Reviewing the literature to 1979, Maniglia et al. (338) found only 56 reported cases (30, 67, 172, 188, 192, 342, 352, 359, 395, 426, 451, 473, 486, 548, 549, 624). Neurinomas of the jugular foramen are classified into 3 types according to the exact tumor origin and to the main direction of growth (255):

- Type-A tumors grow predominantly intracranially.
- Type-B tumors have their main bulk in the jugular foramen.
- Type-C tumors are situated mainly within the neck.

These differences in tumor location explain the variable clinical presentation of the tumors. In Type-A tumors, deafness, vertigo, ataxia and other cerebello-pontine angle symptoms dominate the clinical picture. Facial weakness occurs rarely. Symptoms from palsies of the lower cranial nerves may be absent (255, 445).

Tumors of Types-B and C usually exhibit palsies of the lower cranial nerves, often combined with symptoms of medullary compression (549). Such lower cranial nerve palsies occur earlier in patients in whom the tumor lies primarily within the bone or extracranially (Types-B and C, respectively). The combination of vocal cord palsy, weakness of the trapezius and sternocleidomastoid muscles and occipito-nuchal headache is especially suggestive of a jugular foramen tumor (64, 70, 97, 352, 445).

Since the clinical presentation is often misleading, jugular foramen neurinomas are frequently misinterpreted as acoustic neurinomas or as chemodectomas.

2 Conventional Radiology

Conventional X-ray and pluridirectional tomography typically demonstrate enlargement of the pars nervosa of the jugular foramen (63, 101, 123, 149, 211, 265, 544, 590, 618). These conventional radiological techniques have now been replaced by high resolution CT.

Type-A tumors may cause no change on conventional radiologic studies. Type-B tumors are characterized by widening of the jugular foramen. Since jugular neurinomas erode bone by pressure, the enlarged jugular foramen is sharply marginated and often shows a sclerotic rim (101). In contradistinction, chemodectomas that enlarge the jugular foramen often infiltrate and destroy the bone, leaving an indistinct irregular margin. In patients with jugular foramen neurinomas, vertebral angiography demonstrates an avascular mass that displaces the anterior inferior and posterior inferior cerebellar arteries away from the jugular fossa (131, 255, 445). Superselective external carotid angiography may show a tumor blush in the cerebello-pontine angle and the jugular foramen (71, 212, 255).

3 Computed Tomography

The CT appearance of jugular foramen neurinomas is identical with that of other neurinomas, except for location.

Tumor Density and Contrast Enhancement

Jugular neurinomas are usually iso- or slightly hyperdense masses. There is prominent contrast enhancement, which may be homogeneous or irregular, depending on the degree of cystic tumor alteration (Figs. 109 and 110) (71, 131, 212, 255, 257, 333).

Tumor Shape and Location

The center of Type-A tumors is located in the caudal part of the pontocerebellar cistern, i.e. more caudally than in most cases of acoustic neurinoma. Since the pontocerebellar cistern is wider than is the lateral cerebellomedullary cistern, Type-A jugular foramen neurinomas assume a rounder shape than do hypoglossal neurinomas (70).

Osseous Changes

Bony changes consist in widening and pressure erosion of the jugular foramen (Figs. 109 and 110). Type-A or mixed Type-A/B tumors may also erode the posterior surface of the petrous bone. Bone infiltration is not observed. Widening of the internal auditory canal is unusual (70). However, a single report documents widening of the internal auditory canal by a jugular foramen neurinoma (397). In that case widening may have resulted from a cerebro-spinal fluid entrapment cyst, such as is known to occur with meningiomas of the posterior surface of the petrous bone.

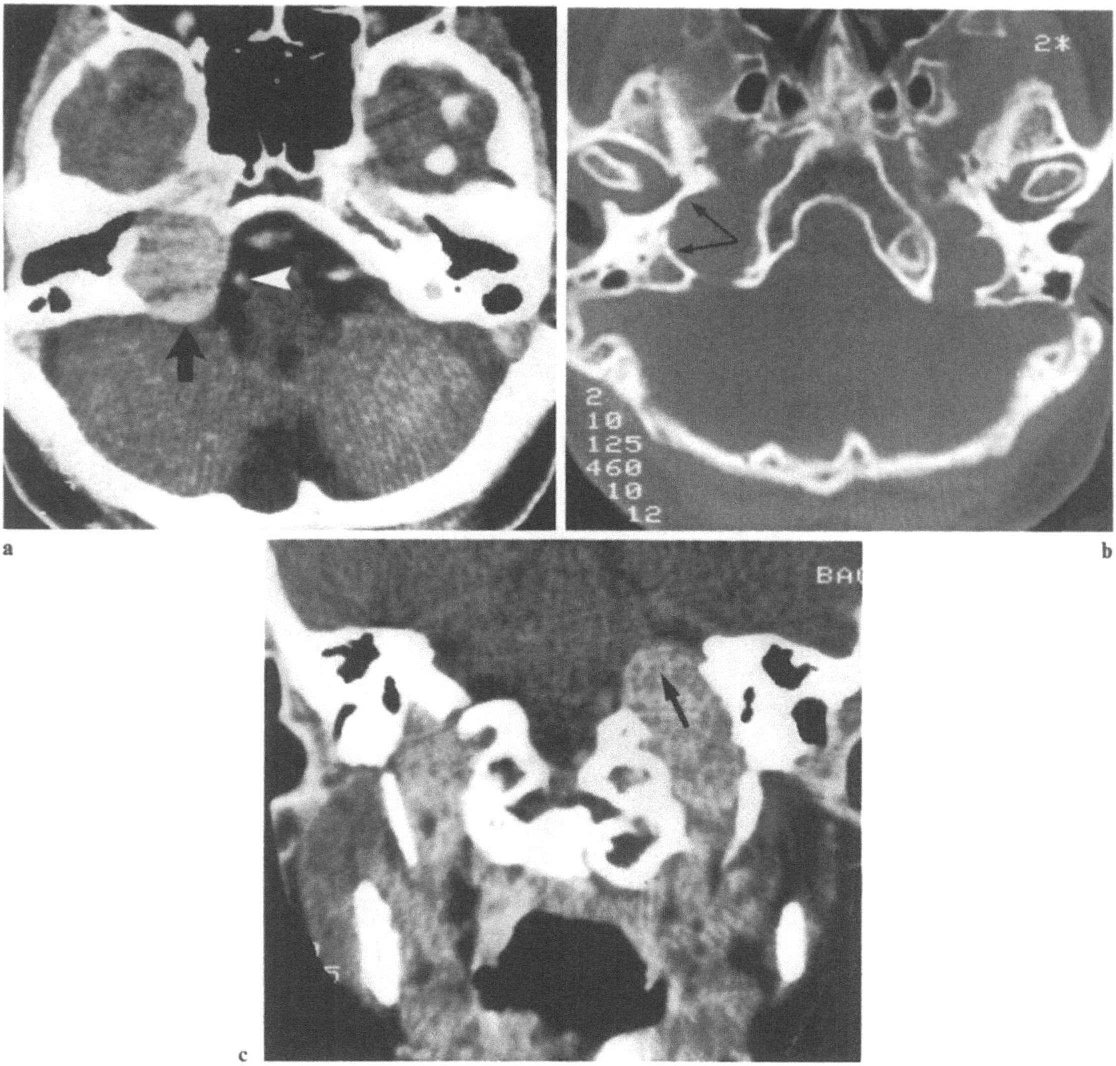

a b c

Fig. 109a–c. Jugular foramen neurinoma, Type-B. **a** Axial post contrast CT shows a homogeneously enhancing lesion in the jugular foramen with minimal extradural intracranial extension. The medial tumor border is covered by enhancing dura (*arrow*). The tumor is clearly separated from the vertebral artery (*arrowhead*). **b** Axial high resolution section shows significant enlargement of the jugular foramen with characteristic sharp contours (*arrows*), caused by pressure and not by infiltration. There is also pressure erosion of the right hypoglossal canal. **c** Coronal post contrast CT shows the oval shape of the tumor with beginning intracranial extradural extension through the jugular foramen (*arrow*)

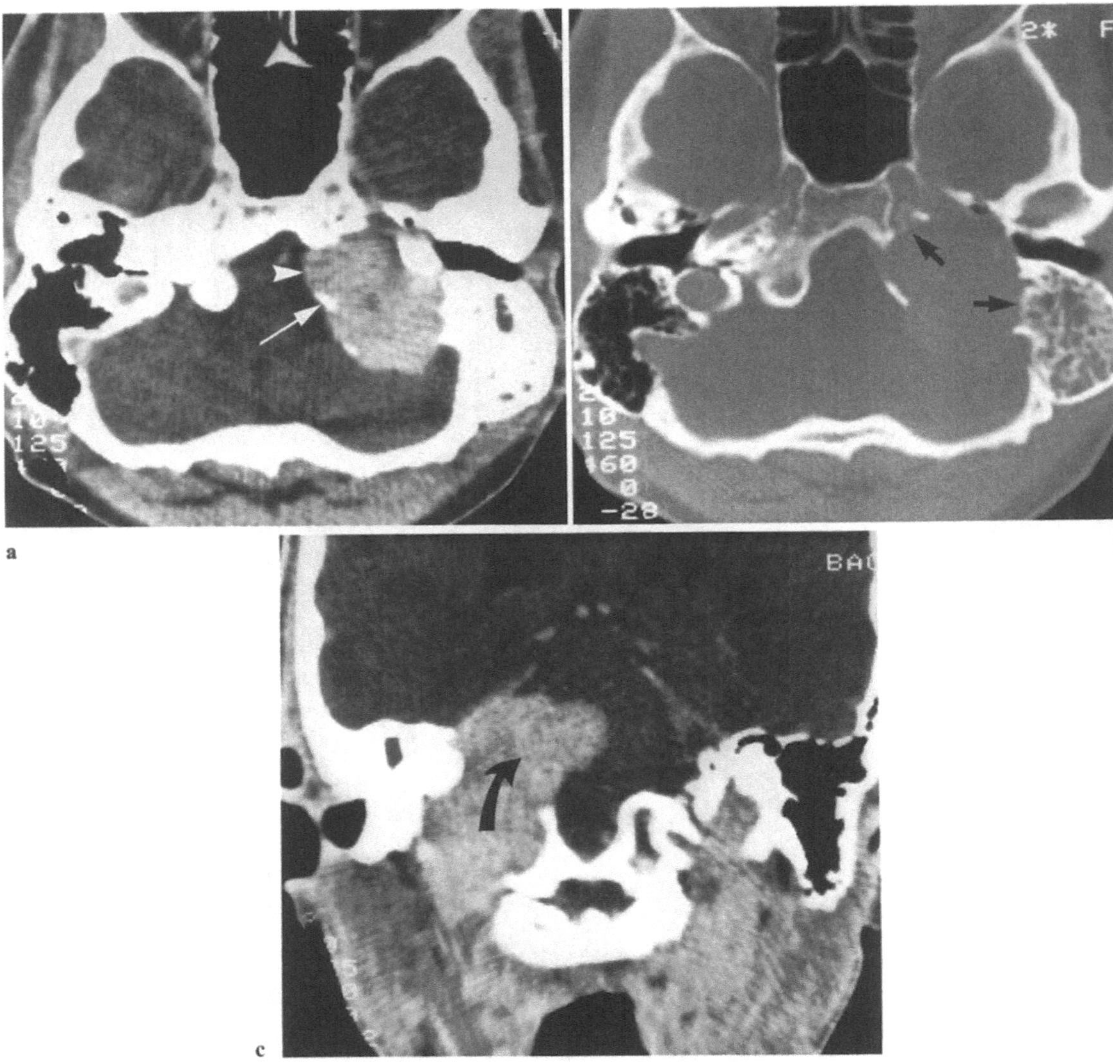

Fig. 110a–c. Jugular foramen (vagal) neurinoma Type-A/B. **a** Axial post contrast scan shows homogeneous and intense enhancement of the tumor. The tumor occupies the lower portion of the pontocerebellar cistern. Its medial border is covered by dura (*arrowhead*). A small peripheral calcification (*arrow*) is also seen. **b** High resolution CT section at the same level shows typical sharp demarcation of the enlarged jugular foramen (*arrows*). **c** In coronal CT section the growth pattern of the tumor from the jugular foramen into the cerebello-pontine angle is seen (*curved arrow*)

4 Differential Diagnosis

The major differential diagnosis of Type-A tumors without enlargement of the jugular foramen is a medial type of acoustic neurinoma. The acoustic neurinoma is usually located more rostrally than is the jugular neurinoma. Widening of the jugular foramen is unusual with acoustic neurinomas. However, an acoustic neurinoma may cause widening of the jugular foramen in very rare instances (101). Type-B tumors may usually be differentiated from chemodectomas by the smooth, sclerotic border of the eroded jugular foramen. Chemodectomas more frequently exhibit invasive bone destruction with irregular margins. Chordomas calcify in nearly 50% of cases and may often be differentiated by that feature.

Neurinomas of the Facial Nerve

1 General Considerations

Neurinomas of the facial nerve are among the rarest tumors of the petrous bone and of the cerebello-pontine angle. The first report of facial nerve neurinomas was published by Schmidt in 1930 (511). Since then, more than 100 cases have been reported (270, 400, 457). In Fisch's series (144) of 53 petrous bone and cerebello-pontine angle tumors presenting with facial nerve palsy, 12 of the 53 (23%) were facial neurinomas. Facial nerve neurinomas and primary cholesteatomas are the most common tumors to present with a progressive peripheral facial nerve palsy, and constitute about 25% of such tumors each. However, the vast majority (80%) of facial nerve palsies are idiopathic, i.e. Bell's palsy (239, 398). Only about 20% of facial nerve palsies are caused by tumor, trauma, herpes zoster oticus or otitis media combined.

Facial nerve neurinomas are much more common in otoneurosurgical practice than in neurosurgical practice. They constitute only 0.4% of cerebello-pontine angle tumors operated upon by the suboccipital approach (629). Facial nerve neurinomas usually originate in the region of the geniculate ganglion and from there extend secondarily into the internal auditory canal and into the cerebello-pontine angle (142, 144). Tumors may also grow from the geniculate ganglion through the middle ear cavity into the extratemporal space.

Neurinomas and other mesenchymal tumors (hemangioma, meningioma) of the facial nerve originate from the region of the geniculate ganglion with striking frequency. Fisch (144) believes that microscopic structural changes of the facial nerve, known to occur at the level of the geniculate ganglion, predispose to tumor formation. Facial nerve neurinomas rarely originate within the cerebello-pontine angle cistern. Therefore, facial nerve neurinomas found within the cerebello-pontine angle more commonly represent secondary extension of geniculate neurinomas into the cerebello-pontine angle than primary tumors of the cisternal segment of the facial nerve (144, 224, 298, 400).

Facial nerve neurinomas are classified according to their growth pattern into three groups:

- tumors with purely intratemporal extension,
- tumors with intratemporal and intracranial extension,
- tumors with intratemporal and extracranial (extratemporal) extension.

The typical clinical presentation of facial nerve neurinoma is progressive peripheral facial nerve palsy (144). Hearing loss, tinnitus and vertigo and other less specific symptoms may erroneously be misinterpreted as signs of an acoustic neurinoma

(400). In Nelson and House's series (400) of 13 facial nerve neurinomas with intracranial extension, 85% presented with hearing loss, 62% with tinnitus and 46% with vertigo.

2 Conventional Radiology

Intratemporal facial nerve neurinomas can be suspected when Stenvers or anteroposterior transorbital views show bone erosion localized in the region of the geniculate fossa. Bone destruction and tumor extension into the middle ear can be demonstrated by conventional tomography (144, 588). Before the introduction of CT, Pantopaque meatocisternography was the preferred method for detection of intracranial extension (144).

3 Computed Tomography

Density and Contrast Enhancement

Since facial nerve neurinomas and acoustic neurinomas are identical tumors histologically, they present nearly the same appearance on CT. Depending on the extent of regressive changes, a facial nerve neurinoma will present as an iso- or slightly hyperdense, sharply marginated lesion with homogeneous or inhomogeneous enhancement. In one personal case, the tumor was predominantly hypodense on non contrast CT and showed no enhancement. Histology showed a facial nerve neurinoma with fatty degeneration.

Gas CT cisternography is as helpful for assessing purely intracanalicular extension of facial neurinomas as it is for intracanalicular acoustic neurinomas (Fig. 111).

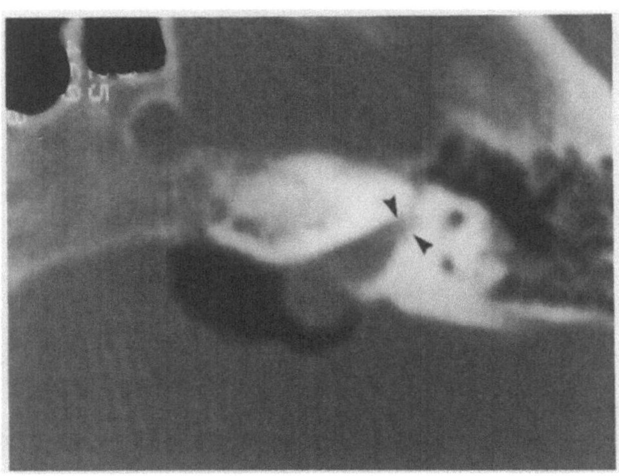

Fig. 111. Gas CT cisternography in a case of surgically proven facial neurinoma. The tumor is indistinguishable from acoustic neurinoma. However, slight dilatation of the labyrinthine segment of the Fallopian canal (*arrowheads*) suggests a facial neurinoma

Osseous Changes

High resolution CT demonstrates the intrapetrous course of the facial nerve canal. Axial sections depict the labyrinthine segment of the facial canal including the foramen meatale (i.e. the origin of the facial nerve canal from the antero-superior compartment of the internal auditory canal) (298, 578). The meatal foramen is the narrowest portion of the Fallopian canal and has a mean diameter of only 0.68 mm (578). The labyrinthine segment of the facial nerve canal courses antero-laterally. At the cochlear level it forms an anterior genu and ends at the geniculate ganglion. On coronal slices the geniculate ganglion presents as two punctate hypodensities ("snake-eyes") situated immediately supero-lateral to the cochlea. The medial hypodensity represents the labyrinthine part of the geniculate fossa. The lateral hypodensity represents the tympanic part of the geniculate fossa. The tympanic (horizontal) segment of the facial canal begins at the geniculate ganglion and courses dorsally around the vestibule and beneath the lateral semicircular canal to reach the mastoid bone. Just behind the external auditory canal, the facial nerve forms a posterior genu and turns downward as the descending (vertical) segment of the facial nerve canal. This extends from the posterior genu to the stylomastoid foramen. The greater superficial petrosal nerve arises from the geniculate ganglion and, coursing antero-medially through the pterygoid canal, reaches the sphenopalatine ganglion in the pterygopalatine fossa.

Facial neurinomas that originate from the geniculate ganglion initially enlarge the geniculate ganglion fossa. With increasing size, these tumors extend into the labyrinthine or tympanic segment, as well as along the greater superficial petrosal nerve. These extensions widen the labyrinthine and tympanic segments of the facial nerve canal respectively (Fig. 112).

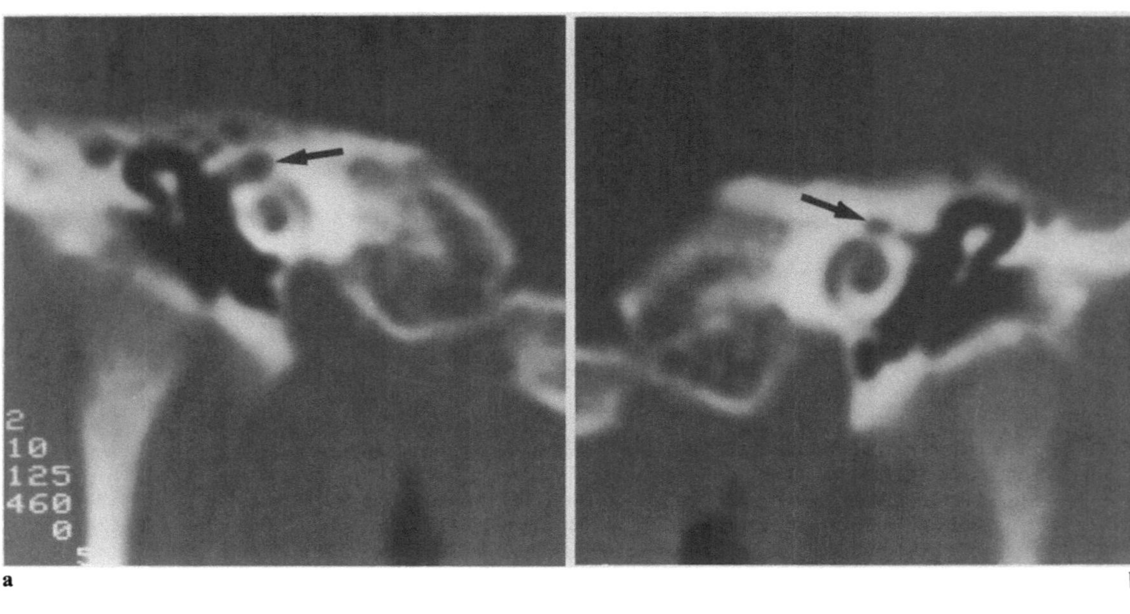

a b

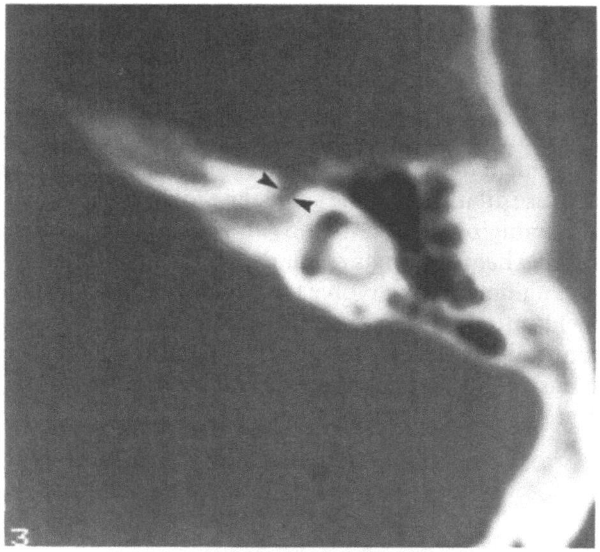

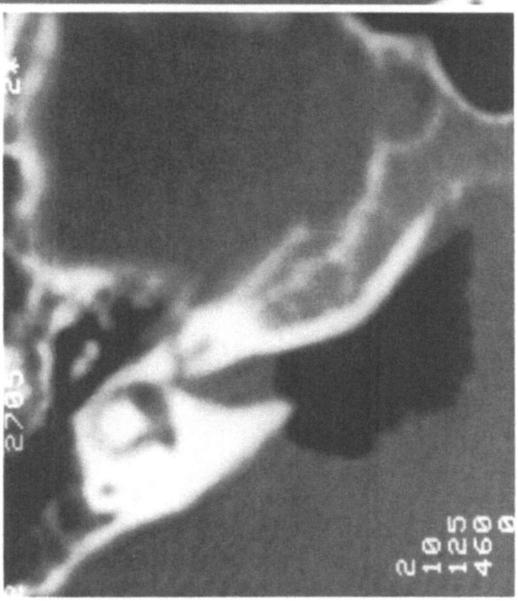

d

Fig. 112a–d. Facial nerve neurinoma of the left Fallopian canal. **a** Coronal high resolution CT section shows enlargement of the geniculate ganglion fossa (*arrow*). **b** Comparison view of the normal right geniculate ganglion fossa (*arrow*). **c** Axial high resolution CT section shows widening of the labyrinthine segment of the Fallopian canal (*arrowheads*) indicating extension of the tumor towards the internal auditory canal. **d** Intracanalicular cavernous hemangioma. Gas CT cisternography shows a small mass obliterating and slightly enlarging the internal auditory canal. Note enlargement of the labyrinthine segment of the Fallopian canal, indicating tumor extension along the facial nerve. In contradistinction to acoustic neurinomas, meningiomas and facial nerve neurinomas, the tumor exhibits a flat medial border

4 Differential Diagnosis

The main differential diagnosis of facial nerve neurinoma is acoustic neurinoma. Facial neurinomas that originate in or extend secondarily into the internal auditory canal can be differentiated from intracanalicular acoustic neurinomas by virtue of the associated enlargement of the labyrinthine segment of the facial canal (298, 591). Other tumors that cause dilatation of the geniculate fossa are cavernous or ossifying hemangioma and meningioma (142, 144, 577). Meningiomas often infiltrate the bone directly. Ossifying hemangiomas regularly exhibit intratumoral calcifications.

Cavernous hemangiomas may involve the geniculate fossa, extend through the labyrinthine segment into the internal auditory canal and thus mimic facial nerve neurinoma. In contradistinction to facial nerve neurinomas, cavernous hemangiomas exhibit intense contrast enhancement and more importantly a flat medial tumor border on gas CT cisternography (Fig. 112d).

Vascular Lesions of the Cerebello-Pontine Angle

Vascular lesions of the cerebello-pontine angle are among the rarest angle lesions and include aneurysms, vascular malformations and ectasia of the basilar artery. Yaşargil (629) found only 9 aneurysms and 5 arteriovenous malformations among 248 operated lesions of the cerebello-pontine angle. Vascular lesions may compress the neurovascular bundle within the angle and therefore may mimic the clinical signs of true neoplasms. Since most cerebello-pontine angle tumors are now operated upon without angiography, it is essential to appreciate the presence of a vascular lesion on CT prior to operation.

A. Berry Aneurysms of the Cerebello-Pontine Angle

Aneurysms of the cerebello-pontine angle are extremely rare (56, 199, 223, 245, 277, 354, 452, 629). They may originate from vessels coursing through the cerebello-pontine angle or may extend into the pontocerebellar cistern secondarily. The first group includes aneurysms of the peripheral portions of the anterior inferior and posterior inferior cerebellar arteries. The second group includes giant aneurysms that originate from the vertebral and basilar arteries and extend secondarily into the cerebello-pontine angle.

1 General Considerations

Aneurysms are usually diagnosed before they reach 1.5 cm in diameter. These aneurysms present as subarachnoid hemorrhage and usually do not pose diagnostic problems. However, signs of compression of the seventh and eighth cranial nerves may occur even with small aneurysms that originate from the loop of the anterior inferior cerebellar artery. Analysis of 11 patients with aneurysms of the anterior inferior cerebellar artery reported in the literature reveals that a cerebello-pontine angle tumor was suspected in 5 patients and that 2 of these 5 were operated upon for the erroneous diagnosis of a cerebello-pontine angle tumor (245). The other 8 patients presented with subarachnoid hemorrhage. In this series, 91% of the patients had facial palsy; 82% had hearing loss. Since cerebello-pontine angle tumors may rarely present with subarachnoid hemorrhage, correct differential diagnosis can be difficult (628, 632).

2 Conventional Radiology

Plain radiographs and pluridirectional tomography may demonstrate misleading enlargement of the internal auditory canal. Thus, pressure erosion and enlargement of the porus of the internal auditory canal were found in 4 of 10 cases reported in the literature (245). Pantopaque meatocisternography may show non filling of the canal that is indistinguishable from the non filling caused by tumor (245). Vertebral angiography is the only *conventional* technique able to establish the correct diagnosis (277, 332).

3 Computed Tomography

To our knowledge, no case of aneurysm of the anterior inferior cerebellar artery has been reported in the CT literature. An aneurysm of the cerebello-pontine angle can be expected to present as an intensely enhancing, sharply demarcated lesion. However, one may expect to miss some small aneurysms on CT because of the known limitations of CT. It can be assumed that gas CT cisternography may demonstrate a filling defect not distinguishable from a tumor. Dynamic CT may be the only CT method capable of diagnosing an angle aneurysm correctly. This may be combined with gas CT cisternography for finer resolution.

B. Giant Cerebello-Pontine Angle Aneurysms

1 General Considerations

Giant aneurysms are defined as intracranial aneurysms that exceed 2.5 cm in diameter. Giant aneurysms present different clinical signs than do the smaller aneurysms. The common mode of presentation is that of a space occupying lesion. Subarachnoid hemorrhage is encountered only rarely (2, 114, 240, 277, 369, 372, 409, 502, 604, 631). Giant intracranial aneurysms that originate from the basilar or vertebral arteries may extend secondarily into the cerebello-pontine angle and cause cerebello-pontine angle symptoms that mimic a tumor.

Giant intracranial aneurysms are partially thrombosed in 50% of the cases, totally thrombosed in 10% of cases and not thrombosed in 40% of cases (436, 442, 516).

2 Conventional Radiology

Conventional radiographs may show shell-like calcification, typically occurring in the wall of the aneurysm. Definitive diagnosis of a giant cerebello-pontine angle aneurysm can only be established angiographically. However, angiography demonstrates just the patent, blood containing portion of the aneurysm. The real size of the aneurysm has to be deduced from the displacement of adjacent vessels.

Totally thrombosed giant intracranial aneurysms present angiographically as avascular masses. With this type of aneurysm, the artery from which the aneurysm originates is often occluded (48, 502, 547).

3 Computed Tomography

Giant aneurysms of the cerebello-pontine angle exhibit the same CT features as do giant aneurysms at other locations. The CT morphology depends mainly upon the degree of thrombosis present (51, 157, 198, 377, 436, 442, 516, 564, 635).

Partially Thrombosed Giant Cerebello-Pontine Angle Aneurysms

Partially thrombosed giant intracranial aneurysms appear as iso- or slightly hyperdense, sharply marginated extraaxial lesions and often exhibit shell-like or interrupted curvilinear calcifications at or near their periphery (436, 442, 516). The nature of the lesions may be suspected on the non contrast scan, if the density of the thrombosed portion differs significantly from that of the circulating blood. After contrast enhancement, a sharply demarcated region *inside* the lesion shows a very intense, homogeneous enhancement. This region corresponds to the residual, patent lumen of the aneurysm. Additional curvilinear enhancement is seen at the periphery of the aneurysm (Fig. 113 and 114). Since the wall of giant intracranial aneurysms may show impressive hypervascularity at operation, the peripheral ring enhancement was first thought to represent vascular enhancement (516). More recently dynamic CT has shown that part of the enhancement is extravascular

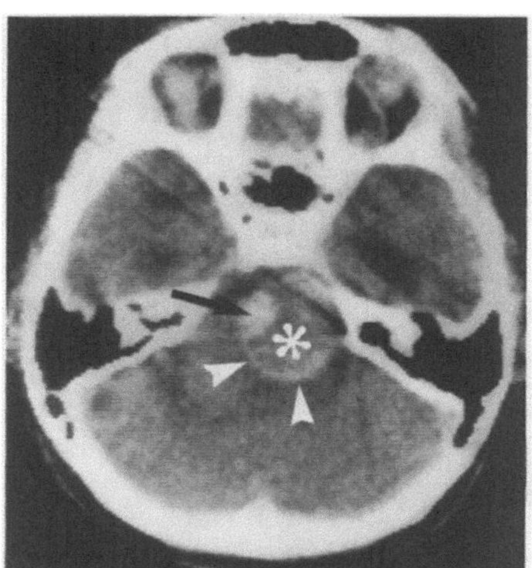

Fig. 113. Partially thrombosed giant intracranial aneurysm originating from the basilar artery. Post contrast axial CT section. The aneurysm occupies the anterior portion of the left pontocerebellar cistern. The open part of the aneurysm presents as a homogeneously enhancing nodule (*arrow*). The thrombosed portion of the aneurysm does not enhance (*asterisk*). There is also curvilinear enhancement of the aneurysmal wall (*arrowheads*)

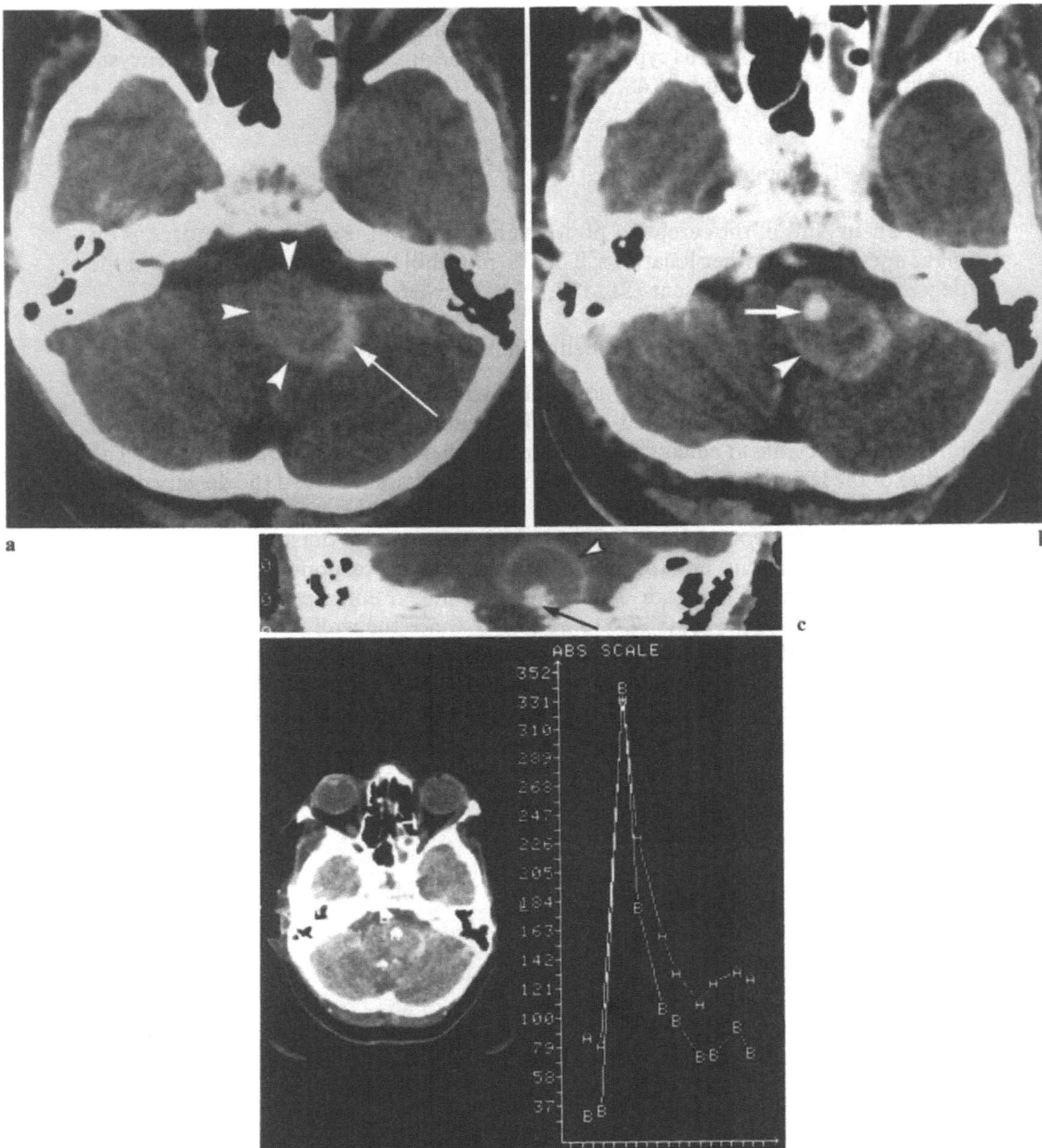

a b c d

Fig. 114a–d. Partially thrombosed giant intracranial aneurysm originating from the posterior inferior cerebellar artery. **a** Non contrast axial CT shows a mass embedded inbetween the medulla and the cerebellar hemisphere (*arrowheads*) and partially occupying the pontocerebellar cistern. The mass itself is slightly hyperdense. Its lateral border contains a dense area which represents a fresh clot (*arrow*). **b** Post contrast axial CT shows the patent portion of the aneurysm as a homogeneously enhancing nodule (*arrow*) (target sign). The thrombosed portion and the fresh

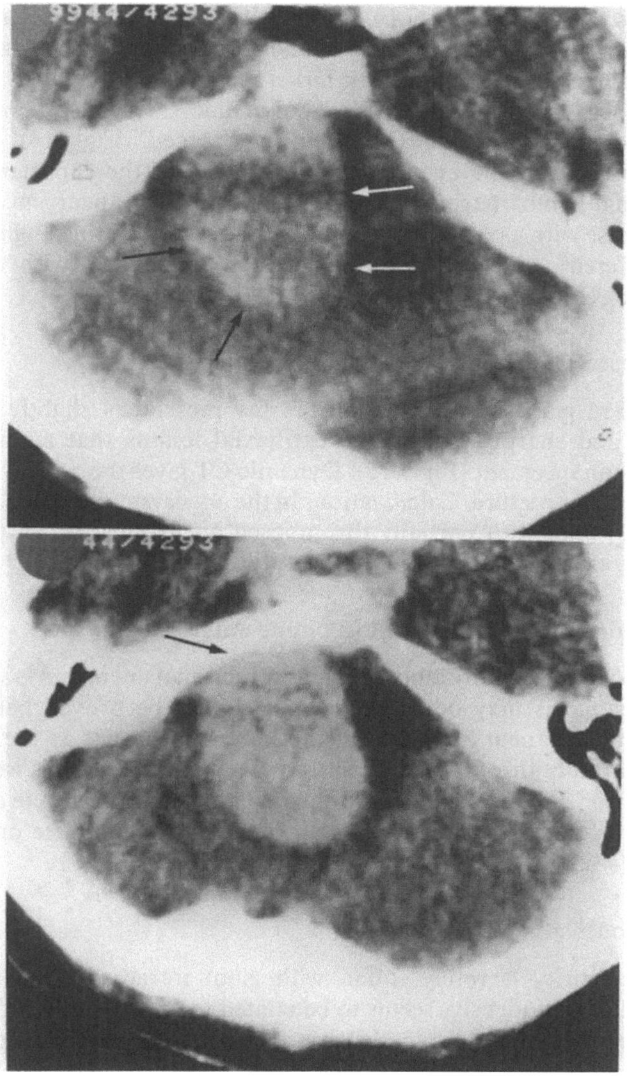

a

b

Fig. 115a, b. Non thrombosed giant basilar artery aneurysm. **a** Non contrast axial CT shows a sharply marginated extraaxial lesion occupying the anterior portion of the pontocerebellar cistern (*arrows*). **b** Post contrast CT shows homogeneous enhancement of the lesion. Note pressure erosion at the petrous apex (*arrow*)

◄———

clot do not enhance. The aneurysmal wall shows slight curvilinear enhancement (*arrowhead*). **c** Coronal reformation shows the inferiorly located open portion of the aneurysm (*arrow*). The larger thrombosed portion is well defined by curvilinear enhancement of the aneurysm wall (*arrowhead*). **d** Dynamic CT performed at the level of the open portion of the aneurysm (*A*) and at the basilar artery (*B*) demonstrates identically shaped time-density curves. This indicates similar flow behaviour between the basilar artery and the open portion of the aneurysm

(Huber P., personal communication). That is, the aneurysm wall behaves like dura mater. Together, the intensely enhancing lumen, non enhancing clot and peripheral ring enhancement create a characteristic *target sign*. The CT diagnosis of a partially thrombosed aneurysm can be verified by dynamic CT, which shows a typical vascular time-density curve over the enhancing "target" (Fig. 114).

Hypervascularity of the aneurysm wall, rupture of the capsular vessels and intra-aneurysmal hemorrhage seem to be responsible for aneurysm growth (10). One personal case with a partially thrombosed cerebello-pontine angle giant PICA aneurysm suffered acute clinical deterioration associated with acute intra-aneurysmal clot (Fig. 114) (513).

Non Thrombosed Giant Cerebello-Pontine Angle Aneurysms

Non thrombosed giant intracranial aneurysms present as slightly hyperdense, homogeneous and sharply marginated extraaxial lesions that manifest intense, homogeneous enhancement (Fig. 115). Dynamic CT gives the typical time-density curve of a vascular structure. Calcifications in the aneurysmal wall are encountered much less often than with partially thrombosed aneurysms. When present, they usually appear as small, punctate hyperdensities (442, 516).

Totally Thrombosed Giant Cerebello-Pontine Angle Aneurysms

The diagnosis of a totally thrombosed giant intracranial aneurysm is very difficult. The correct diagnosis may be suspected but cannot be proven before surgery. Totally thrombosed aneurysms present the same appearance as the thrombosed portion of a partially thrombosed aneurysm. That is, the lesion is iso- or slightly hyperdense, is non enhancing and is extraaxial in location. Shell-like calcifications may be encountered. The aneurysmal wall often shows complete or partial ring enhancement (442, 516).

Perifocal Hypodensity

Perifocal hypodensity is rarely found with giant intracranial aneurysms. The frequency of such hypodensity seems to be related to aneurysm size (516). It is not known whether the perifocal hypodensity represents edema or atrophy.

Osseous Changes

Like other slowly growing space occupying lesions, giant aneurysms may cause pressure erosion of the posterior surface of the petrous bone (Fig. 115). Bone infiltration and bone destruction do not occur.

Topographical Relationship of the Aneurysm to the Pontocerebellar Cistern

Although criteria for identifying the extraaxial location of mass lesions have proved fairly reliable (387), extraaxial masses may still be misinterpreted as intraaxial lesions. This is especially true for aneurysms with peripheral origin (357). The aneurysm may be nearly completely surrounded by the pons, medulla and the cerebellar hemisphere and therefore may be misinterpreted as an intraaxial lesion (Fig. 114).

The precise origin of a giant intracranial aneurysm usually cannot be identified on CT. However, the origin may be *suspected* from the location of the aneurysm in the pontocerebellar cistern. Aneurysms originating from the basilar artery tip may extend caudo-laterally into the premeatal part of the pontocerebellar cistern. Aneurysms originating from the basilar trunk usually involve the central portion of the pontocerebellar cistern. Aneurysms originating from the vertebral artery may extend into the retro- or inframeatal portion of the cistern.

4 Differential Diagnosis

The CT appearance of partially thrombosed giant cerebello-pontine angle aneurysms is usually pathognomonic. In doubtful cases, dynamic CT helps to establish the diagnosis. Non thrombosed aneurysms may be mistaken for enhancing tumors such as meningiomas, medial acoustic neurinomas or neurinomas of other cranial nerves. The intensity and homogeneity of the luminal enhancement usually indicate that the lesion is a non thrombosed aneurysm. If present, shell-like calcification of the aneurysmal wall helps to establish the diagnosis. Non thrombosed giant cerebello-pontine angle aneurysms may also be mistaken for a hyperdense epidermoid.

C. Megadolichobasilar Anomaly

1 General Considerations

The megadolichobasilar anomaly consists in dilatation, elongation and tortuosity of the basilar artery. It was first described by Morgagni in 1761 (368). Later on, Stopford (543) recognized the relationship between dilated, elongated vertebral and basilar arteries and symptoms of nerve compression in the cerebello-pontine angle. During a posterior fossa operation, Wells (606) observed a dilated and tortuous basilar artery that compressed cranial nerves six, seven and eight and that caused hydrocephalus by aqueductal obstruction.

Many reports of the megadolichobasilar anomaly followed these first descriptions (34, 41, 53, 72, 84, 178, 287, 371, 495, 567). It is widely believed that megadolichobasilar anomaly represents a pathologic condition and not merely an extreme of the normal range as could be suggested by the term anomaly. Therefore, the term basilar ectasia would be more appropriate. Despite that, the term megadolichobasilar anomaly is widely accepted.

The etiology of megadolichobasilar anomaly remains unknown. It seems likely that this arteriopathy results from deficiencies in the muscularis and the internal elastic lamina (169).

Although basilar ectasia is probably secondary to congenital defects in the arterial wall, symptoms do not usually develop until the patient reaches middle or old age. The arteries then appear to dilate and elongate under the stress of elevated blood pressure and superimposed atherosclerotic disease.

The clinical presentation of megadolichobasilar anomaly is not uniform (34). The most common symptoms, found in about 15 to 20% of cases each, include headache, facial spasm, gait disturbance, facial pain and symptoms of bulbar palsy (371). Infrequently diplopia, vertigo, hearing loss, episodes of hemiparesis and even dementia occur. Clinical examination commonly reveals palsies of the seventh and eighth cranial nerves. Palsies of the fifth, sixth, ninth and tenth nerves are less common. Moseley and Holland (371) found cerebellar signs in 45% of cases, pyramidal signs in 37.5% and dementia in 17.5% of cases.

The multiple clinical signs associated with megadolichobasilar anomaly may be classified into three groups (343): 1. ischemic signs, 2. signs of cranial nerve compression, and 3. pseudotumoral symptoms. The combination of different signs including hydrocephalus, lower cranial nerve lesions and cerebellar and pyramidal signs in a hypertensive male should raise the suspicion of megadolichobasilar anomaly.

2 Conventional Radiology

Conventional radiographs and tomograms are usually normal. Rarely, calcifications may be seen in the vascular wall (371). Dilatation of the porus of the internal auditory canal has been reported in only two cases (16, 463).

Pantopaque meatocisternography demonstrates the dilated basilar artery as a curvilinear filling defect in the pontocerebellar cistern (178, 205).

With conventional techniques, the definitive diagnosis relies upon angiography (34, 90, 178, 261, 277, 343, 489, 533). By definition, the basilar artery is ectatic if the lumen of the basilar trunk measures greater than 5.3 mm at a point 3 mm distal to the union of the vertebral arteries to form the basilar artery (621). In patients with megadolichobasilar anomaly, antero-posterior views show the ectatic basilar trunk crossing the pons and reaching the cerebello-pontine angle (432). The lateral projection demonstrates elongation of the basilar artery. The bifurcation of the basilar artery lies within the interpeduncular cistern and indents the floor of the third ventricle. In rare instances it may compress the dorsal portion of the third ventricle (34, 178).

Variations in vessel size, irregularities of the vessel wall and other alterations which are commonly found in atherosclerotic vessels are also regularly demonstrated in cases of megadolichobasilar anomaly. These atherosclerotic alterations are usually not confined to the basilar trunk, but also involve the vertebral and carotid arteries (34).

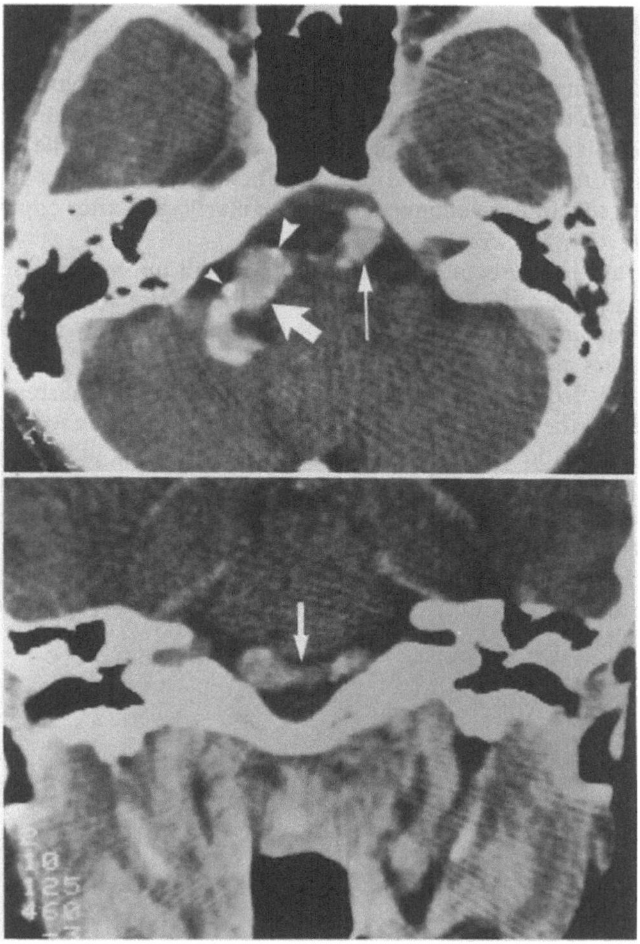

a

b

Fig. 116a, b. Megadolichobasilar anomaly. Post contrast CT. **a** Axial CT demonstrates a serpiginous cerebello-pontine angle lesion (*thick arrow*) with punctate peripheral calcifications (*arrowheads*). The scanning plane almost parallels the upper loop of the ectatic basilar artery which appears as band-like structure. Before reaching the opposite side (*small arrow*) the basilar artery swings downwards and is therefore not included in the slice, producing the false impression of separate right and left cerebello-pontine angle lesions. **b** Direct coronal scanning demonstrates the elongated ectatic basilar artery as horizontal band crossing the midline anterior to the pons (*arrow*)

3 Computed Tomography

On CT, megadolichobasilar anomaly presents as a hyperdense, band-like (Figs. 116 and 117) and often tubular (Fig. 118) lesion that extends from widened prepontine and pontocerebellar cisterns into the interpeduncular cistern. The lesion appears serpiginous and often exhibits band-like or punctate calcifications at its periphery (Figs. 116 and 117). Intense enhancement is regularly seen after contrast administration (16, 96, 194, 371, 523).

The appearance of the ectatic basilar trunk depends upon its course with respect to the scanning plane. As the distal portion of the ectatic artery swings from the cerebello-pontine angle to the midline, it usually lies in or near the axial scanning plane and appears as a band-like or serpiginous structure. The presence of such a band that courses from the lateral part of the pontocerebellar cistern towards the midline or even to the opposite side is pathognomonic for the megadolichobasilar anomaly (Figs. 116 and 117) (22, 96, 351, 371, 432, 523). At other scanning levels, the basilar trunk courses more nearly perpendicular to the scanning plane and appears as a round or oval lesion on axial CT sections. In such cases, the true nature of the lesion can be appreciated by performing coronal CT scans or reformatted coronal images to show that the series of round, oval and band-like enhancing lesions conforms to the course of an ectatic basilar artery (Figs. 116 and 118).

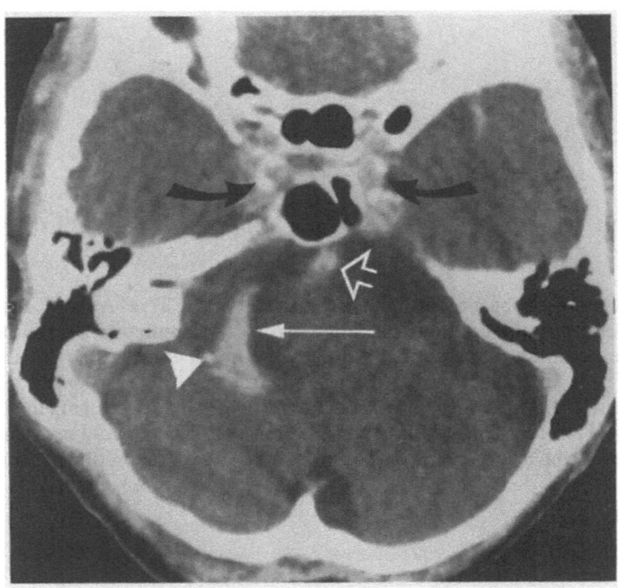

Fig. 117. Megadolichobasilar anomaly. Axial post contrast CT. The medial portion of the dilated pontocerebellar cistern harbours a tubular, homogeneously enhancing structure (*arrow*) with a small peripheral calcification (*arrowhead*). The ascending portion of the basilar artery (*open arrow*) is medially located between pons and clivus. Note also bilateral ectatic carotid arteries with mural calcifications (*curved arrows*)

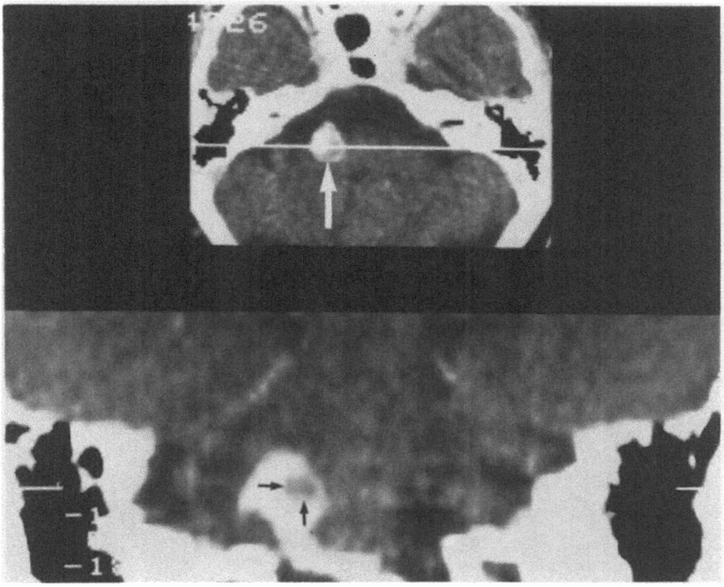

Fig. 118. Megadolichobasilar anomaly with partial thrombosis. On the axial post contrast scan (*upper image*) a nodular, partially enhancing lesion is seen in the right cerebello-pontine angle (*white arrow*). Coronal reformation (*lower image*) demonstrates that this lesion represents the basilar artery coursing laterally into the pontocerebellar cistern. The thrombosed portion of the basilar artery (*short black arrows*) presents as a non enhancing marginal defect which is confined by the enhancing arterial wall

In rare instances, partial enhancement of the basilar artery is caused by partial thrombosis of the vessel (371). Partial thrombosis of the megadolichobasilar artery causes a target sign similar to that seen with partially thrombosed giant intracranial aneurysms (Fig. 118) (516). Partial thrombosis is only rarely seen on CT. The common angiographic assumption that a free space between the ectatic basilar artery and the clivus represents thrombosis is probably wrong in the majority of cases. CT shows that the ectatic basilar artery often courses along the pons in the dilated prepontine and pontocerebellar cisterns and that the space between artery and clivus contains cerebro-spinal fluid, not thrombus (371).

4 Hydrocephalus

In 1956, Greitz and Löfstedt (178) published a classic pneumoencephalographic and angiographic study on the relationship between the tip of the basilar artery and the floor of the third ventricle. The relationship can also be demonstrated by reformatted sagittal CT scans (Fig. 119). Development of hydrocephalus is related to the indentation of the floor of the third ventricle by the ectatic basilar tip. In rare instances, the indentation is severe enough to cause complete obliteration of the dorsal third ventricle and obstructive hydrocephalus (485). Much more commonly, hydrocephalus develops without complete obstruction of the cerebro-spinal fluid

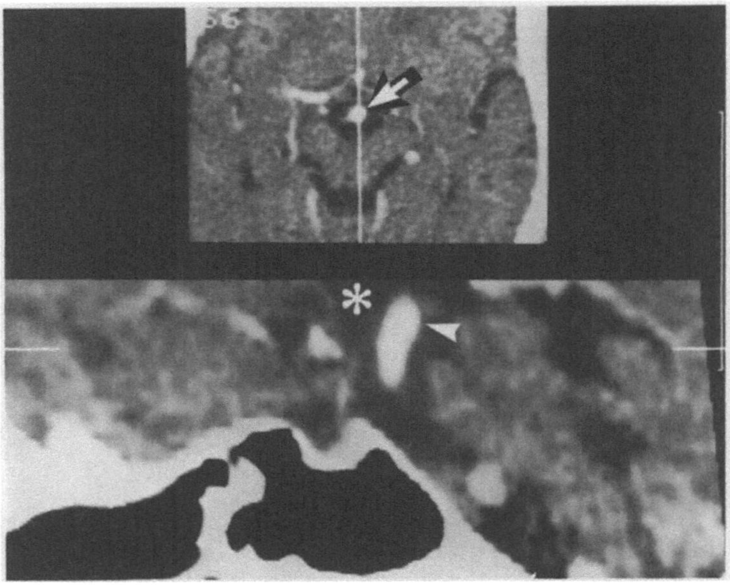

Fig. 119. Megadolichobasilar anomaly with hydrocephalus. The axial section (*upper image*) shows the ectatic basilar artery tip (*arrow*) in the interpeduncular cistern. Sagittal reformation (*lower image*) shows to better advantage the high position of the basilar artery tip (*arrowhead*) causing indentation of the floor of the third ventricle (*asterisk*)

pathways. Breig et al. (40) explained the development of non obstructive hydrocephalus by the arterial pulsations against the floor of the third ventricle. These pulsations are transferred to the cerebro-spinal fluid circulation at the level of the foramina of Monro. Despite the impaired cerebro-spinal fluid circulation, the intraventricular pressure is not elevated, as proved later by intraventricular pressure monitoring (119, 180).

Periventricular hypodensity may be encountered in these patients. The origin of the hypodensity is unknown in the individual case. The hypodensity could be the expression of transependymal cerebro-spinal fluid resorption or of hypertensive leukoencephalopathy (371).

D. Vascular Malformations of the Cerebello-Pontine Angle

1 General Considerations

Arteriovenous malformations are extremely rare in the cerebello-pontine angle. Arteriovenous malformations of the pons and the cerebellar hemispheres are more common and may extend secondarily into the cerebello-pontine angle (50, 100, 109, 118, 175, 254, 595, 629).

Arteriovenous malformations may be classified into leptomeningeal, dural and mixed types. Dural arteriovenous malformations are the most frequent type encountered in the cerebello-pontine angle. They are probably acquired lesions and originate in the wall of a dural sinus such as the sigmoid, superior and inferior petrosal sinus (102, 232, 236, 288, 347, 405, 412). They are more correctly designated fistulas.

2 Conventional Radiology

Angiography is the method of choice for evaluation of all types of vascular malformations. In cases of dural arteriovenous malformations, selective injection of the potential feeders including the occipital, ascending pharyngeal, middle meningeal and posterior auricular arteries is mandatory. In addition to the meningeal branches of the external carotid artery, dural arteriovenous malformations may be supplied from meningeal branches of the internal carotid and vertebral arteries.

Dural arteriovenous fistulas are classified into 4 types according to their different patterns of drainage (102):

- Type 1 fistulas drain directly into a venous sinus or into a meningeal vein,
- Type 2 fistulas drain into a sinus, but also show retrograde drainage into a cortical vein,
- Type 3 fistulas drain directly into a cortical vein, and
- Type 4 fistulas drain into varicose venous structures, which may exert pressure on the neighbouring structures. Therefore, this type of dural arteriovenous malformation is called pseudotumoral.

3 Computed Tomography

On CT, arteriovenous malformations of the cerebello-pontine angle have the same appearance as arteriovenous malformations in other locations (258, 299, 560). On non contrast CT scans, arteriovenous malformations present as lesions of mixed density; in rare instances they may be isodense. On the post contrast scan the enhancement is characteristically inhomogeneous, punctate, tubular and serpiginous (Figs. 120 and 121). Dilated draining veins, especially the petrosal vein of Dandy, may be visible (254).

On gas CT cisternography arteriovenous malformations appear as a network of structures that partially fill out the pontocerebellar cistern (254). The CT appearance of dural fistulas depends upon the specific type of fistula present. Small Type 1 to 3 fistulas are usually not visible on CT. However, the dilated cortical veins in Type 2 and 3 fistulas may be visible (Fig. 122). The dilated, space occupying draining veins of Type 4 fistulas are regularly seen on CT (Fig. 123). Pressure erosion of the petrous bone may be present (Fig. 121) and in all types of fistulas, high resolution CT may show dilated arterial foramina at the base of the skull. These indicate the transosseous course of the feeding and draining vessels.

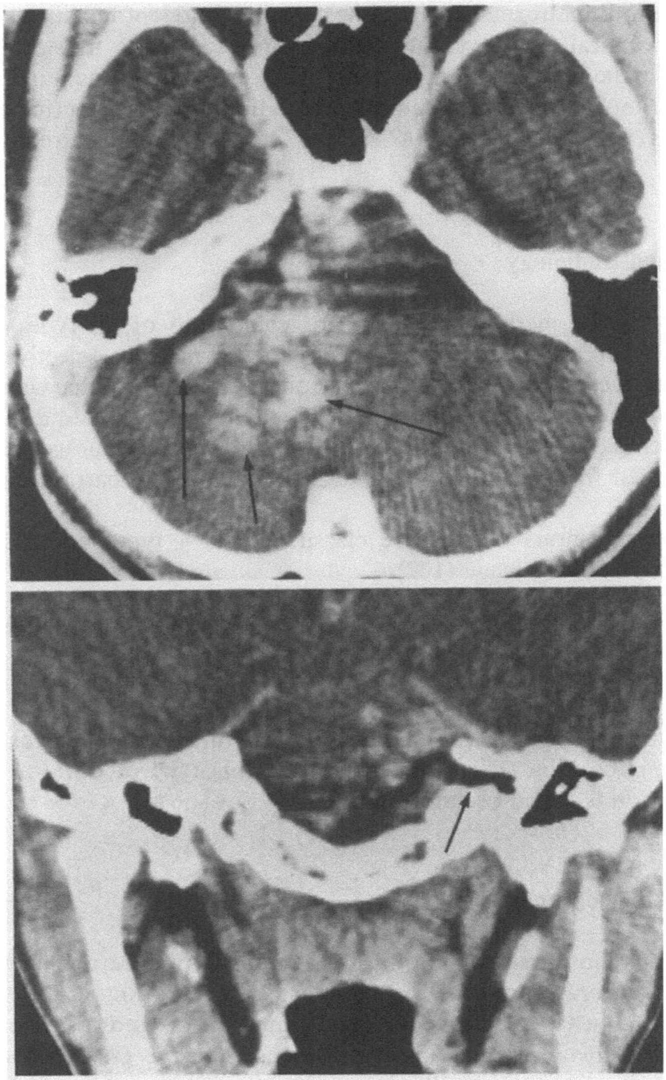

a

b

Fig. 120a, b. Arteriovenous malformation of the cerebello-pontine angle. Post contrast CT. **a** Axial CT demonstrates multiple nodular and serpiginous enhancing structures (*arrows*) within the cerebello-pontine angle as well as in the adjacent cerebellar parenchyma – an appearance typical for arteriovenous malformation. Angiography (not shown) proved the presence of an arteriovenous malformation and showed that the nodular and serpiginous structures seen on CT represent draining veins. **b** Coronal CT shows slight dilatation of the internal auditory canal (*arrow*)

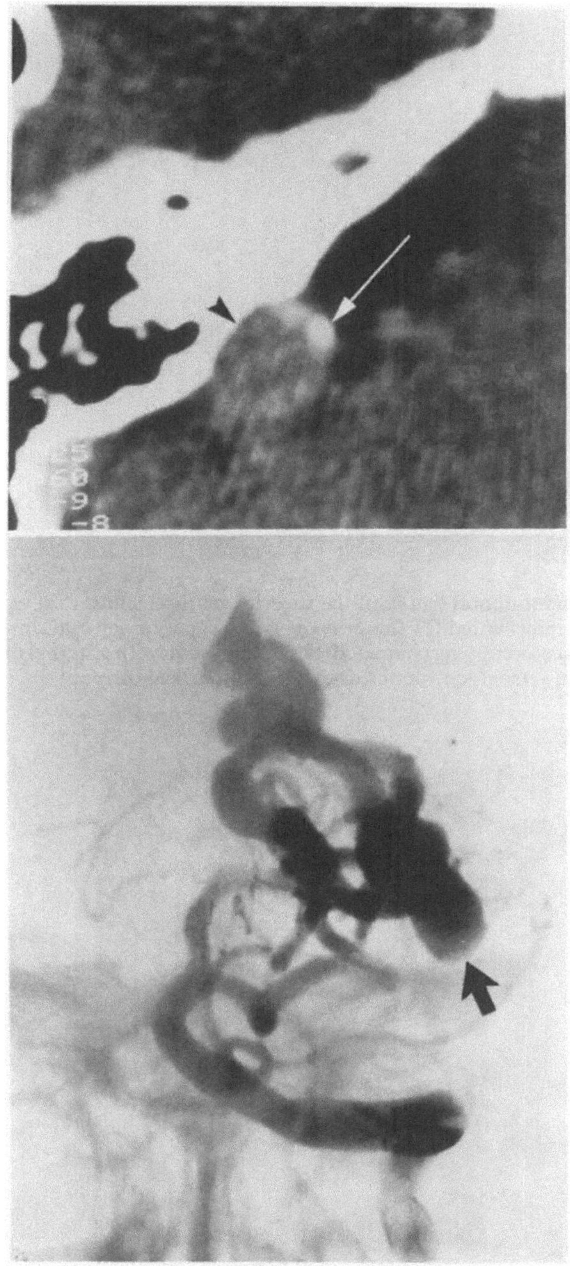

a

b

Fig. 121 a, b. Varix-node in the cerebello-pontine angle. **a** Axial post contrast CT shows a homogeneously enhancing nodular lesion in the pontocerebellar cistern causing pressure erosion of the posterior surface of the petrous bone (*arrowhead*). Note a punctate calcification (*arrow*). **b** Angiography shows the presence of an arteriovenous malformation. The nodular lesion seen on CT represents a varicose draining vein (*arrow*)

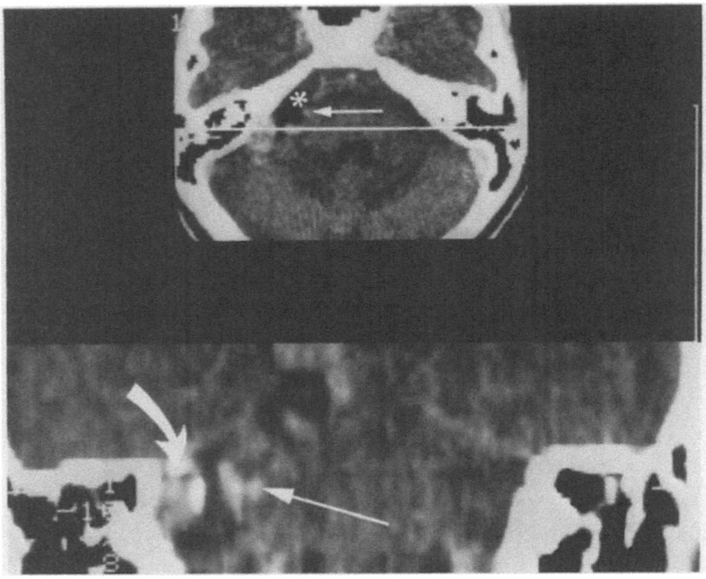

Fig. 122. Dural pseudotumoral fistula of the superior petrosal sinus. Post contrast axial (*upper image*) and coronal reformatted CT (*lower image*). The superior petrosal sinus is dilated (*curved arrow*). Note the space-occupying characteristics of this lesion with cisternal dilatation (*asterisk*). Note also additional retrograde venous drainage into cortical (*arrows*)

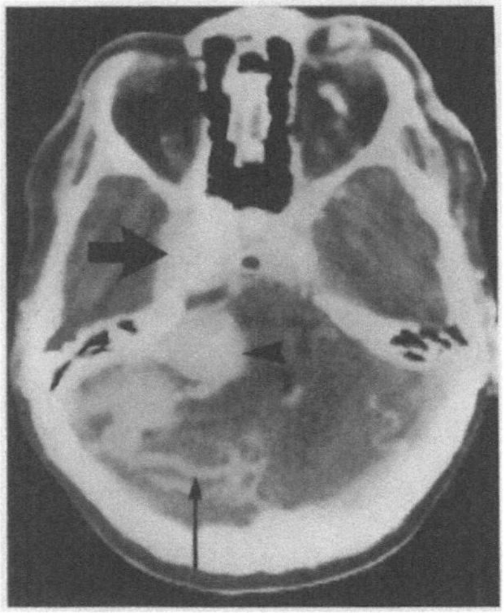

Fig. 123. Carotid-cavernous fistula with posterior drainage. Post contrast axial CT. The carotid-cavernous fistula (*thick arrow*) drains into the dilated petrosal vein (*arrowhead*). There is also retrograde drainage into dilated cerebellar cortical veins (*thin arrow*). Courtesy E.J. Russell, Chicago

Secondary Tumors of the Cerebello-Pontine Angle

The cerebello-pontine angle may be involved by secondary extension of tumors that originate in neighbouring structures. Some of the tumors that extend into the cerebello-pontine angle have been discussed in earlier chapters. Other, usually malignant tumors with exophytic or infiltrative growth characteristics may also extend into the cerebello-pontine angle. It is beyond the scope of this book to describe all the possible tumors. However, recognition of tumor extension into the cerebello-pontine angle is important for operative planning.

Intraaxial tumors are the tumors most likely to cause secondary extension into the cerebello-pontine angle. Included in this group are cerebellar astrocytomas, ependymomas, medulloblastomas, hemangioblastomas, papillomas, sarcomas, lymphomas (Fig. 124) and pontine gliomas (120, 222, 271, 391, 394, 576, 629, 636, 637). Characteristically, ependymomas extend into the pontocerebellar cistern through the preformed pathway of the lateral recess of the fourth ventricle (120, 391, 629). They may also grow from the fourth ventricle into cisterna magna and, from there, they may extend further under the cerebellar hemisphere to reach the cerebello-pontine angle. In rare cases, demonstration of extension of intraaxial tumors into the cerebello-pontine angle may be impossible, because the tumors are isodense and exhibit minimal or no contrast enhancement.

Extra-axial tumors may reach the cerebello-pontine angle from different locations.

1. Sellar, parasellar, suprasellar and clival tumors may invade the premeatal part of the pontocerebellar cistern. Included in this group are invasive pituitary adenomas (Fig. 125), clival chordomas and parasellar meningiomas.
2. Extra-axial tumors and tumors of the base of the posterior fossa may extend into the cerebello-pontine angle through the jugular foramen (Fig. 126). Included in this group are jugular chemodectomas, rhabdomyosarcomas, nasopharyngeal carcinomas and chondrosarcomas.
3. Petrous bone tumors may infiltrate the bone and extend directly into the cerebello-pontine angle. Included in this group are carcinomas of the external and middle ear, rhabdomyosarcomas and malignant ceruminoma (Fig. 127). Primary cholesteatoma of the petrous apex often involves the cerebello-pontine angle.

The cerebello-pontine angle may also be involved by hematogeneous or subarachnoid (1) spread of malignancies (Figs. 128–130). This diagnosis is suggested in patients with known metastatic primary tumor, but may be impossible to establish in cases with no known primary tumor and without other metastases. Lack of bone erosion is typical for secondary cerebello-pontine angle tumors and may be a helpful, but often not reliable differential diagnostic criterion.

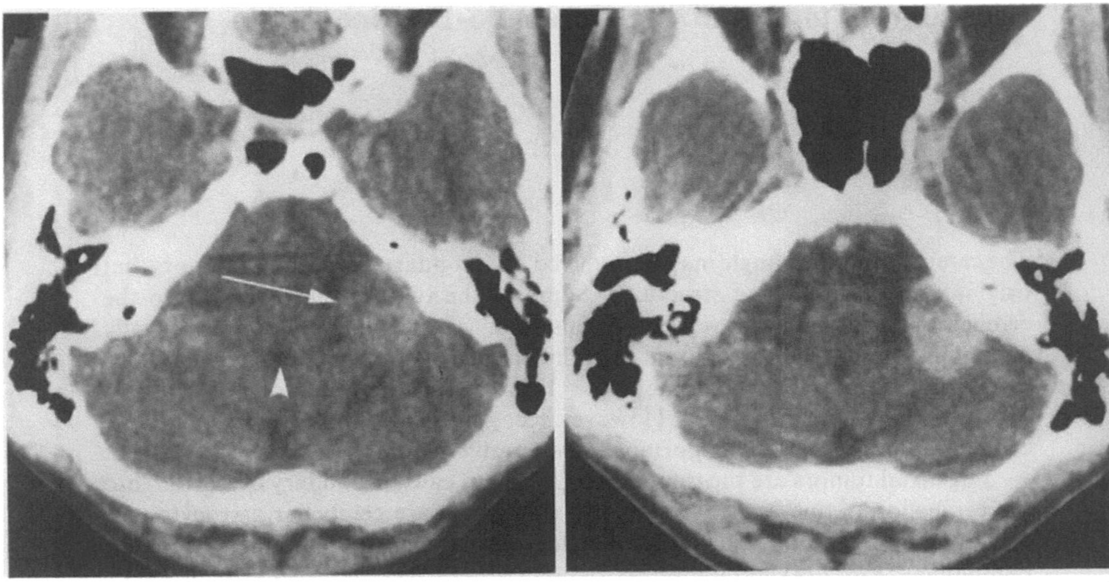

a b

Fig. 124a, b. Lymphoma of the cerebello-pontine angle. **a** Non contrast axial CT. A slightly hyperdense mass occupies the left cerebello-pontine angle (*arrow*). The fourth ventricle is only minimally compressed (*arrowhead*). High resolution CT (not shown) showed symmetrical, normal internal auditory canals. **b** Post contrast axial CT shows homogeneous, intense contrast enhancement. The almost round shape with the acute angle formed between the lateral tumor border and the posterior surface of the petrous bone suggests the misdiagnosis of a medial type of acoustic neurinoma. Surgery disclosed a primary cerebello-pontine angle lymphoma

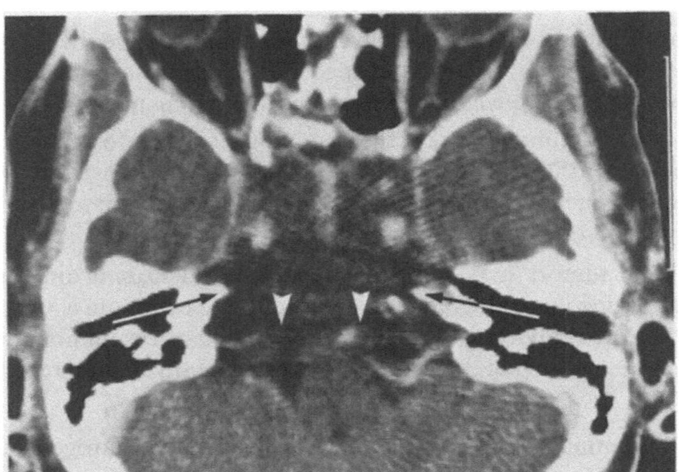

Fig. 125. Invasive pituitary adenoma. Axial post contrast CT. The mostly hypodense pituitary adenoma destroys both petrous apices (*arrows*) and invades the anterior portion of the pontocerebellar cisterns (*arrowheads*)

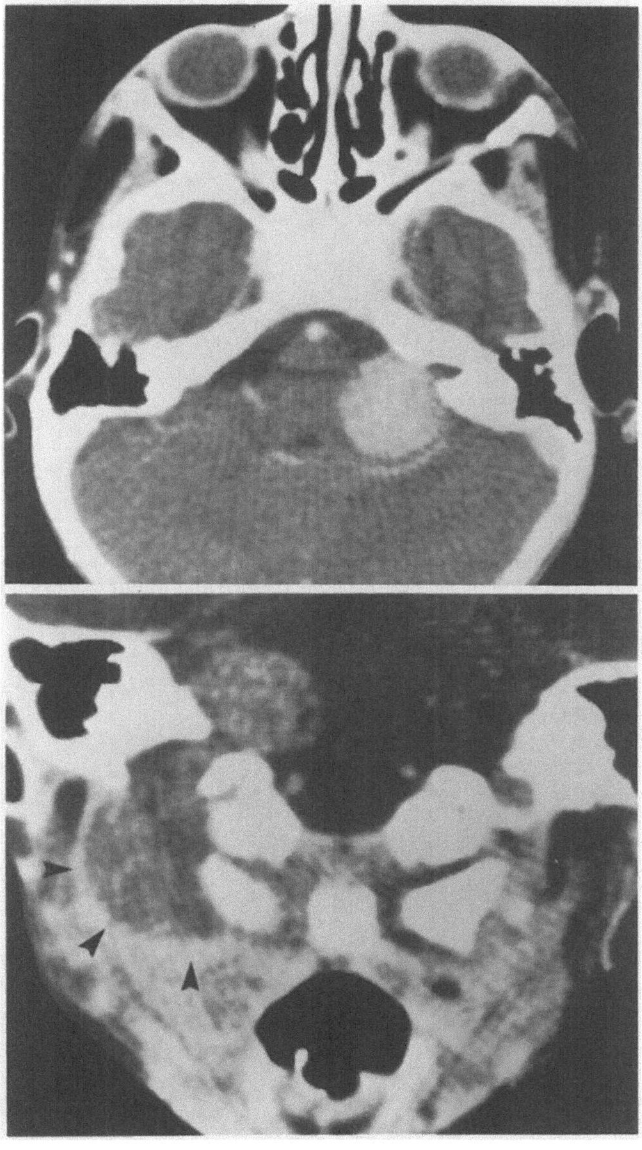

a

b

Fig. 126a, b. Parapharyngeal histiocytoma with secondary invasion of the cerebello-pontine angle. Post contrast CT. **a** Axial section shows a round, sharply delineated and homogeneously enhancing tumor of the cerebello-pontine angle. **b** Coronal section shows the real extent of the dumbbell-shaped tumor with the main tumor bulk situated in the infratemporal parapharyngeal space. The extracranial portion presents as hypodense tumor with ring enhancement (*arrowheads*). In contradistinction to typical jugular foramen tumors (e.g. neurinomas) the foramen is only minimally dilated

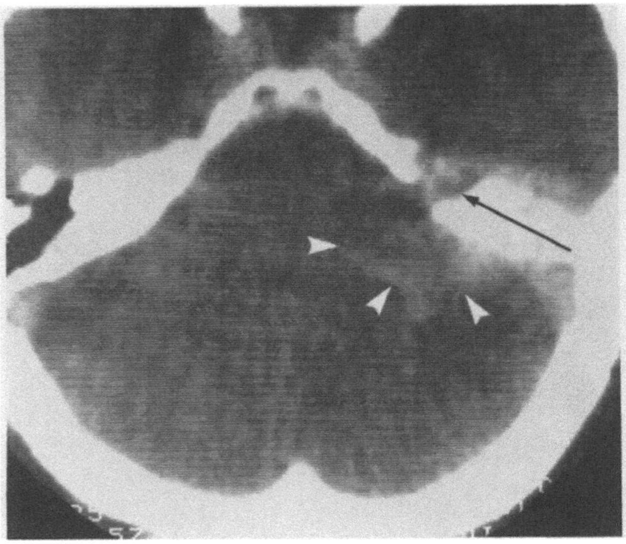

Fig. 127. Malignant ceruminoma of the petrous bone with secondary invasion into the cerebello-pontine angle. Note infiltration of the petrous bone (*arrow*) and tumor extension into the upper portion of the pontocerebellar cistern (*arrowheads*)

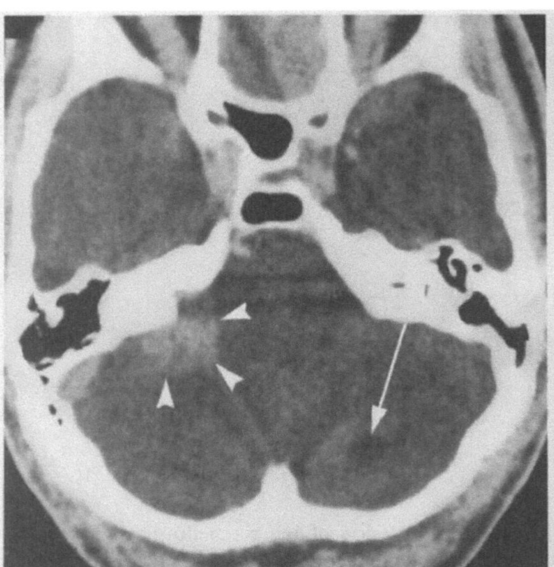

Fig. 128.

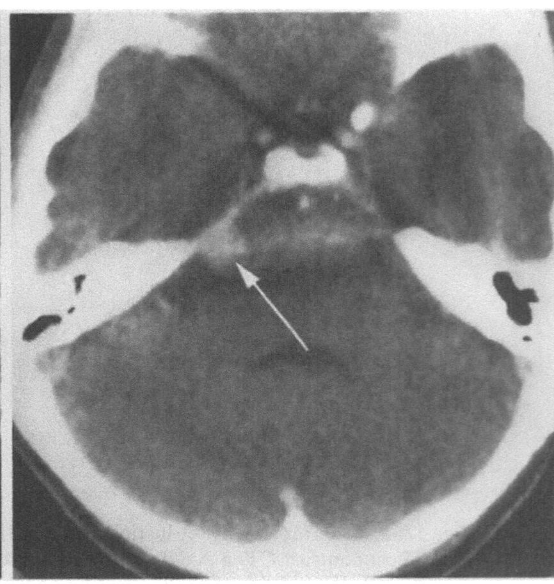

Fig. 129.

Fig. 128. Cerebello-pontine angle metastasis (primary tumor: bronchogenic carcinoma). Axial post contrast CT. Despite the fact that the porus acusticus internus is slightly enlarged, the false diagnosis of an acoustic neurinoma can be avoided by appreciating the retromeatal location of the tumor center and the irregular tumor margins (*arrowheads*). Note also a second necrotic metastatic nodule in the left cerebellar hemisphere (*arrow*)

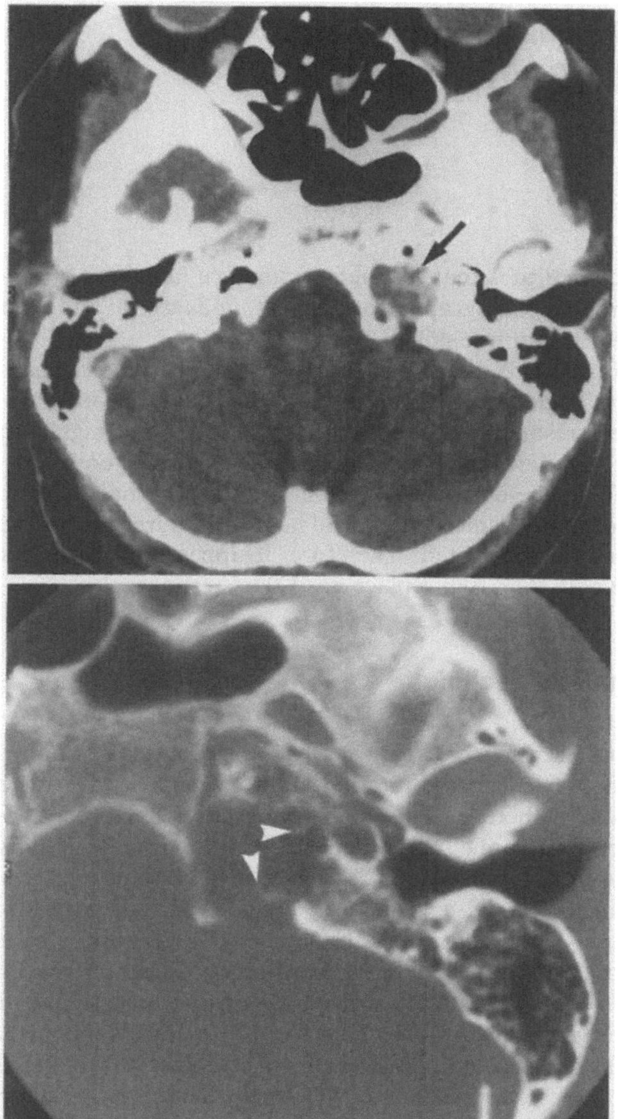

a

b

Fig. 130a, b. Jugular foramen metastasis (primary tumor: bronchogenic carcinoma). Post contrast CT. **a** Axial section shows enhancing tumor (*arrow*) within the dilated and eroded jugular foramen. **b** High resolution CT shows typical malignant bone invasion with unsharp margins and small bone fragments within the tumor (*arrowheads*)

◄———

Fig. 129. Metastasis at the trigeminal root (primary tumor: breast carcinoma). Axial post contrast CT. In this patient presenting with facial hypesthesia, a metastasis was found at the trigeminal root (*arrow*)

Magnetic Resonance Imaging of the Cerebello-Pontine Angle

Initial experience indicates that magnetic resonance imaging (MRI) is at least as sensitive as computed tomography for delineating anatomy and detecting pathology of the cerebello-pontine angle.

Further improvements in demonstrating the anatomy and the pathology of the cerebello-pontine angle and the internal auditory canal have followed improvements in magnetic resonance technology such as the use of higher-strength static magnetic fields, new developments in the design of surface coils and reduction in slice thickness. With these new MRI techniques the cisternal and intracanalicular courses of the vestibulocochlear and facial nerve and purely intracanalicular mass lesions have been demonstrated. Therefore, it appears probable that high field strength surface coil MRI will replace gas CT cisternography.

MRI Examination Technique

Thin sections are essential to display very small structures normally found in the cerebello-pontine angle and the internal auditory canal and to detect the small lesions that may arise there. The detectability of individual structures and contrast between different anatomic parts depend mainly upon the pulse sequences employed. No uniform, widely accepted series of pulse sequences has yet evolved.

Currently available pulse sequences include partial saturation, inversion recovery and spin-echo sequences. Of these, the inversion recovery sequences produce the poorest contrast between the vestibulocochlear nerve complex and the surrounding cerebro-spinal fluid, since both exhibit low signal intensity with inversion recovery sequences (403). Therefore, present inversion recovery pulse sequences should not be used for MRI of the cerebello-pontine angle.

Spin-echo pulse sequences demonstrate satisfactorily the cerebello-pontine angle, even with low-strength static magnetic fields. Improved contrast between the nerves and cerebrospinal fluid can be achieved in a high field-strength of 1.5 Tesla by use of T1-weighted partial saturation pulse sequences, with a repetition time (TR) of approximately 400 ms (87). At present, partial saturation pulse sequences in a 1.5 Tesla static magnetic field appear to provide the best demonstration of the cerebello-pontine angle and the internal auditory canal.

T1-weighted spin-echo images resemble partial saturation images, but the contrast between cerebro-spinal fluid and the vestibulocochlear-facial nerve bundle is not as high as with the partial saturation pulse sequence. T2-weighted spin-echo images with TR longer than 1500 ms and TE longer than 60 ms have the advantage of enhancing the signal obtained from cerebro-spinal fluid. These images resemble water soluble positive-contrast CT cisternograms and define well the size and shape of the cerebello-pontine angle. However, the vestibulocochlear and facial nerves are partially obscured by the high signal intensity of the cerebro-spinal fluid and are more difficult to identify on the T2-weighted series than on T1-weighted partial saturation images (87).

Significant improvement in displaying the pontocerebellar cistern and the internal auditory canal can be achieved by using surface coils in conjunction with high-strength static magnetic fields to improve the signal-to-noise ratios (14, 87, 506). The signal-to-noise and the contrast-to-noise ratios of the image are both increased in high-strength fields (greater than 1.0 Tesla) as compared with lower-strength fields (32).

Surface coils can also be used to produce a high signal-to-noise ratio in a selected small volume of anatomy and to eliminate most of the noise contributed by tissues that lie outside the sensitive volume of the surface coil. Overall image noise is reduced (88, 506). Selection of a small field of view such as 13 cm and use of sections as thin as 3 mm further improve spatial resolution (88). To date, the best results in imaging the internal auditory canal have been achieved by combining the benefits of surface coils and of high-strength static magnetic fields and by using a partial saturation pulse sequence with short TR (300–400 ms) and short TE (20 ms) (88).

MRI Anatomy

The petrous bone has almost negligible signal intensity because of its low fraction of mobile protons. It appears dark to black regardless of the pulse sequence used.

Although the petrous bone and the walls of the internal auditory canal do not produce a MR signal on any of the pulse sequences, the size of the internal auditory canal can still be determined readily on MRI (Fig. 131).

The arteries exhibit very low signal intensity because of their rapid blood flow. The loop of the anterior inferior cerebellar artery may be visualized within the high signal intensity pontocerebellar cistern on T2-weighted thin-section spin-echo images (Fig. 132).

The signal intensities of the pontocerebellar cistern, the cistern of the internal auditory canal and their contents depend primarily on the pulse sequence used.

The cerebro-spinal fluid within the pontocerebellar cistern and the internal auditory canal behaves like intraventricular fluid. It has low signal intensity on partial saturation and on T1-weighted spin-echo images, but exhibits high signal intensity on T2-weighted, long TE, spin-echo images (Fig. 131). These latter images closely resemble water soluble positive-contrast CT cisternograms. As a general rule, the nerves in the pontocerebellar cistern and in the internal auditory canal behave like white matter. Without surface coils the vestibulocochlear and facial nerves usually cannot be demonstrated separately; they appear together as a single nerve bundle.

On T1-weighted spin-echo images, this nerve bundle exhibits higher signal intensity than the surrounding hypointense cerebro-spinal fluid, and is therefore visible within the pontocerebellar cistern. Depending on the slice thickness and

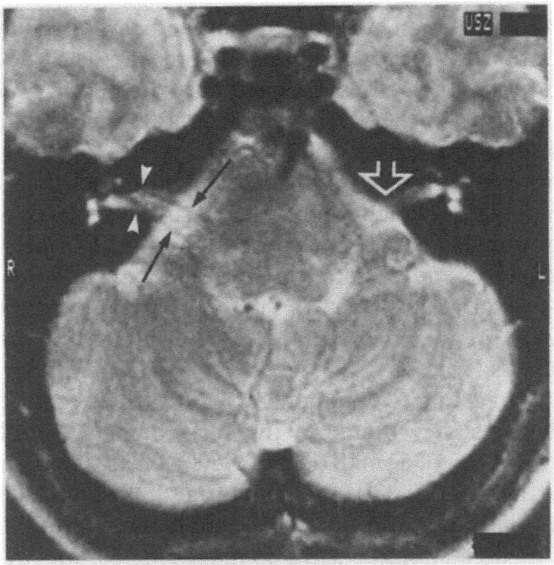

Fig. 131. T2-weighted spin-echo image (1.5 Tesla, TR 2000 ms, TE 100 ms) of normal internal auditory canal and pontocerebellar cistern. With this pulse sequence the signal of the cerebrospinal fluid is increased. Because of partial volume averaging cerebro-spinal fluid within the internal auditory canal (*open arrow*) appears darker than the CSF within the pontocerebellar cistern. Note excellent delineation of the facial and vestibulocochlear nerves (*arrows*) in their cisternal and intracanalicular segments. Note also absent signal from petrous bone, but excellent delineation of the anterior and posterior walls of the internal auditory canal (*arrowheads*), as well as of the fundus

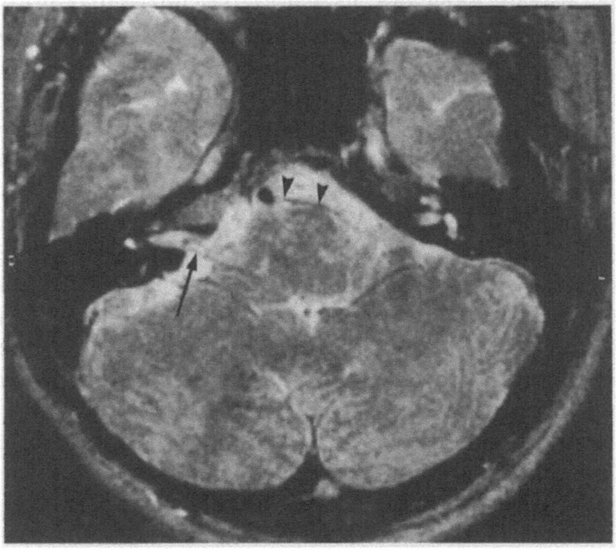

Fig. 132. T2-weighted spin-echo image (1.5 Tesla, TR 2000 ms, TE 100 ms) of the cerebellopontine angle shows the low signal intensity AICA-loop (*arrow*) at the porus of the right internal auditory canal. Note also the origin of the left AICA (*arrowheads*) from the basilar artery

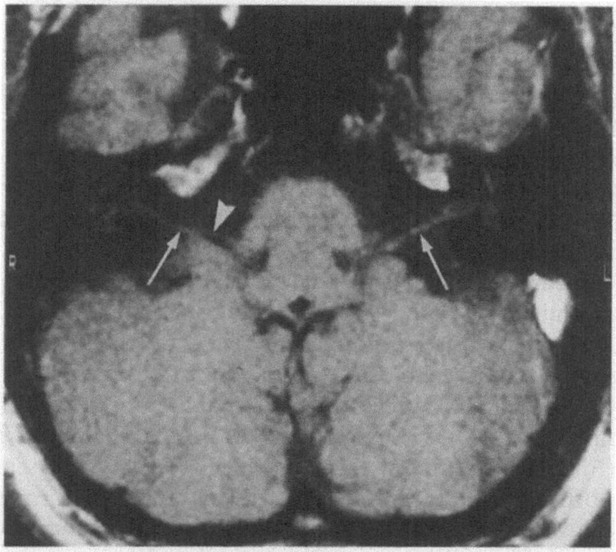

Fig. 133. 3 mm thin, T1-weighted axial spin-echo image (1.5 Tesla, TR 600 ms, TE 30 ms) of the normal internal auditory canal and pontocerebellar cistern. On this axial image, the entire course of the vestibulocochlear nerve is visible (*arrows*). It exhibits the same signal intensity as the brain parenchyma but contrasts clearly to the low intensity cerebro-spinal fluid. On the right side the cisternal portion of the facial nerve is visible (*arrowhead*). It is thinner than the vestibulocochlear nerve and lies in front of it

partial volume contribution, the bundle may also be discernible within the internal auditory canal (Fig. 133). Spin-echo sequences with TR of 1500 ms or longer and with TE of 60 ms or longer may obscure the medial part of the nerve bundle, since the nerve bundle and the cerebro-spinal fluid have almost identical signal intensity (403). The medial part of the nerve bundle can be demonstrated successfully by sequences with relatively short TR of 500 to 1000 ms and TE of 30 ms (403).

T2-weighted spin-echo images provide good contrast between cerebro-spinal fluid and the nerve bundle. With T2-weighted techniques, the nerve bundle within the pontocerebellar cistern appears hypointense relative to the high signal cerebro-spinal fluid (Fig. 131). Within the internal auditory canal, however, the intense signal of the cerebro-spinal fluid may obscure the nerve bundle (403).

Surface-coil high-field partial saturation images provide excellent differentiation between the nerves and the cerebro-spinal fluid. With this imaging technique, the cisternal and intracanalicular segments of the nerves are both well delineated as high signal structures surrounded by low signal cerebro-spinal fluid.

MRI of Acoustic Neurinoma

Accumulated experience indicates that MRI is at least as sensitive as routine contrast enhanced CT in detecting large and medium-sized acoustic neurinomas. With the use of surface coils, purely intracanalicular acoustic neurinomas have also been demonstrated. It appears probable that MRI will replace routine contrast enhanced CT as well as gas CT cisternography for the evaluation of patients with possible acoustic neurinoma.

The MRI appearance of acoustic neurinoma depends upon the pulse sequence used, and is determined by changes in the relaxation times T1 and T2. The majority of acoustic neurinomas cause prolongation of T2 and slight shortening of T1.

On T1-weighted spin-echo and partial saturation images, medium-sized acoustic neurinomas usually appear as masses that are isointense (Figs. 134–136) or slightly hypointense (Fig. 137) relative to brain parenchyma. Large acoustic neurinomas (Fig. 138) mostly present as mixed density masses with iso- and hypointense portions. These represent regressive and cystic transformations of Antoni-A into Antoni-B tumors. Since large acoustic neurinomas completely obliterate the pontocerebellar cistern, the nerve bundle cannot be distinguished.

Smaller acoustic neurinomas typically exhibit slightly greater signal intensity than cerebro-spinal fluid. With surface coils the cisternal portion of the vestibulocochlear-facial nerve bundle can be seen to merge with the convex medial border of the tumor. Occasionally, small acoustic neurinomas may produce rather inhomogeneous signals on T1-weighted partial saturation surface coil images. This inhomogeneity has been attributed to the less intense neurovascular structures that pass through the tumor within the internal auditory canal (87).

On T2-weighted spin-echo images, small acoustic neurinomas characteristically exhibit lower signal intensity than the cerebro-spinal fluid and slightly greater signal intensity than the brain parenchyma (Fig. 137). In the authors' experience, the intensity difference between tumor and cerebro-spinal fluid is often only minimal; small acoustic neurinomas that do not distort and compress the adjacent pons and cerebellum may thus not be seen. T2-weighted spin-echo images are therefore of limited value in the diagnosis of small and medium-sized acoustic neurinomas. In patients with small acoustic neurinomas, the vestibulocochlear-facial nerve bundle may be identified as a low intensity linear structure that merges with the convex medial border of the tumor within the high intensity cisternal cerebro-spinal fluid.

Occasionally, a regularly shaped ring of low signal intensity or punctate low intensity structures may be observed at the periphery of acoustic neurinomas. These ring or punctate low intensity structures are thought to represent capsular veins (639) (Fig. 136).

Arachnoid cysts are occasionally observed in association with larger acoustic neurinomas. As a rule their signal intensity behaves like cerebro-spinal fluid. Since arachnoid cysts appear isointense with cerebro-spinal fluid on the various pulse sequences used, they can be differentiated from acoustic neurinomas reliably.

Experimental studies in animals and preliminary clinical trials in human patients with intracranial tumors have shown that Gadolinium-DTPA (Gd-DTPA) is an effective paramagnetic contrast agent for MRI. The agent causes minimal

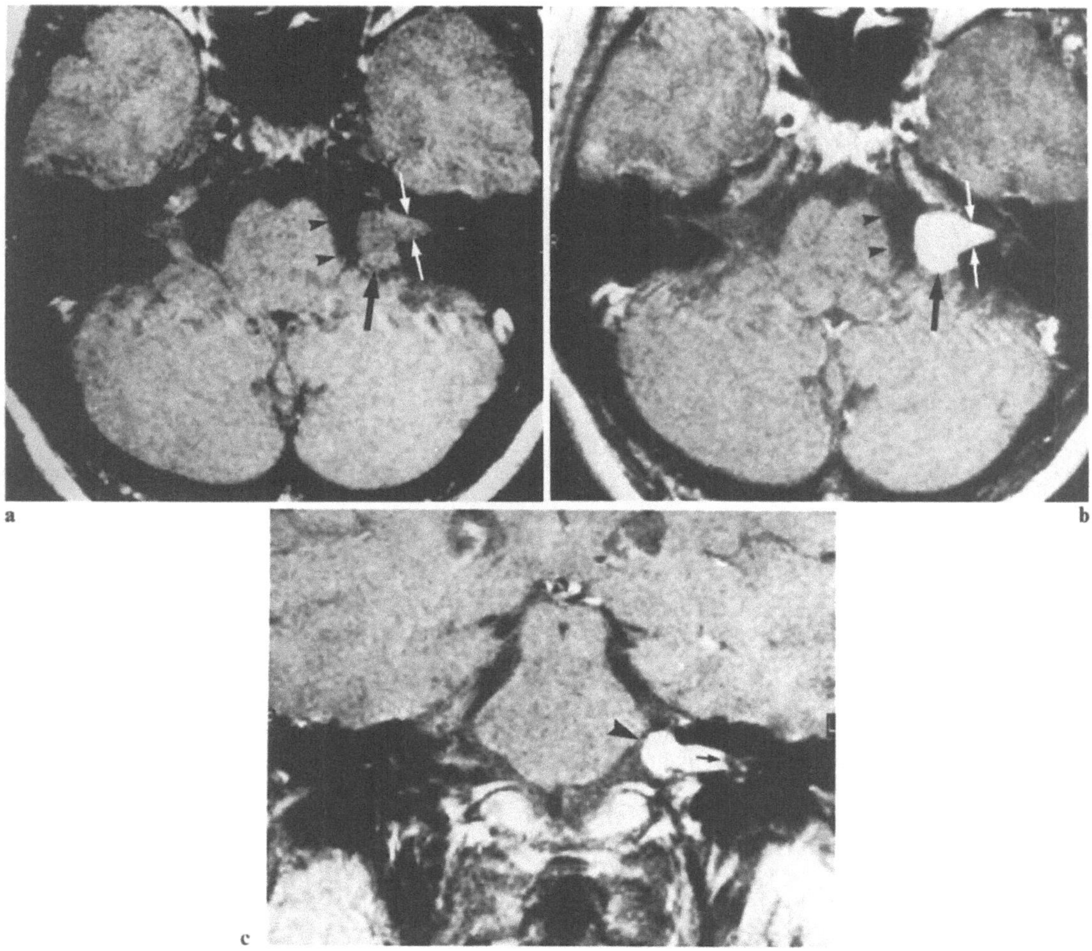

Fig. 134a–c. Small left-sided acoustic neurinoma. Axial T1-weighted spin-echo MR section (1.5 Tesla, TR 500 ms, TE 30 ms) before **a** and after **b** enhancement with Gd-DTPA. The tumor (*arrow*) shows homogeneous and intense contrast enhancement. Its sharply demarcated medial border is surrounded by low-intensity cerebro-spinal fluid (*arrowheads*), separating the tumor from the pons. No intervening low-density cerebro-spinal fluid is seen posterior to the cisternal portion of the tumor, indicating that the mass reaches the flocculus. The intracanalicular portion of the tumor is also perfectly depicted. Note excellent delineation of the anterior and posterior walls of the significantly dilated internal auditory canal (*thin arrows*). **c** The coronal Gd-DTPA enhanced T1-weighted spin-echo section also shows both the intracanalicular portion of the tumor and its cisternal extension. Note low-intensity cerebro-spinal fluid (*arrowhead*) separating the tumor from the pons. The small indentation on the lateral end of the tumor near the fundus of the internal auditory canal (*thin arrow*) is probably caused by the falciform crest

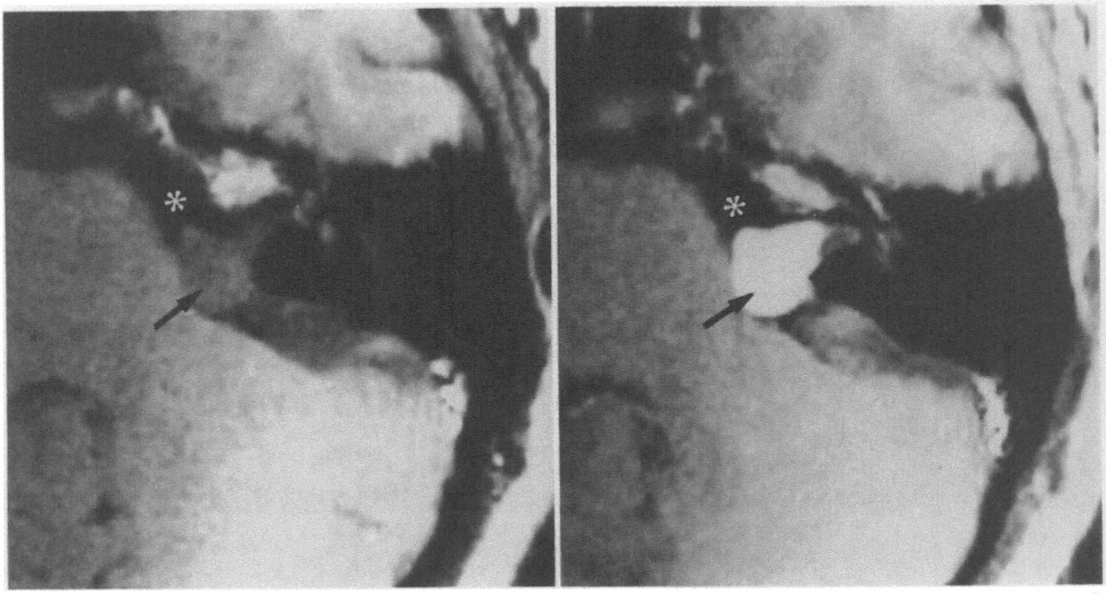

a b

Fig. 135a, b. Medium-sized, left-sided acoustic neurinoma. T1-weighted axial spin-echo, surface coil images (1.5 Tesla, TR 500 ms, TE 30 ms) before **a** and after **b** intravenous administration of Gd-DTPA. On the non contrast image the isointense cerebello-pontine angle tumor (*arrow*) stands out in contrast to the hypointense cerebro-spinal fluid (*asterisk*). The intracanalicular portion of the tumor is not discernible. After intravenous administration of Gd-DTPA the image shows homogeneous and intense enhancement of the tumor. The tumor (*arrow*) occupies only the medial portion of the internal auditory canal

→

Fig. 136a–e. Medium-sized, right-sided acoustic neurinoma. **a** Axial postcontrast CT. The slightly enlarged internal auditory canal contains a moderately enhancing mass (*arrow*) that extends into the pontocerebellar cistern. **b–e** T1-weighted spin-echo images (1.5 Tesla, TR 650 ms, TE 30 ms). **b, c** On the non contrast images, the tumor (*arrowhead*) exhibits slightly decreased signal intensity compared to brain parenchyma but contrasts clearly with the low intensity cerebro-spinal fluid (*asterisk*). **d, e** The tumor (*arrowhead*) exhibits intense and homogeneous contrast enhancement after intravenous administration of Gd-DTPA. On both, axial **d** and coronal **e** images the tumor is seen to be completely surrounded by cerebro-spinal fluid (*asterisk*). The small, round signal void (*open arrow* in **d**) at the medial border of the tumor probably represents a capsular vessel. Note the proximity of the tumor to the trigeminal nerve (*arrows* in **c** and **e**)

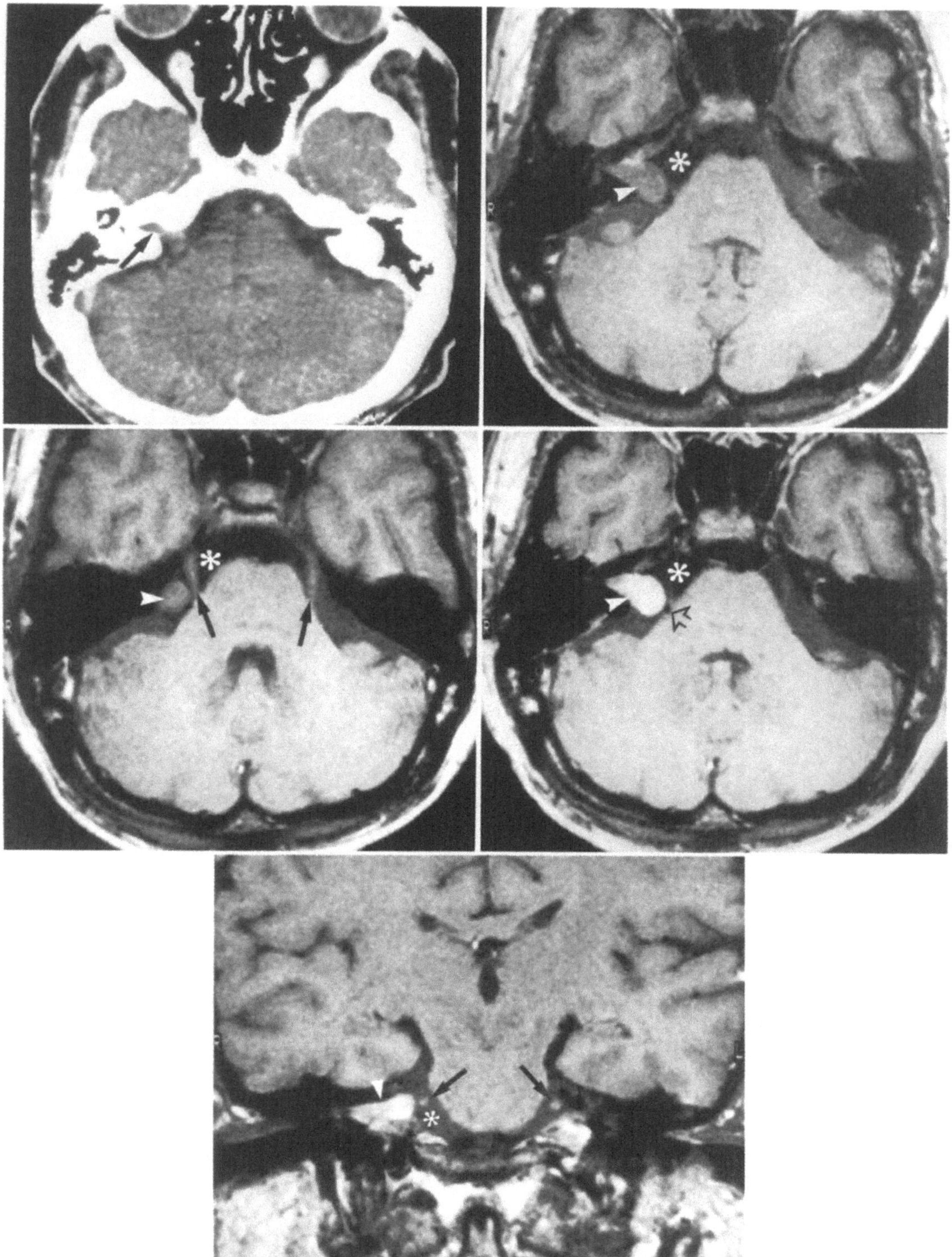

a b c d e

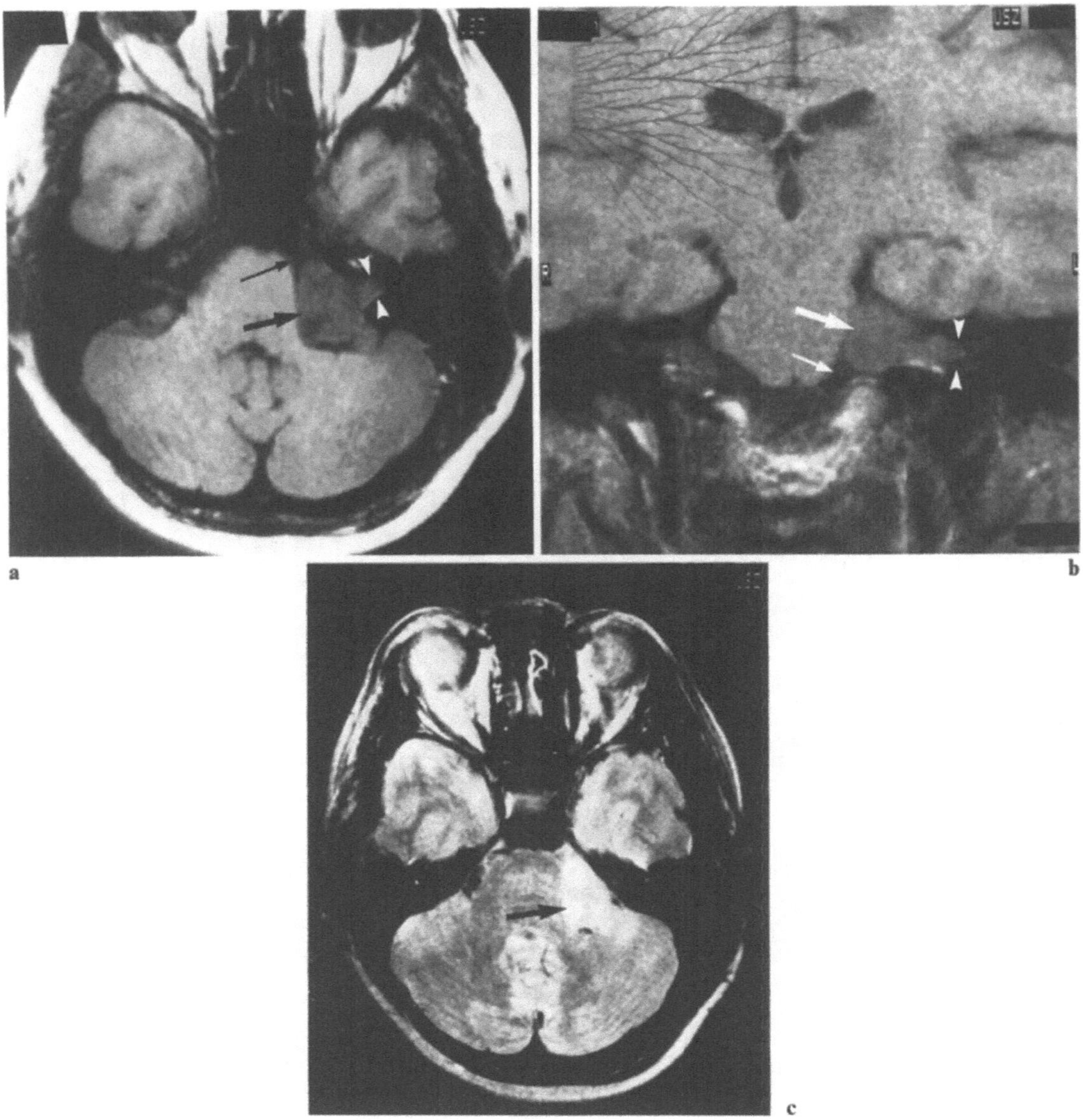

Fig. 137a–c. Medium-sized left-sided acoustic neurinoma. T1-weighted spin-echo, axial **a** and coronal **b** MR-sections (1.5 Tesla, TR 600 ms, TE 30 ms). The tumor (*arrow*) exhibits lower signal intensity than brain parenchyma. Note displacement of the pons and cerebellum and ipsilateral cisternal widening (*thin arrow*) indicating extraaxial origin and location of the mass. The tumor also occupies the internal auditory canal (*arrowheads*), which is significantly dilated compared to the normal contralateral side. **c** T2-weighted spin-echo axial MR section (1.5 Tesla, TR 2250 ms, TE 50 ms). The tumor (*arrow*) now exhibits greater signal intensity than brain parenchyma

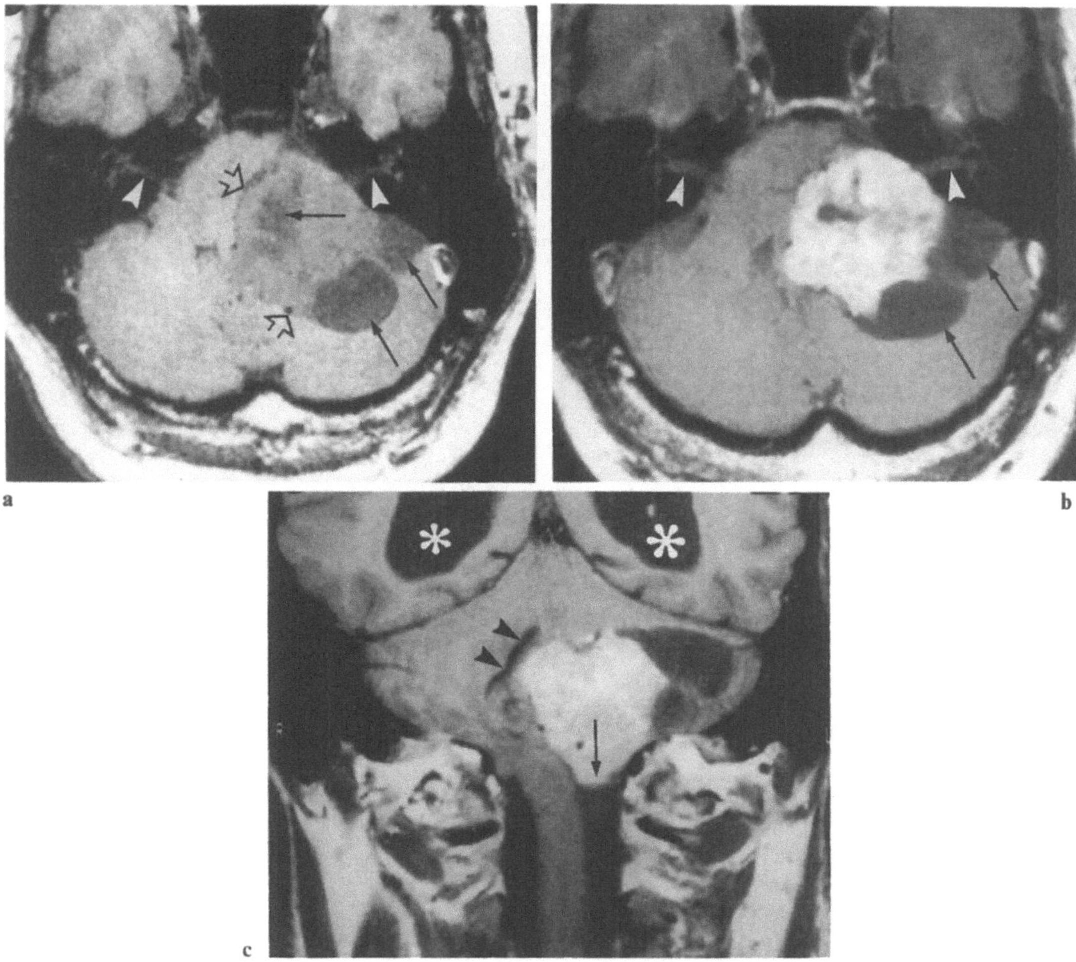

Fig. 138a–c. Medial type of left-sided acoustic neurinoma. T1-weighted spin-echo images (1.5 Tesla, TR 600 ms, TE 30 ms). **a** The axial, non contrast section shows symmetric, non enlarged internal auditory canals (*arrowheads*). The tumor exhibits inhomogeneous signal intensity with peripheral and eccentric zones of low intensity (*arrows*). Several small capsular vessels (*open arrows*) are seen at the periphery of the tumor. **b** Axial, Gd-DTPA enhanced section at the same level shows intense, but inhomogeneous enhancement of the solid portion of the tumor. The cystic parts (*arrows*) exhibit low signal intensity identical with the cerebro-spinal fluid. **c** Coronal, Gd-DTPA enhanced section posterior to the level of the internal auditory canal shows caudal extension of tumor (*arrow*) towards foramen magnum, causing displacement and compression of the upper medulla. The fourth ventricle (*arrowheads*) is compressed and displaced, causing obstructive hydrocephalus (*asterisks*)

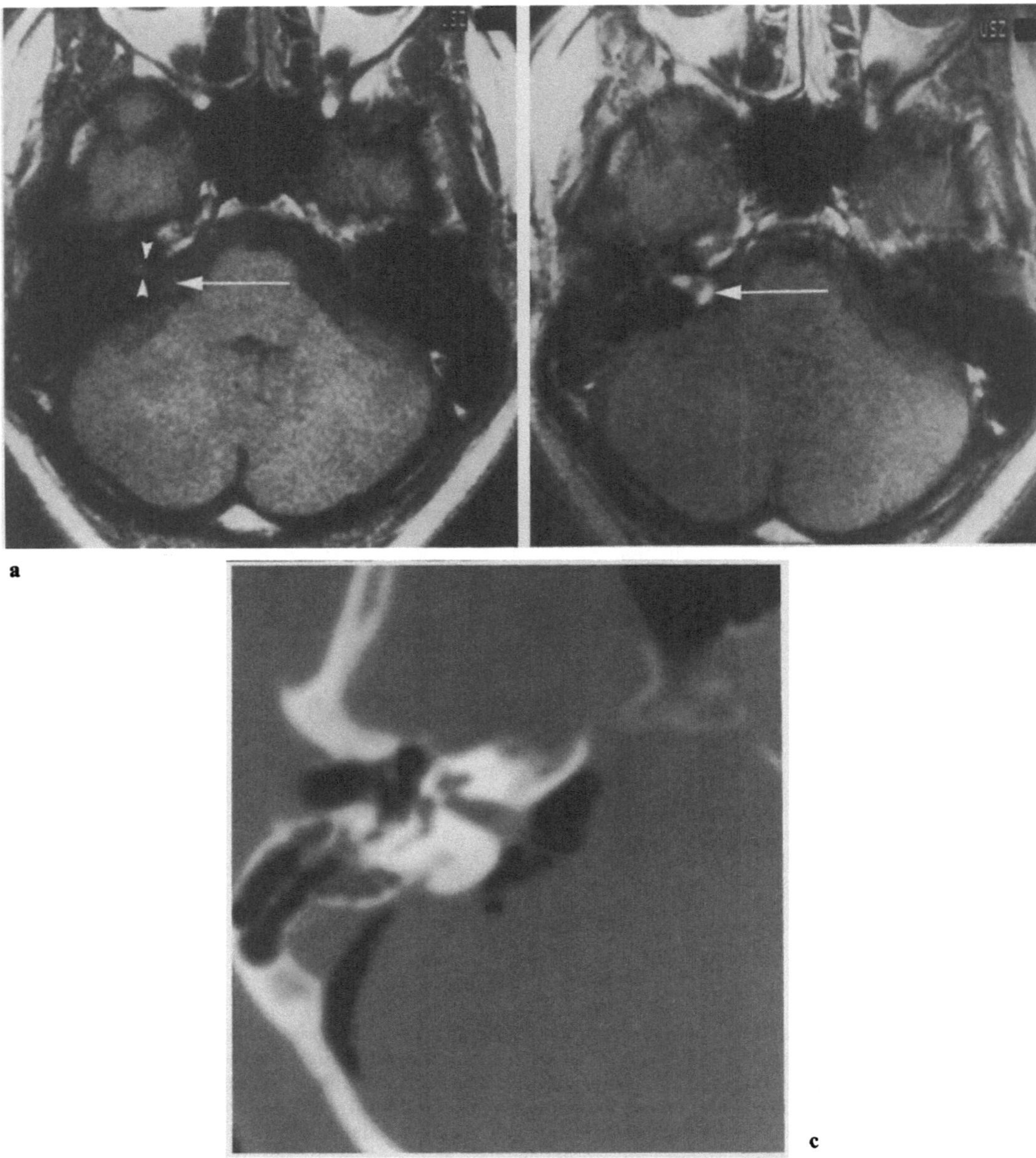

a b c

Fig. 139a–c. Small, mainly intracanalicular right-sided acoustic neurinoma. T1-weighted spin-echo axial MR sections before **a** and after **b** enhancement with Gd-DTPA. On the unenhanced image **a** the tumor (*arrow*) exhibits only slightly increased signal intensity compared to the low-intensity cerebro-spinal fluid. The internal auditory canal is dilated (*arrowheads*), compared to the normal left side. **b** The tumor (*arrow*) exhibits intense, but inhomogeneous enhancement. **c** Gas CT cisternography in the same case toxicity and has excellent patient tolerance (37, 129). The enhancement of Gd-DTPA results from paramagnetic shortening of both the T1- and T2-relaxation times (512). The mechanism of contrast enhancement of Gd-DTPA is assumed to be analogous to that of iodinated contrast agents in CT (129).

In a recent clinical study, including 40 patients with intracranial tumors, it was shown that the best pulse sequence to display the contrast enhancing effect of Gd-DTPA is a T1-weighted spin-echo sequence (129).

In extraaxial tumors, like acoustic neurinomas, significant enhancement of tumor contrast was reported to occur on T1-weighted spin-echo images after intravenous injection of 0.1 mmol/kg body weight of Gd-DTPA (129). In the authors' experience acoustic neurinomas show significant contrast enhancement on T1-weighted spin-echo images (Figs. 134–136, 138). As a result, axial and coronal Gd-DTPA enhanced MR sections display small neurinomas as markedly hyperintense masses surrounded by relatively hypointense cerebro-spinal fluid. The strong contrast between the low intensity walls of the internal auditory canal and the enhancing tumor permits accurate estimation of the size of the intracanalicular portion of the neurinoma (Figs. 135 and 139). Gd-DTPA enhanced images, especially when combined with the use of surface coils (Fig. 135), show even small intracanalicular neurinomas that are not clearly discernible on T1-weighted images (Fig. 139). Therefore it can be expected that Gd-DTPA enhanced MRI will completely replace gas CT cisternography.

MRI of Other Cerebello-Pontine Angle Masses

Other tumors of the cerebello-pontine angle are detected by MRI as sensitively as by CT. However, MR seems to be less specific than CT for characterizing lesion histology. The precise MR appearance of the diverse masses will depend on the pulse sequence selected as well as on lesion histology.

Meningiomas of the cerebello-pontine angle are expected to behave like meningiomas at other intracranial sites (639). On T1-weighted images (Figs. 140 and 141) meningiomas usually appear as masses that are isointense or slightly hypointense relative to brain parenchyma. On T2-weighted images the tumors appear isointense or slightly hyperintense relative to brain parenchyma. In a recently reported series that included two meningiomas of the cerebello-pontine angle, both tumors exhibited high signal intensity and high contrast with respect to the surrounding cerebellum on both T1- and T2-weighted spin-echo images (639). In the authors' experience, a malignant meningioma presented with inhomogeneous hyperintensity on T1- (Fig. 142) and T2-weighted images.

On T1-weighted images it may be possible to separate the meningioma from the adjacent displaced nerve bundle (356). The venous capsule surrounding meningiomas is frequently seen as a peripheral rim of low signal intensity (639) (Figs. 140 and 141).

Since the intensity differences of meningiomas on T1- and T2-weighted images are often minimal compared to brain parenchyma, small meningiomas which cause no distortion and compression of the adjacent pons and cerebellum may be missed

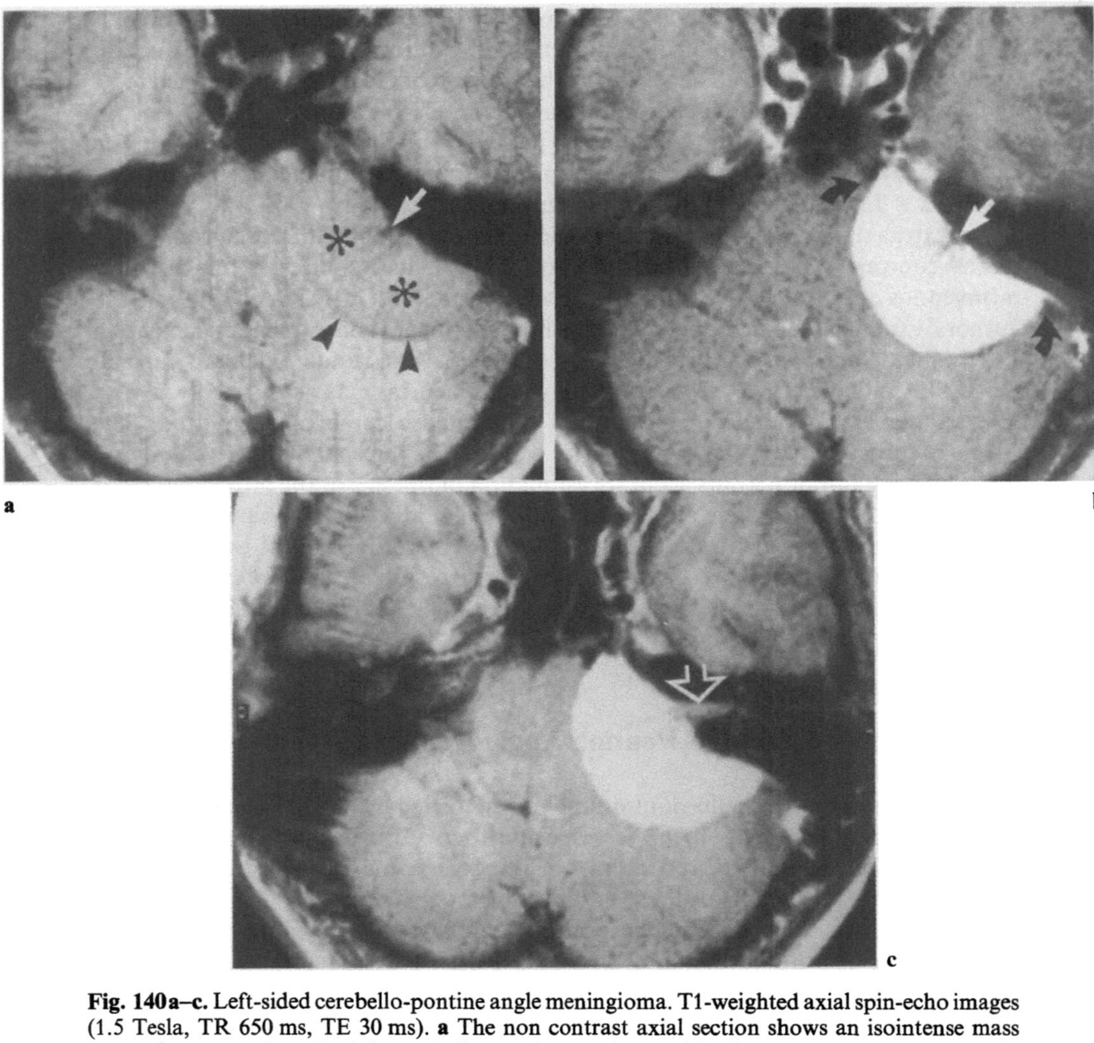

Fig. 140a–c. Left-sided cerebello-pontine angle meningioma. T1-weighted axial spin-echo images (1.5 Tesla, TR 650 ms, TE 30 ms). **a** The non contrast axial section shows an isointense mass (*asterisks*) occupying the left cerebello-pontine angle. A thin linear structure (*arrowheads*) representing the tumor capsule separates the tumor from the surrounding brain. At the tumor base, a small low intensity linear structure (*arrow*) projects from the posterior surface of the petrous bone into the tumor mass. As evidenced by angiography (not shown), this structure represents dural vascular supply of the tumor. **b** The Gd-DTPA enhanced section shows intense and homogeneous enhancement of the tumor as well as the typical obtuse angle sign (*curved arrows*). Note again the signal void within the tumor vessels (*arrow*). **c** The axial Gd-DTPA enhanced section at the level of the internal auditory canal shows no enhancement of the contents of the non dilated internal auditory canal (*open arrow*). This finding suggests that the tumor does not extend intracanalicularly

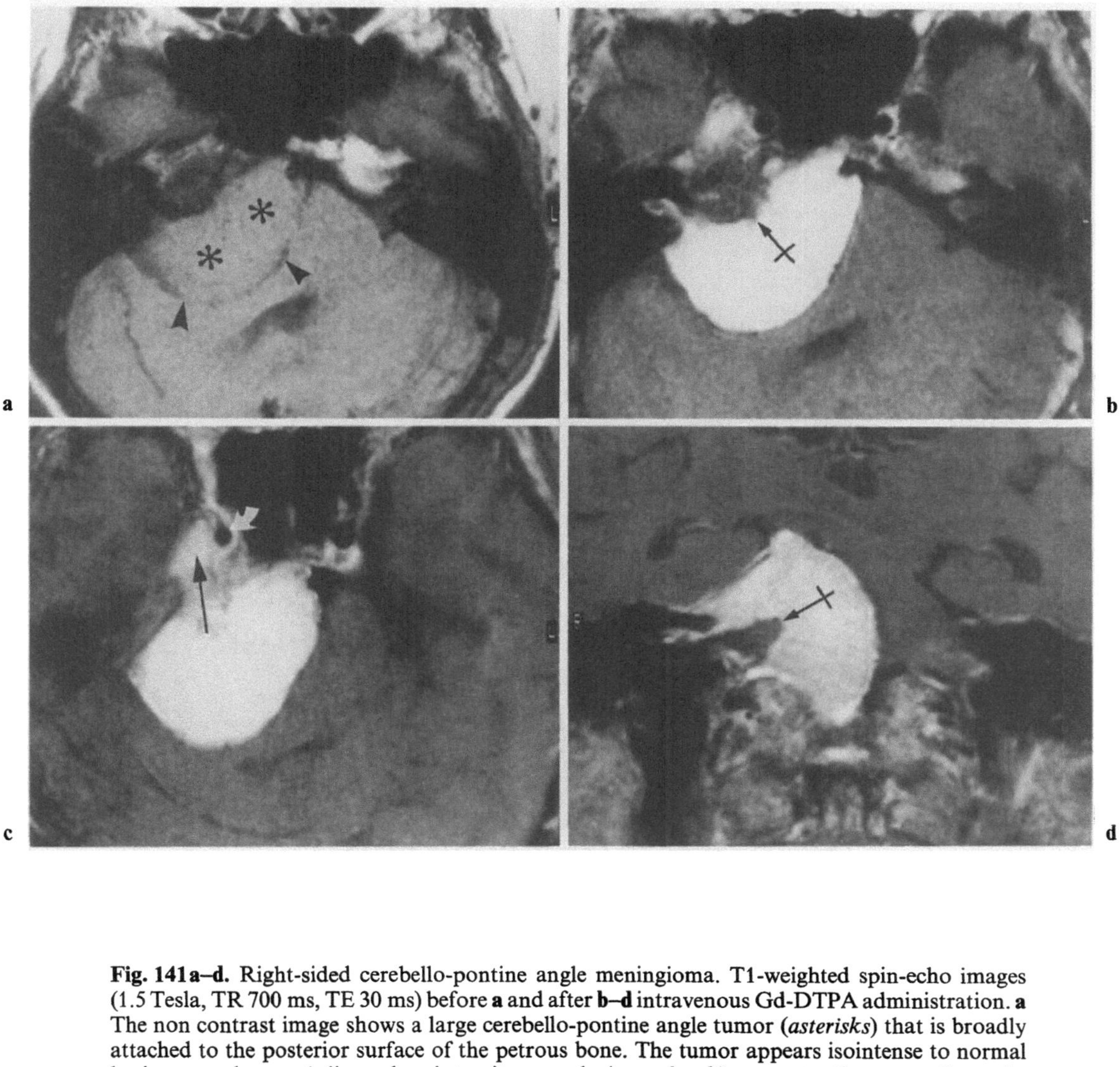

Fig. 141 a–d. Right-sided cerebello-pontine angle meningioma. T1-weighted spin-echo images (1.5 Tesla, TR 700 ms, TE 30 ms) before **a** and after **b–d** intravenous Gd-DTPA administration. **a** The non contrast image shows a large cerebello-pontine angle tumor (*asterisks*) that is broadly attached to the posterior surface of the petrous bone. The tumor appears isointense to normal brain parenchyma. A linear low intensity capsule (*arrowheads*) separates the tumor from the compressed brain. **b** After administration of Gd-DTPA the tumor exhibits intense and homogeneous contrast enhancement. **c** A higher axial section shows destruction of the petrous apex and invasion of the cavernous sinus (*arrow*). The tumor surrounds the internal carotid artery (*curved arrow*). Note the focal large exostosis at the antero-inferior portion of the porus of the internal auditory canal (*crossed arrow*), seen on both axial **b** and coronal **d** sections. On all axial images the tumor exhibits the obtuse angle sign characteristic of meningiomas

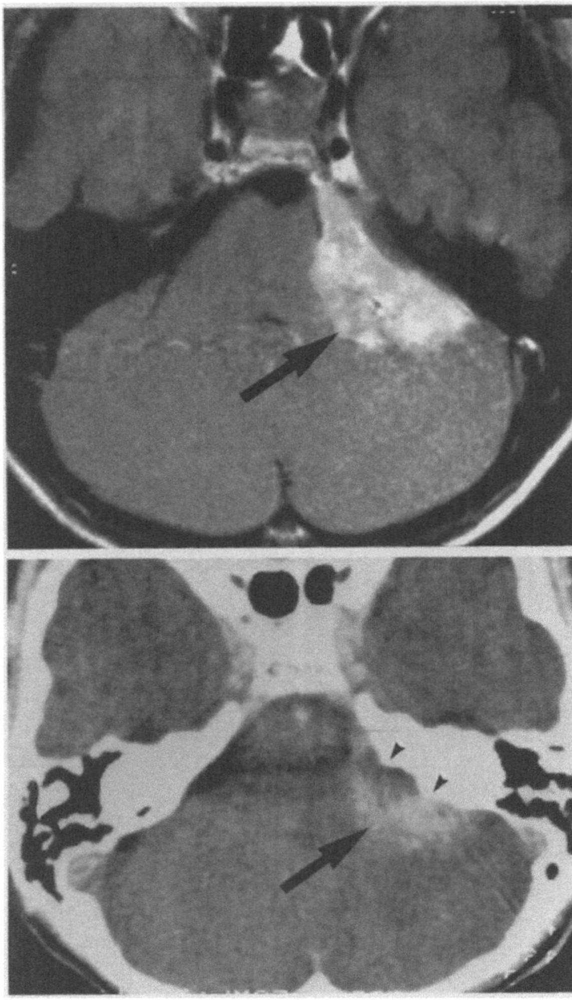

a

b

Fig. 142a, b. Malignant meningioma of the cerebello-pontine angle. **a** On the T1-weighted spin-echo axial section (1.5 Tesla, TR 750 ms, TE 30 ms) the tumor (*arrow*) exhibits high signal intensity. Note the typical broad attachment of its lateral border to the posterior surface of the petrous bone. **b** Axial contrast enhanced CT shows moderate contrast enhancement of the tumor (*arrow*). Note the better demonstration of hyperostosis (*arrowheads*) on the CT image

Fig. 143a–d. Dermoid tumor of the cerebello-pontine angle. **a** Axial contrast enhanced CT shows a hypodense mass (*arrowheads*) occupying the right cerebello-pontine angle and extending ventral to the pons toward the left cerebello-pontine angle (*arrow*). **b** On the T1-weighted spin-echo axial section (1.5 Tesla, TR 650 ms, TE 30 ms), the tumor appears as a low intensity mass occupying the right cerebello-pontine angle. It displaces the lateral contour of the pons medially (*arrowheads*). The tumor extends anterior to the belly of the pons into the anterior compartment of the contralateral cerebello-pontine angle (*arrow*). Note that the basilar artery has been displaced

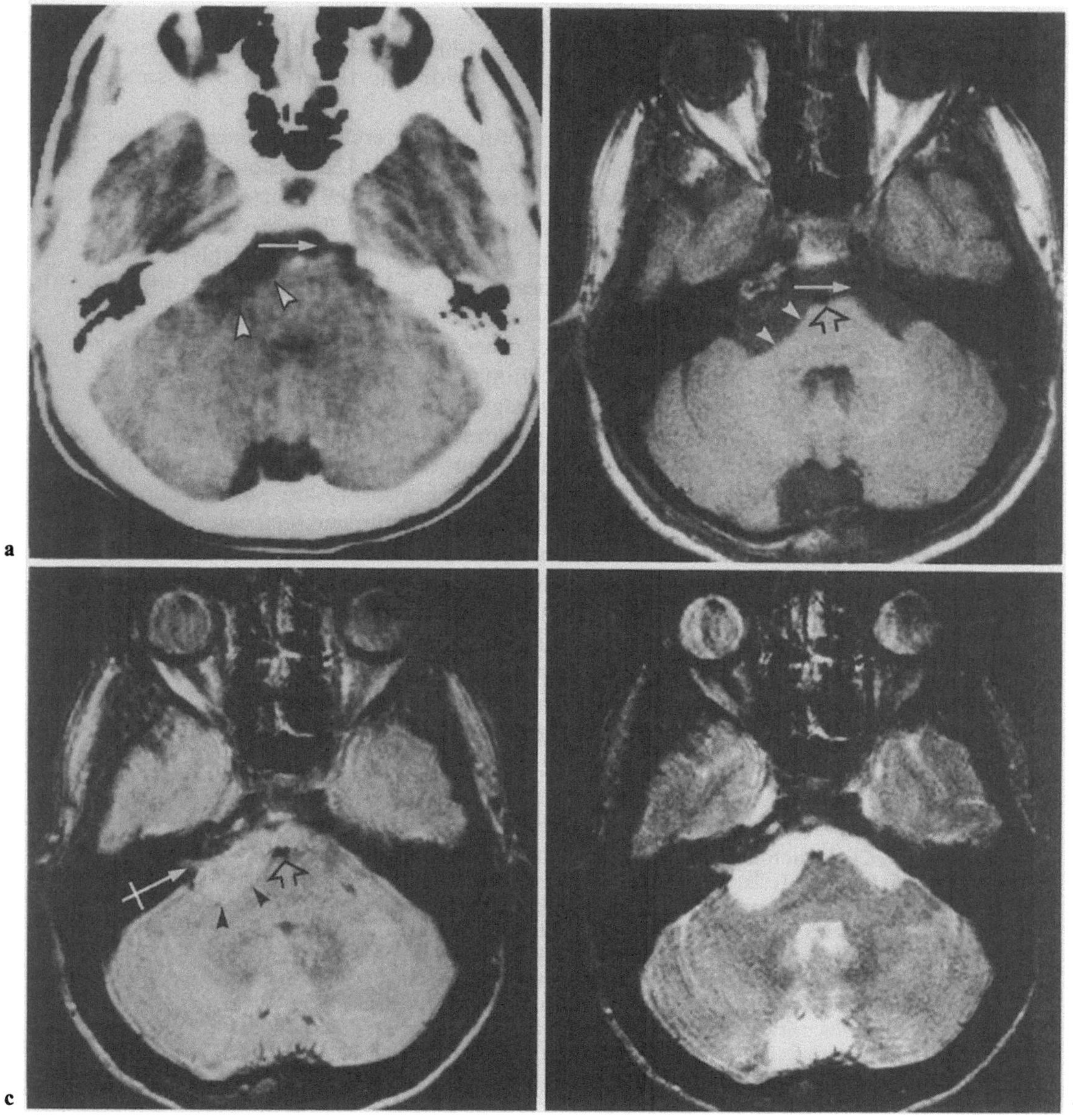

posteriorly (*open arrow*). **c, d** T2-weighted spin-echo axial sections (1.5 Tesla, TR 2000 ms, TE 50 ms (**c**), TE 100 ms (**d**)). **c** On the first echo image, the tumor (*arrowheads*) shows minimally increased signal intensity compared to both cerebro-spinal fluid and brain parenchyma. The contents of the internal auditory canal (*crossed arrow*) have slightly lower intensity than the tumor and behave like cerebro-spinal fluid. This finding excludes intracanalicular tumor extension. **d** The intensity of the tumor increases markedly on the second echo image and becomes isointense with cerebro-spinal fluid. The exact tumor margin on the left side cannot be assessed on MRI. However, meningiomas regularly show significant enhancement after intravenous administration of Gd-DTPA (Figs. 140 and 141). The enhancement is best seen on T1-weighted spin-echo images. With this technique, even small meningiomas are discernible with MRI.

The obtuse angle sign is also very helpful for differentiating meningiomas from other cerebello-pontine angle tumors (Figs. 140–142). Despite the poor demonstration of bone changes on MR, large exostoses may be detected (Fig. 141). Such exostoses are nearly pathognomonic for meningiomas. Tumor vessels which originate from the site of tumor attachment to the posterior surface of the petrous bone may also be visible on MRI as linear flow void structures (Fig. 140). If present, these linear flow voids are nearly specific for meningiomas.

Experience with the MRI appearance of other primary tumors of the cerebello-pontine angle is limited. At present, the location and shape of the mass seem to help characterize the lesion better than does its signal intensity (639).

The signal intensity of dermoids and epidermoids (Fig. 143) varies with their chemical composition. The higher their fat content, the higher their signal intensity will be on T1-weighted images. The choice of the appropriate pulse sequence depends on the chemical composition of the tumor. In one personal case in which the tumor contained only minimal amounts of fat, the best tumor delineation was achieved with a long TR, short TE spin-echo sequence. On T1-weighted and heavily T2-weighted images, the tumor was isointense compared to cerebro-spinal fluid.

A chordoma (Fig. 144) appeared hypointense on T1-weighted and hyperintense on T2-weighted images. This appearance is not characteristic; other tumors, especially metastases, may not be differentiable from chordomas. If present, hypointense calcifications suggest that the lesion may be a chordoma rather than another tumor.

Fig. 144a, b. Clival chordoma extending into both cerebello-pontine angles. **a** T1-weighted spin-echo axial image (1.5 Tesla, TR 600 ms, TE 30 ms). The tumor occupies the sellar (*thick arrow*) and parasellar (*curved arrow*) area and extends through the incisura into both cerebello-pontine angles (*open arrows*). It exhibits mixed high and low signal intensity. On this pulse sequence, the borders of the tumor are not clearly discernible. **b** T2-weighted spin-echo axial image (1.5 Tesla, TR 1800 ms, TE 50 ms). The tumor exhibits inhomogeneous high signal intensity. Several low signal intensities (*arrowheads*) dispersed within the tumor represent calcifications. With this pulse sequence, a low intensity tumor capsule (*thin arrows*) becomes visible and allows separation of the tumor from the pons. The venous angioma in the right cerebellar hemisphere (*crossed arrow*) represents an incidental finding

Fig. 145a–d. Type-C-3, De-2, Di-1 left-sided chemodectoma. **a, b** T1-weighted axial **a** and coronal **b** spin-echo images (1.5 Tesla, TR 750 ms, TE 30 ms) show the tumor (*arrow*) occupying the jugular foramen and extending medially into the cerebello-pontine angle. The isointense tumor contains multiple low intensity linear and round structures (*arrowheads*) representing flow voids within intratumoral vessels. The tumor displaces pons and cerebellum. **c, d** T1-weighted Gd-DTPA enhanced axial **c** and coronal **d** images (1.5 Tesla, TR 750 ms, TE 30 ms). The tumor exhibits intense contrast enhancement. The multiple flow voids are again seen within and at the periphery of the tumor. The tumor surrounds the vertical segment of the carotid canal (*asterisks*) and reaches the inner border of the horizontal segment of the carotid canal. The dura is interrupted focally, indicating intradural extension of a small tumor nodule (*curved arrow*). The small jugular chemodectoma on the right side (*open arrow*) is an associated finding

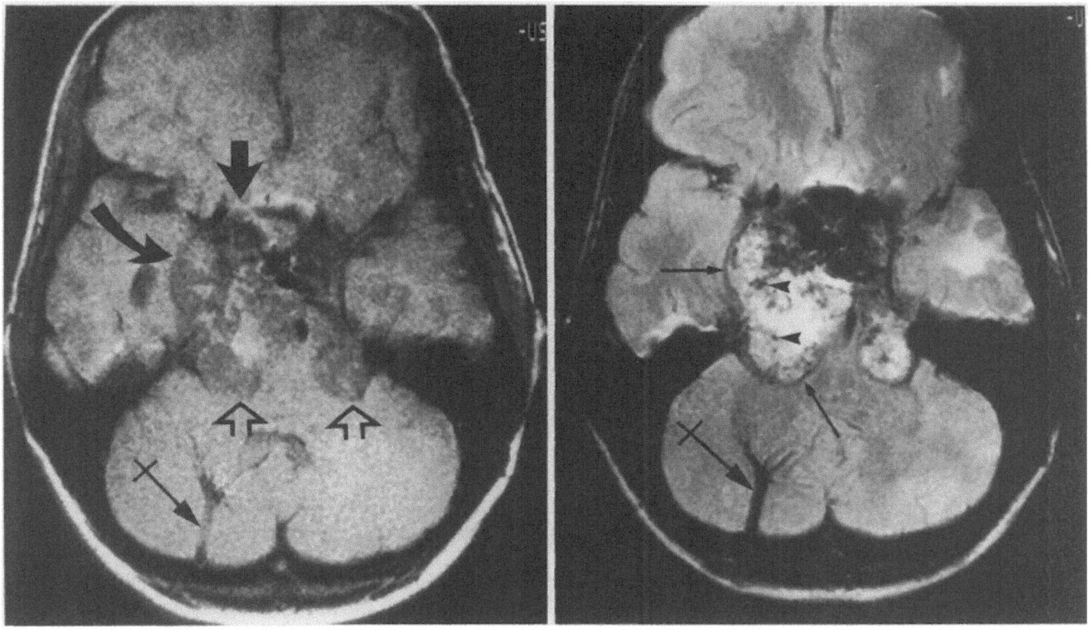

144
a
b

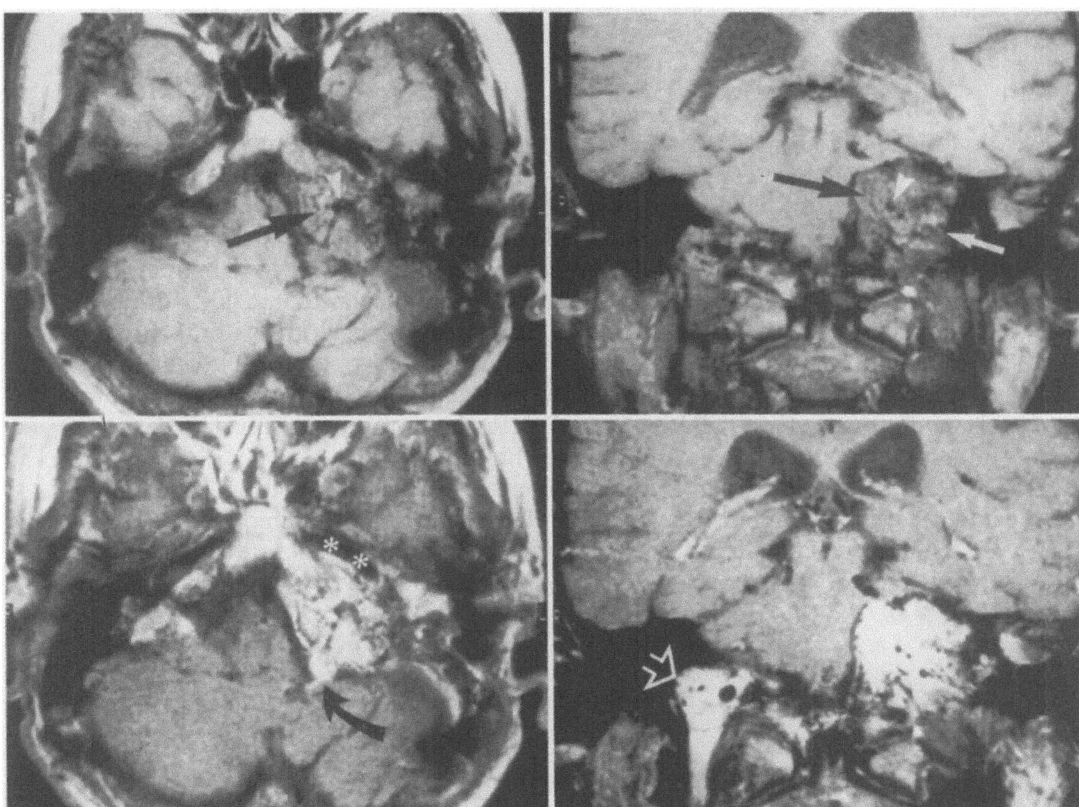

145
a
c
d

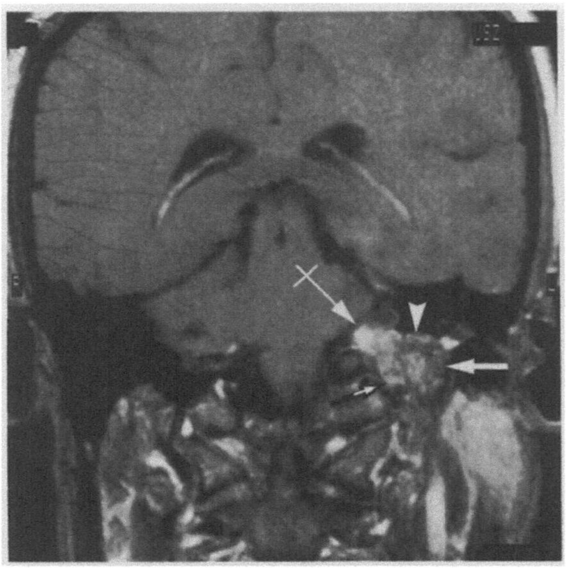

Fig. 146. Type-C-2, De-1 chemodectoma. Coronal, T1-weighted spin-echo (1.5 Tesla, TR 300 ms, TE 30 ms), Gd-DTPA enhanced MR section. The tumor (*arrows*) shows inhomogeneous contrast enhancement. Note enlargement and erosion of the jugular foramen and of the infralabyrinthine compartment of the temporal bone (*arrowhead*). Small intracranial extradural tumor extension (*crossed arrow*)

Chemodectomas (Figs. 145 and 146) present as mixed intensity masses on T1- and T2-weighted images. The blood pools and the tumor vessels contained in the tumor produce flow void signal loss on both T1- and T2-weighted pulse sequences. The solid portions of the tumor show enhancement after Gd-DTPA administration (Fig. 145). Since the precise classification of chemodectomas relies on bone changes that are poorly shown on MRI, the most effective diagnostic modality presently remains high resolution CT. However, MRI may be helpful for differentiating chemodectomas from other jugular foramen tumors, especially neurinomas (Fig. 147). Most neurinomas do not show the signal voids that are characteristic for chemodectomas. Gd-DTPA enhanced MRI has proved sensitive in detecting intradural extension of chemodectomas (Fig. 145).

MRI is also sensitive in detecting secondary extension of petrous bone tumors into the cerebello-pontine angle and in detecting secondary tumors.

Small vascular malformations of the cerebello-pontine angle are easily detected by MRI because of their characteristic low signal and typical "vermiform" pattern (Fig. 148).

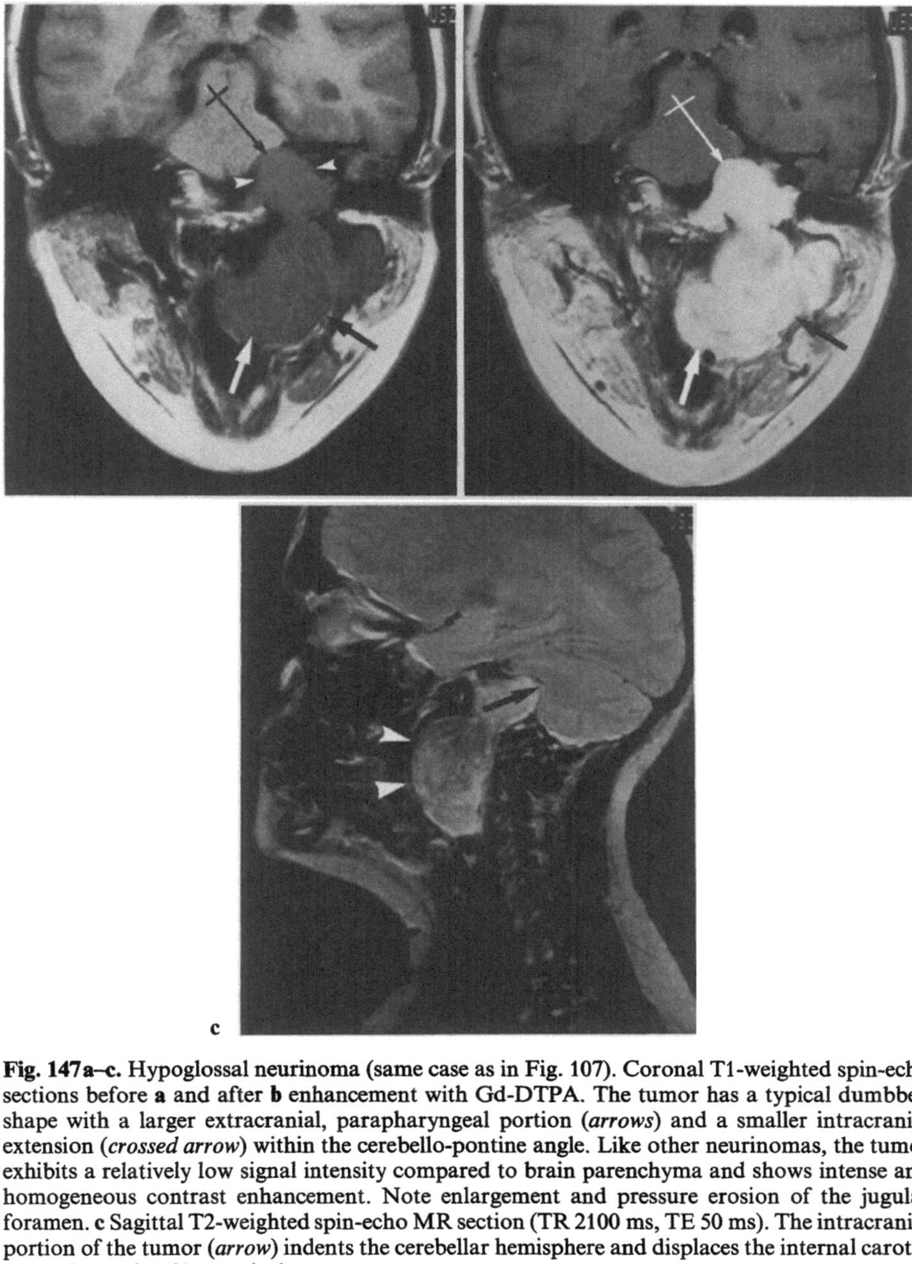

a b c

Fig. 147a–c. Hypoglossal neurinoma (same case as in Fig. 107). Coronal T1-weighted spin-echo sections before **a** and after **b** enhancement with Gd-DTPA. The tumor has a typical dumbbell shape with a larger extracranial, parapharyngeal portion (*arrows*) and a smaller intracranial extension (*crossed arrow*) within the cerebello-pontine angle. Like other neurinomas, the tumor exhibits a relatively low signal intensity compared to brain parenchyma and shows intense and homogeneous contrast enhancement. Note enlargement and pressure erosion of the jugular foramen. **c** Sagittal T2-weighted spin-echo MR section (TR 2100 ms, TE 50 ms). The intracranial portion of the tumor (*arrow*) indents the cerebellar hemisphere and displaces the internal carotid artery (*arrowheads*) anteriorly

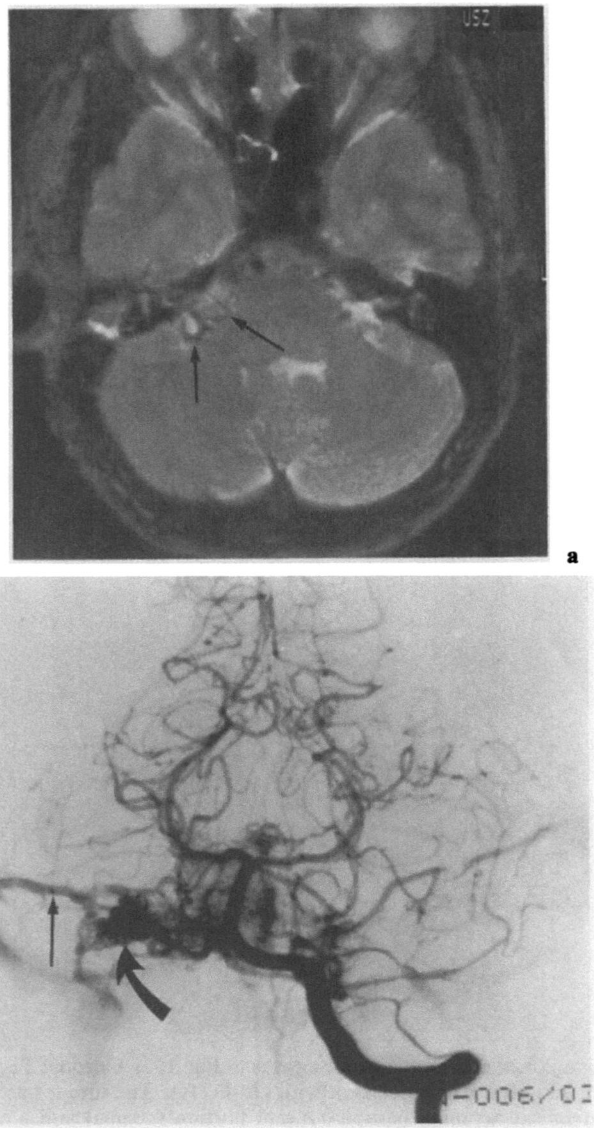

a

b

Fig. 148a, b. Arteriovenous malformation of the cerebello-pontine angle. **a** Axial, T2-weighted MR section (1.5 Tesla, TR 2000 ms, TE 100 ms) shows dilated, hypointense vascular loops (*arrows*) within the pontocerebellar cistern. **b** Digital subtraction vertebral angiography confirms the presence of an AVM. The nidus (*curved arrow*) is located within the cerebello-pontine angle. It is supplied by the dilated AICA. A laterally coursing dilated draining vein (*arrow*) is also seen

References

1. Aguila LA, Chou SM, Bay JW (1984) Primary intracranial germinoma presenting as lower cranial nerve involvement: case report and review of the literature. Neurosurgery 14:475–479
2. Alajouanine T, Le Beau J, Houdart R (1948) La symptomatologie tumorale des volumineux anévrysmes des artères vertebrales et basilaires. Rev Neurol (Paris) 80:321–337
3. Alford BR, Guilford FR (1962) A comprehensive study of tumors of the glomus jugulare. Laryngoscope 72:765–787
4. Altmann F (1928) Zur Kenntnis der primären Geschwülste des Trigeminus und des Ganglion Gasseri. Beitr Path Anat 80:361–404
5. Ambrose J (1973) Computerized transverse axial scanning (tomography): Part 2. Clinical application. Br J Radiol 46:1023–1047
6. Anderson FM, Segall HD, Caton WL (1979) Use of computerized tomography scanning in supratentorial arachnoid cysts. J Neurosurg 50:333–338
7. Anderson R, Olson J, Dowart R, Merkle M, Schaefer S (1982) CT air-contrast scanning of the internal auditory canal. Ann Otol Rhinol Laryngol 91:501–505
8. Aoyagi T, Kyuno K (1912) Ueber die endothelialen Zellzapfen in der Dura mater cerebri und ihre Lokalisation in derselben, nebst ihrer Beziehung zur Geschwulstbildung in der Dura mater. Neurologia 11:1–12
9. Applebaum EL, Valvassori GE (1984) Auditory and vestibular system findings in patients with vascular loops in the internal auditory canal. Ann Otol Rhinol Laryngol Suppl. 112:63–70
10. Artmann H, Vonofakos D, Müller H, Grau H (1984) Neuroradiologic and neuropathologic findings with growing giant intracranial aneurysm. Surg Neurol 21:391–401
11. Arumugaramay N, Rudralingam V, Sarvanathan K, Pillay DRP (1972) Intracranial hypoglossal neurinoma: a report of two cases. Med J Malaysia 26:168–172
12. Atkinson WJ (1949) The anterior inferior cerebellar artery; its variations, pontine distribution, and significance in surgery of cerebello-pontine angle tumours. J Neurol Neurosurg Psychiatry 12:137–151
13. Aubaniac R (1951) Les variations du canal déchiré postérieur. Trav Lab Anat Fac Med Alger, p 23–33
14. Axel L (1984) Surface coil magnetic resonance imaging. J Comput Ass Tomogr 8:831–834
15. Axmann K, Danes K (1959) Beitrag zur Röntgendiagnostik der Neurinome des N. Trigeminus. Röntgenologische und klinische Symptomatologie. RÖFO 91:273–277
16. Azar-Kia B, Palacios E, Spak M (1976) The megadolichobasilar artery anomaly and expansion of the internal auditory meatus. Neuroradiology 11:109–111
17. Bailey P, Bagdasar B (1929) Intracranial chordoblastoma. Am J Pathol 5:439–449
18. Bailey P, Buchanan DN, Bucy PC (1939) Intracranial tumors of infancy and childhood. University of Chicago Press, Chicago, p 277
19. Baker HL (1963) Myelographic examination of the posterior fossa with positive contrast medium. Radiology 81:791–801
20. Baker HL (1972) Cerebellopontine angle myelography. J Neurosurg 36:614–624
21. Banna M (1976) Arachnoid cysts on computed tomography. AJR 127:979–982
22. Banna M, Romeo MA (1979) Cerebral arterial ectasia on computed tomography. J Can Assoc Radiol 30:259–260
23. Barrs DM, Brackmann DE, Olson JE, House WF (1985) Changing concepts of acoustic neuroma diagnosis. Arch Otolaryngol. 111:17–21
24. Bartel AD, Djaldetti MM, Mandel EM, Lerner MA (1973) Dumb-bell neurinoma of the hypoglossal nerve. J Neurol Neurosurg Psychiatry 36:592–595

25. Bebin J (1979) Pathophysiology of acoustic tumors. In: House WF, Luetje CM (eds) Acoustic tumors, vol I: Diagnosis and treatment. University Park Press, Baltimore, pp 45–83
26. Bentson JR, Mancuso AA, Winter J, Hanafee WN (1980) Combined gas cisternography and edge-enhanced computed tomography of the internal auditory canal. Radiology 136:777–779
27. Bergvall U (1975) Temporal course of contrast medium enhancement in differential diagnosis of intracranial lesions with computer tomography. In: Salamon G (ed) Advances in cerebral angiography. Springer, Berlin Heidelberg New York, pp 346–348
28. Berkmen YM, Brucher J, Salmon JH (1969) Congenital arachnoid cysts. AJR 105:298–304
29. Bernasconi V (1953) Tomografia cranica nei neurinomi del nervo acustico. Chir Patol Sper 8:310–320
30. Bernasconi V, Columella F, D'Andrea E (1955) Sindrome dell'angolo pontocerebellare da neurinome dei nervi IX, X, XI. Chir Patol Sper 10:447–451
31. Bettoni L, Baldi P, Bertolino G (1985) CT diagnosis of intracranial neurinoma of the hypoglossal nerve. J Comput Ass Tomogr 9:827–828
32. Bilaniuk LT, Zimmerman RA, Wehrli FW et al. (1985) Cerebral magnetic resonance: comparison of high- and low-field strength imaging. Radiology 153:409–414
33. Bird CR, Hasso AN, Drayer BP, Hinshaw DB, Thompson JR (1985) The cerebellopontine angle and internal auditory canal: neurovascular anatomy on gas CT cisternograms. Radiology 154:667–670
34. Boeri R, Passerini A (1964) The megadolichobasilar anomaly. J Neurol Sci 1:475–484
35. Bonafé A, Manelfe C, Clanet M, Fraysse B, Soulier MJ, de Kersaint-Gilly A, Raphalen JP, Legent F, Massot M (1985) Electrophysiology – CT correlations in exploration for acoustic neurinoma. J Neuroradiol 12:61–70
36. Boussens J, Caillé JM, Koehler R, Boyer M, Piton J, Bisch X, Martin PL (1972) A propos de la vascularisation du conduit auditif interne. Cah ORL (Montpellier) 7:763–774
37. Brasch RC, Weinmann HJ, Wesbey GE (1984) Contrast-enhanced NMR imaging: animal studies using gadolinium-DTPA complex. AJR 142:625–630
38. Braun IF, Naidich TP, Leeds NE, Koslow M, Zimmerman HM, Chase NE (1977) Dense intracranial epidermoid tumors. Radiology 122:717–719
39. Braun JP, Tournade A, Adynowski J (1984) A comparative anatomical CT study of the vascular and nervous structures of the cerebello-pontine angle. Neuroradiology 26:3–7
40. Breig A, Ekbom K, Greitz T, Kugelberg E (1967) Hydrocephalus due to elongated basilar artery. A new clinico-radiological syndrome. Lancet 1967:874–875
41. Brihaye J, Périer O, Smulders J, Franken L (1956) Glossopharyngeal neuralgia caused by compression of the nerve by an atheromatous vertebral artery. J Neurosurg 13:294–302
42. Britton BH, Hitselberger WE, Hurley BJ (1968) Iophendylate examination of posterior fossa in diagnosis of cerebello-pontine angle tumors. Arch Otolaryngol 88:608–617
43. Britton BH (1974) Glomus tympanicum and glomus jugulare tumors. Radiol Clin North Am 12:543–551
44. Brooks RA, Di Chiro G (1976) Beam hardening in X-ray reconstructive tomography. Phys Med Biol 21:390–398
45. Brunner H (1935) Zur Diagnose der Akustikustumoren. Monatsschr Ohrenheilkd 69: 549–561
46. Budka H (1974) Intracranial lipomatous hamartomas (intracranial "lipomas"). Acta Neuropathol (Berl) 28:205–222
47. Bull JW (1969) Tentorium cerebelli. Proc R Soc Med 62:1301–1310
48. Bull J (1969) Massive aneurysms at the base of the brain. Brain 92:535–570
49. Bull J, Kozlowski P (1970) The angiographic pattern of the petrosal veins in the normal and pathological. Neuroradiology 1:20–26
50. Bunts A (1949) Malformations vasculaires du cerveau. Rev Neurol 81:442–452
51. Byrd SE, Bentson JR, Winter J, Wilson GH, Joyce PW, O'Connor L (1978) Giant intracranial aneurysms simulating brain neoplasms on computed tomography. J Comput Ass Tomogr 2:303–307
52. Camp JO, Cilley EJL (1939) Significance of asymmetry of pori acustici as an aid in diagnosis of eighth nerve tumors. AJR 41:713–718

53. Campbell EH, Keedy C (1947) Hemifacial spasm: note on etiolgy in 2 cases. J Neurosurg 4:342–347
54. Campbell E, Wittfield RD (1948) Posterior fossa meningiomas. J Neurosurg 5:131–153
55. Canigiani G (1978) Nativdiagnostik mit Tomographie der Kleinhirnbrückenwinkeltumoren. In: Plester D, Wende S, Nakayama N (eds) Kleinhirnbrückenwinkeltumoren. Diagnostik und Therapie. Springer, Berlin Heidelberg New York, pp 92–120
56. Castaigne P, Pertuiset B, Cambier J, Brunet P (1967) Anévrysme de l'artère auditive interne révélé par une paralysie faciale récidivante. Cure radicale. Presse Méd 75:2493–2496
57. Castellano F, Ruggiero G (1953) Meningiomas of the posterior fossa. Acta Radiol [Suppl] (Stockh) 104:1–177
58. Castillo R, Watts C, Pulliam M (1982) Sudden hemorrhage in an acoustic neurinoma. Case report. J Neurosurg 56:417–419
59. Caughran M, White TJ, Gerald B, Gardner G (1980) Computed tomography of jugulotympanic paragangliomas. J Comput Ass Tomogr 4:194–198
60. Cecchini A (1960) Il quadro radiologico del neurinoma del nervo acustico: Considerazioni su 68 casi. Radiol Med (Torino) 44:183–199
61. Cervos-Navarro J, Matakas F, Lazaro MC (1968) Das Bauprinzip der Neurinome. Ein Beitrag zur Histogenese der Nerventumoren. Virchows Arch [A] 345:276–291
62. Chambers AA, Lukin RR, Tomsick TA (1977) Cranial epidermoid tumors: diagnosis by computed tomography. Neurosurgery 1:276–280
63. Chaussé C (1950) Trois incidences pour l'examen du rocher. Acta Radiol 34:274–287
64. Christoferson LA, Leech RW, Grossman M (1982) Intracranial neurilemmoma of the accessory nerve. Surg Neurol 18:18–20
65. Clark WC, Acker JD, Robertson JH, Gardner G, Dusseau JJ, Moretz W (1982) Neuroradiological detection of small and intracanalicular acoustic tumors: an emphysis on CO_2 contrast-enhanced computed tomographic cisternography. Neurosurgery 11:733–738
66. Clemis JD, Mc Gee T (1979) Brain stem electric response audiometry in the differential diagnosis of acoustic tumors. Laryngoscope 89:31–42
67. Cohen H (1937) Glosso-pharyngeal neuralgia. J Laryngol Otol 52:527–536
68. Cohen WA, Pinto RS, Kricheff II (1982) Value of dynamic scanning. Radiol Clin North Am 20:23–35
69. Coin CG, Coin T (1980) Contact enhancement by xenon gas in computed tomography of the spinal cord and brain: preliminary observations. J Comput Ass Tomogr 4:217–221
70. Columella F, Delzanno GB, Nicola GC (1959) Les neurinomes des quatre derniers nerf craniens. Neurochirurgie 5:280–295
71. Courtheoux P, Da Silva DC, Houtheville JP, Valdazo A, Lechevalier B, Théron J (1982) Schwannome du foramen jugulaire. Aspect angiographique et tomodensitométrique. J Radiol 63:557–561
72. Courville CB (1962) Arteriosclerotic aneurysms of the circle of Willis. Some notes on their morphology and pathogenesis. Bull Los Angeles Neurol Soc 27:1–13
73. Crabtree JA, Gardner G (1979) Radiographic findings in cerebellopontine angle tumors. In: House WF, Luetje CM (eds) Acoustic tumors, vol. I: Diagnosis. University Park Press, Baltimore, pp 241–252
74. Cravioto H (1969) The ultrastructure of acoustic nerve tumors. Acta Neuropathol 12: 116–140
75. Crouzet G, Dorland P, Doyon D, Jeanmart JL, Legre J, Metzger J, Simon J, Sterkers JM, Trujillo M, Vignaud J (1974) Results of 514 opaque cisternograms. Fortschr Hals-Nas-Ohrenheilkd 21:76–81
76. Cushing H (1917) Tumors of nervus acusticus and syndrome of cerebellopontine angle. W.B. Saunders, Philadelphia
77. Cushing H (1932) Intracranial tumors. C.C. Thomas, Springfield
78. Cushing H, Eisenhardt L (1938) Meningiomas, their classification, regional behaviour, life history and surgical end results. C.C. Thomas, Springfield
79. Cushing H (1963) Tumors of the nervus acusticus and the syndrome of the cerebellopontine angle. Hafner Publishing Co., New York
80. Dalle OA, Godina A (1957) Tumori dell'acustico. Considerazioni radiologiche. Minerva Neurochir 1:92

81. Dandy WE (1919) Roentgenography of the brain after the injection of air into the spinal canal. Ann Surg 70:397–403
82. Dandy WE (1919) Ventriculography following the injection of air into the cerebral ventricles. AJR 6:26–36
83. Dandy WE (1922) An operation for the total extirpation of tumors of the cerebellopontine angle. A preliminary report. Bull Johns Hopk Hosp 33:344–345
84. Dandy WE (1934) Concerning the cause of trigeminal neuralgia. Am J Surg 24:447–455
85. Daniels DL, Haughton VM, Williams AL, Berns TF (1981) The flocculus in computed tomography. AJNR 2:227–229
86. Daniels DL, Williams AL, Haughton VM (1983) Jugular foramen: Anatomic and computed tomographic study. AJNR 4:1227–1232
87. Daniels DL, Herfkins R, Koehler PR, Millen SJ, Shaffer KA, Williams AL, Haughton VM (1984) Magnetic resonance imaging of the internal auditory canal. Radiology 151:105–108
88. Daniels DL, Schenk JF, Foster T et al. (1985) Surface-coil magnetic resonance imaging of the internal auditory canal. AJNR 6:487–490
89. Danziger J, Allen KL, Bloch S (1974) Intracranial chordomas. Clin Radiol 25:309–316
90. Danziger J, Bloch S (1975) The radiology of arachnoid pouches. Clin Radiol 26:275–283
91. Danziger J, Bloch S (1975) Intracranial aneurysms presenting as mass lesions. Clin Radiol 26:267–273
92. Davis JM, Davis KR, Hesselink JR, Greene R (1980) Malignant glomus jugulare tumor: A case with two unusual radiographic features. J Comput Ass Tomogr 4:415–417
93. Davis KR, Roberson GH, Taveras JM, New PFJ, Trevor R (1976) Diagnosis of epidermoid tumor by computed tomography. Analysis and evaluation of findings. Radiology 119: 347–353
94. Davis KR, Parker SW, New PFJ, Roberson GH, Taveras JM, Ojemann RJ, Weiss AD (1977) Computed tomography of acoustic neuroma. Radiology 124:81–86
95. Davis KR, Parker SW, New PFJ (1979) Cerebello-pontine angle masses. In: Wolpert SM (ed) Multiple imaging procedures, vol 2: Central nervous system. Grune & Stratton, New York San Francisco London, pp 83–93
96. Deeb ZL, Jannetta PJ, Rosenbaum AE, Kerber CW, Drayer BP (1979) Tortuous vertebrobasilar arteries causing cranial nerve syndromes: screening by computed tomography. J Comput Ass Tomogr 3:774–778
97. De Martel T, Subirana A, Guillaume J (1933) Voluminoso neurinoma del hipoglosso con desarrollo juxto-bulbo-proteberancial. Ars Med Barcelona 9:416–419
98. De Moura L (1967) Inner ear pathology in acoustic neurinoma. Arch Otolaryngol 85: 125–134
99. D'Enrico A (1950) Meningiomas of the posterior fossa. J Neurosurg 7:227–232
100. Dereux J, Deberdt R (1960) Syndromes de l'angle ponto-cérébelleux par lésions et malformations vasculaires. Sem Hôp Paris 36:1849–1851
101. Di Chiro G, Fisher RL, Nelson KB (1964) The jugular foramen. J Neurosurg 21:447–460
102. Djindjian R, Merland J-J (1978) Superselective arteriography of the external carotid artery. Springer, Berlin Heidelberg New York
103. Dilenge D, David M (1967) L'angiographie vertébrale. Neuro-Chirurgie 13:121–156
104. Dobben GD, Valvassori GE, Mafee MF, Berninger WH (1979) Evaluation of brain circulation by rapid rotational computed tomography. Radiology 133:105–111
105. Dolan EJ, Tucker WS, Rotenberg D, Chui M (1982) Intracranial hypoglossal schwannoma as an unusual cause of facial nerve palsy. J Neurosurg 56:420–423
106. Dosch JC, Wackenheim A (1978) Hypodense meningioma: Computer tomographic examination of a meningioma. J Belge Radiol 61:325–334
107. Dossetor RS, De Winter J, Nurick S (1979) Diagnosis of a small acoustic neuroma by metrizamide computer-assisted cisternography. Br J Radiol 52:667–668
108. Downey EF, Buck DR, Ray JW (1981) Arachnoiditis simulating acoustic neuroma on air-CT cisternography. AJNR 2:470–471
109. Drake CG (1978) Cerebellopontine angle arterio-venous malformations. In: Krayenbühl H (ed) Advances and technical standards in neurosurgery. Springer, Wien New York, p 265
110. Drayer BP, Rosenbaum AE, Maroon JC, Bank WO, Woodford JE (1977) Posterior fossa extraaxial cyst: diagnosis with metrizamide CT cisternography. AJR 128:431–436

111. Dubois PJ, Drayer BP, Bank WO, Deeb ZL, Rosenbaum AE (1978) An evaluation of current diagnostic radiologic modalities in the investigation of acoustic neurilemmomas. Radiology 126:173–179
112. Du Boulay GH (1965) Principles of X-ray diagnosis of the skull. Butterworths, London
113. Duncan AW, Lack EE, Deck MF (1979) Radiological evaluation of paragangliomas of the head and neck. Radiology 132:99–105
114. Duvoisin RG, Yahr MD (1965) Posterior fossa aneurysms. Neurology 15:231–241
115. Dykstra PC (1964) The pathology of acoustic neuromas. Arch Otolaryngol 80:605–616
116. Ebenius B (1934) The results of examination of the petrous bone in auditory nerve tumors. Acta Radiol 15:284–290
117. Eiselsberg A (1913) Ueber die chirurgische Behandlung der Hirntumoren. Trans 17th Internat Cong Med Lond Sect 7, p 203–297
118. Eisenbrey AB, Hegarty WM (1956) Trigeminal neuralgia and arteriovenous aneurysms of cerebellopontine angle. J Neurosurg 13:647–649
119. Ekbom K, Greitz T, Kalmér M, López J, Ottosson S (1969) Cerebrospinal fluid pulsations in occult hydrocephalus due to ectasia of basilar artery. Acta Neurochir 2:1–8
120. Enzmann DR, Norman D, Levin V, Wilson C, Newton TH (1978) Computed tomography in the follow-up of medulloblastomas and ependymomas. Radiology 128:57–63
121. Epstein BS (1950) The roentgenologic manifestations of acoustic neuromas. AJR 64: 265–276
122. Epstein BS (1966) Pneumoencephalography and cerebral angiography. Year Book Medical Publ, Chicaco, pp 1–17
123. Eraso ST (1961) Roentgen and clinical diagnosis of glomus jugulare tumors; four cases and a new radiographic technic. Radiology 77:252–256
124. Faerber EN, Wolpert SM (1978) The value of computed tomography in the diagnosis of intracranial lipomata. J Comput Ass Tomogr 2:297–299
125. Falconer MA, Bailey IC, Duchen LW (1968) Surgical treatment of chordoma and chondroma of the skull base. J Neurosurg 29:261–275
126. Farrell VJ, Hawkins D (1967) Glomus jugulare tumors with special reference to their radiological features. Br J Surg 54:789–795
127. Farrior JB, Hymans VJ, Benke RH, Farrior JB (1980) Carcinoid apudoma arising in a glomus jugulare tumor: review of endocrine activity in glomus jugulare tumors. Laryngoscope 9:110–119
128. Fawcitt RA, Isherwood I (1977) Intracranial epidermoid and dermoid tumors. In: Du Boulay GH, Moseley IF (eds) Computerised axial tomography in clinical practice. Springer, Berlin Heidelberg New York, pp 94–101
129. Felix R, Schörner W, Laniado M, Niendord HP, Claussen C, Fiegler W, Speck U (1985) Brain tumors: MR-imaging with gadolinium-DTPA. Radiology 156:681–688
130. Fine R, Williams B, Dowling J (1977) Acoustic neuroma causing subarachnoid hemorrhage. Med J Aust 1:137–139
131. Fink LH, Early CB, Bryan RN (1978) Glossopharyngeal schwannomas. Surg Neurol 9:239–245
132. Firooznia H, Pinto RS, Lin JP, Baruch HH, Zausner J (1976) Chordoma: radiologic evaluation of 20 cases. AJR 127:797–805
133. Fisch U (1968) L'anatomie chirurgicale du système artériel du conduit auditif interne chez l'homme. Rev Laryngol Otol Rhinol (Bord) 89:659–671
134. Fisch U, Yaşargil MG (1968) Der translabyrinthäre Zugang für die Akustikusneurinome. Méd Hyg 26:1190–1191
135. Fisch U, Yaşargil MG (1968) Transtemporale, extrapyramidale Eingriffe am inneren Gehörgang. Pract Oto-Rhino-Laryng 30:377–386
136. Fisch U (1969) Zur Indikation der Pantopaque-Cisternographie. Radiologe 9:473–476
137. Fisch U, Weber J (1972) Der diagnostische Wert der Pantopaque-Cisternographie. Méd Hyg 30:1567–1568
138. Fisch U, Wegmüller A (1974) Early diagnosis of acoustic neuromas. ORL J Otorhinolaryngol Relat Spec 36:129–140
139. Fisch U, Nedzelski J, Wellauer J (1975) Diagnostic value of meatocisternography. Arch Otolaryngol 101:339–343

140. Fisch U (1977) Die Mikrochirurgie des Felsenbeines. HNO 25:193–197
141. Fisch U (1977) Infratemporal fossa approach for extensive tumors of the temporal bone and base of the skull. In: Silverstein H, Norrell H (eds) Neurological surgery of the ear. Aesculapius, Birmingham, pp 34–53
142. Fisch U, Rüttner J (1977) Pathology of intratemporal tumors involving the facial nerve. In: Fisch U (ed) Facial nerve surgery. Aesculapius, Birmingham, pp 448–456
143. Fisch U (1978) Otochirurgische Behandlung des Acusticusneurinoms. In: Plester D, Wende S, Nakayama N (eds) Kleinhirnbrückenwinkel-Tumoren. Springer, Berlin Heidelberg New York, p 196–214
144. Fisch U (1979) Fazialislähmungen im labyrinthären, meatalen und intrakraniellen Bereich. In: Berendes J, Link R, Zöllner F (eds) Hals-Nasen-Ohren-Heilkunde in Praxis und Klinik. Thieme, Stuttgart, pp 2145–2166
145. Fisch U, Pillsbury HC (1979) Infratemporal fossa approach to lesions in the temporal bone and base of the skull. Arch Otolaryngol 105:99–107
146. Fisch U (1980) Management of intratemporal facial palsy. In: Krayenbühl H (ed) Advances and technical standards in neurosurgery. Springer, Wien New York, pp 215–238
147. Fisch U (1982) Infratemporal fossa approach for glomus tumors of the temporal bone. Ann Otol Rhinol Laryngol 91:474–479
148. Fisch U, Fagan P, Valavanis A (1984) The infratemporal fossa approach for the lateral skull base. Otolaryngol Clin North Am 17:513–552
149. Fischgold H, Metzger J, Korach G (1954) Tomographie de la région pétro-sphéno-occipitale: Incidence des quatre dernières paires crâniennes. Acta Radiol 42:56–64
150. Foote EL (1964) Tumors of the glomus jugulare. Am J Clin Pathol 41:72–77
151. Fraser RAR, Carter BL (1975) Unilateral dilatation of the internal auditory canal. Neuroradiology 9:227–229
152. Frey KW (1967) Die Tomographie der Glomustumoren des Ohres. RÖFO 107:775–786
153. Frey KW (1971) Tumors of the glomus jugulare. In: Jensen J, Rovsing H (eds) Fundamentals of ear tomography. C.C: Thomas, Springfield, pp 189–198
154. Fujiwara S, Hachisuga S, Numaguchi Y (1980) Intracranial hypoglossal neurinoma: report of a case. Neuroradiology 20:87–90
155. Fukui M, Tanaka A, Kitamura K, Okudera T (1977) Lipoma of the cerebellopontine angle. Case report. J Neurosurg 46:544–547
156. Gado MH, Phelps ME, Coleman RE (1975) An extravascular component of contrast enhancement in cranial computed tomography. Part I: The tissue-blood ratio of contrast enhancement. Radiology 117:589–593; Part II: Contrast enhancement and the blood-tissue barrier. Radiology 117:595–597
157. Ganti SR, Steniber A, McMurtry JG, Hilal SK (1981) Computed tomographic demonstration of giant aneurysms of the vertebrobasilar system: report of eight cases. Neurosurgery 9:261–267
158. Garcia CA, McGarry PA, Rodriguez F (1981) Primary intracranial squamous cell carcinoma of the right cerebellopontine angle. J Neurosurg 54:824–828
159. Gardeur D, Metzger J (1978) Tomodensitométrie en pathologie tumorale intra-crânienne. Doin Editeurs, Paris, pp 182–189
160. Gardiner G (1980) The early diagnosis of acoustic tumors using posterior fossa cisternography with iophendylate. Laryngoscope 90:181–195
161. Gardner WJ, McCormack LJ, Dohn DF (1960) Embryonal atresia of the fourth ventricle. The cause of "arachnoid cyst" of the cerebellopontine angle. J. Neurosurg. 17:226–237
162. Gejrot T, Laurén T (1964) Retrograde jugularography in diagnosis of glomus tumours in the jugular region. Acta Otolaryngol 58:191–207
163. Glasscock ME (1968) History of the diagnosis and treatment of acoustic neuroma. Arch Otolaryngol 83:578–585
164. Glasscock ME, Jackson CG, Josey AF, Dickins JRE, Wiet RJ (1979) Brain stem evoked response audiometry in a clinical practice. Laryngoscope 89:1021–1034
165. Gleeson RK, Butzer JF, Grin OD (1978) Acoustic neurinoma presenting as subarachnoid hemorrhage. Case report. J Neurosurg 49:602–604
166. Godt P, Stöppler L (1979) Infratentorielle Epidermoide und Dermoide im kranialen Computertomogramm. RÖFO 131:368–371

167. Goldberg R, Byrd S, Winter J, Takahashi M, Joyce P (1980) Varied appearance of trigeminal neuroma on CT. AJR 134:57–60
168. Goldman AM, Martin JE (1970) Tumors involving the temporal bone. Radiol Clin North Am 8:387–402
169. Goldstein SJ, Sacks JG, Lee C, Tibbs PA, McCready RA (1983) Computed tomographic findings in cerebral arterial ectasia. AJNR 4:501–504
170. Gooding CA, Price DC, Newton TH (1972) Experimental studies of falx and tentorial opacification during cerebral angiography. Radiology 102:77–82
171. Gould LV, Cummings CW, Rabuzzi DD, Reed GF, Chung CT (1977) Use of computerized axial tomography of the head and neck region. Laryngoscope 87:1270–1276
172. Graf K (1955) Die Kleinhirnbrückenwinkelgeschwülste. Fortschr Hals-Nas-Ohrenheilkd 2:146–274
173. Graf K, Fisch U (1979) Geschwülste des Ohres und des Felsenbeines. In: Berendes J, Link R, Zöller F (eds) Hals-Nasen-Ohren-Heilkunde in Praxis und Klinik, vol 5: Ohr I. Thieme, Stuttgart, pp 22.1–22.63
174. Graves VB, Schemm GW (1982) Clinical characteristics and CT findings in lipoma of the cerebellopontine angle. Case report. J Neurosurg 57:839–841
175. Green JR, Vaughan RT (1972) Blood vessel tumors and hematomas of the posterior fossa in adolescence. Angiology 23:474–478
176. Greenfield JG (1982) Cytology and cellular pathology of the nervous system. Vol. 3, Penfield W (ed), Hoeber, New York, p 1224
177. Grehn S, Helms J (1976) Der erweiterte "leere" innere Gehörgang. RÖFO 124:150–154
178. Greitz T, Löfstedt S (1954) The relationship between the third ventricle and the basilar artery. Acta Radiol 42:85–100
179. Greitz T, Sjögren SE (1963) The posterior inferior cerebellar artery. Acta Radiol 1:284–297
180. Greitz T, Ekbom K, Kugelberg E, Breig A (1969) Occult hydrocephalus due to ectasia of the basilar artery. Acta Radiol 9:310–316
181. Greitz T, Hindmarsh T (1974) Computer assisted tomography of the intracranial CSF circulation using water-soluble contrast medium. Acta Radiol 15:497–507
182. Greitz T, Möller A, Olivecrona H, Bergström M (1978) Diagnostic efficacy and limitations of computer tomography in posterior fossa lesions. In: Bories J (ed) The diagnostic limitations of computerised axial tomography. Springer, Berlin Heidelberg New York, pp 17–28
183. Gruber (1888) Lehrbuch der Ohrenheilkunde, pp 569–622
184. Gruskin P, Carberry JN (1979) Pathology of acoustic tumors. In: House WF, Luetje CM (eds) Acoustic tumors, vol 1: Diagnosis. University Park Press, Baltimore, pp 85–148
185. Guerrier Y, Villaceque G (1949) Origine et comportement des artères cérébelleuse moyenne et auditive interne. C R Ass Anat 36:377–382
186. Guild SR (1941) A hitherto unrecognized structure, the glomus jugularis, in man. Anat Rec [Suppl] 79 (2), 28
187. Guild SR (1953) The Glomus jugulare, a nonchromaffin paraganglion, in man. Ann Otol Rhinol Laryngol 62:1045–1071
188. Guillain G, Bertrand I, Lereboullet J (1933) Neurinome des nerf mixtes: prolongement extracranien de la tumeur. Rev Neurol 2:56–68
189. Guiot G, Bouche J (1965) Méningiomes et neurinomes intrapétreux. Neuro-Chirurgie 11:361–362
190. Guzowski J, Paprella M, Rao KN, Hoshino T (1976) Meningiomas of the temporal bone. Laryngoscope 86:1141–1146
191. Gyldensted C, Lester J, Thomsen J (1976) Computer tomography in the diagnosis of cerebellopontine angle tumors. Neuroradiology 11:191–197
192. Hakuba A, Hashi K, Fujitani K et al. (1979) Jugular foramen neurinomas. Surg Neurol 11:83–94
193. Hambly WH (1964) The differential diagnosis of acoustic neuroma. Arch Otolaryngol 80:708
194. Hammer B (1979) Computertomographische Diagnose der Megadolichobasilaris. RÖFO 131:255–261

195. Hanafee WN, Mancuso A, Winter J, Jenkins H, Bergstrom L (1980) Edge enhancement computed tomography scanning in inflammatory lesions of the middle ear. Radiology 136:771–775
196. Handa J, Nakano Y, Aii H (1977) CT cisternography with intracranial arachnoidal cyst. Surg Neurol 8:451–454
197. Handa J, Matsuda I, Handa H, Nakano Y, Komuro H, Nakajima K (1978) Extravascular iodine in contrast enhancement with computed tomography. Neuroradiology 15:159–163
198. Handa J, Nakano Y, Aii H, Handa H (1978) Computed tomography with giant intracranial aneurysms. Surg Neurol 9:257–263
199. Harel D, Lavy S, Schwartz A (1967) Aneurysms of basilar artery simulating a cerebellopontine angle tumor. Confin Neurol (Basel) 29:360–364
200. Harner SG, Reese DF (1984) Roentgenographic diagnosis of acoustic neurinoma. Laryngoscope 94:306–309
201. Harper RAK (1957) Glomus jugulare tumors of the temporal bone. J Fac Radiol 8:325–334
202. Hart RG, Davenport J (1981) Diagnosis of acoustic neuroma. Neurosurgery 9:450–463
203. Hart RG, Gardner DP, Howieson J (1983) Acoustic tumors: Atypical features and recent diagnostic tests. Neurology 33:211–221
204. Hastings-James R (1969) Acoustic neuroma – some aspects of the cisternographic investigation. J Can Ass Radiol 20:43–47
205. Hastings-James R (1969) The anatomy of the posterior fossa in relation to positive contrast cisternography. Radiology 92:1065–1072
206. Hasse E (1946) Neurinoma of the twelfth nerve. J Neuropathol Exp Neurol 5:66–71
207. Hatam A, Bergvall U, Lewander R, Larsson S, Lind M (1975) Contrast medium enhancement with time in computer tomography. Differential diagnosis of intracranial lesions. Acta Radiol [Suppl] 346:63–81
208. Hatam A, Bergström M, Möller A, Olivecrona H (1978) Early contrast enhancement of acoustic neuroma. Neuroradiology 17:31–33
209. Hatam A, Möller A, Olivecrona H (1979) Evaluation of the internal auditory meatus with acoustic neuromas using computed tomography. Neuroradiology 17:197–200
210. Hawkins TD (1961) Glomus jugulare and carotid body tumours. Clin Radiol 12:199–213
211. Hawkins TD (1966) Radiological investigation of glomus jugulare tumours. Acta Radiol 5:201–210
212. Healy JF, Goff WB, Bishop JW (1982) Pathologic basis of computed tomographic and angiographic findings in giant ninth nerve neuroma. Comput Radiol 6:227–231
213. Heller M, Wohrle M, Jend HH, Hormann K, Helmke K (1983) Aussagekraft der CT in der Diagnostik von Tumoren der Kleinhirnbrückenwinkelregion. Vergleich der verschiedenen radiologischen, klinischen und otologischen Untersuchungsverfahren. RÖFO 139:48–55
214. Henschen F (1912) Die Acusticustumoren, eine neue Gruppe radiographisch darstellbarer Hirntumoren. RÖFO 18:207–216
215. Higgs WA (1973) Sudden deafness as the presenting symptom of acoustic neurinoma. Arch Otolaryngol 98:73–76
216. Hirsch A, Anderson H (1980) Audiologic test results in 96 patients with tumours affecting the eighth nerve: A clinical study with emphasis on early audiological diagnosis. Acta Otolaryngol [Suppl] (Stockh) 369:1–26
217. Hitselberger WE, House WF (1968) Polytome-Pantopaque: A technique for the diagnosis of small acoustic tumors. Technical note. J Neurosurg 29:214–217
218. Hitselberger WE, Gardner G (1968) Other tumors of the cerebellopontine angle. Arch Otolaryngol 88:164–166
219. Hitselberger WE, House WF (1976) Polytome-Pantopaque: A technique for the diagnosis of small acoustic tumors. Acta Otolaryngol (Stockh) 65:555–564
220. Hodes PJ, Pendergrass EP, Young BR (1949) Eighth nerve tumors: Their roentgen manifestations. Radiology 53:633–665
221. Hodes PJ, Pendergrass EP, Dennis JM (1951) Cerebellopontine angle tumors: Their roentgenologic manifestations. Radiology 57:395–406
222. Hood J, Wilson ER, Alexander CB, Flint A, Ho K-J (1982) Lymphomatoid granulomatosis manifested as a mass in the cerebellopontine angle. Arch Neurol 39:319–320

223. Hori T, Hirakawa K, Jshijima B, Manaka S, Fukushima T, Shimizu N, Sato T (1971) Aneurysm in the internal auditory meatus. Case report. J Neurosurg 35:605–609
224. Horn KL, Crumley RL, Schindler RA (1981) Facial neurilemmomas. Laryngoscope 99:1326–1331
225. Hounsfield GN (1973) Computerized transverse axial scanning (tomography). Part 1. Description of system. Br J Radiol 46:1016–1022
226. Hounsfield GN (1976) Picture quality of computed tomography. AJR 127:3–9
227. House WF (1961) Surgical exposure of the internal auditory canal and its contents through the middle cranial fossa. Laryngoscope 11:1363–1385
228. House WF (1964) Evolution of transtemporal bone removal of acoustic tumors. Arch Otolaryngol 80:731–742
229. House WF (1968) Monograph II. Acoustic neuroma. Arch Otolaryngol 88:576–715
230. House WF, Hitselberger WE (1974) Acoustic tumors. In: Handbook of Clinical Neurology, vol 17/2. North Holland, Amsterdam, pp 666–692
231. House WF (1979) A history of acoustic tumor surgery. 1917–1961. The Dandy era. In: House WF, Luetje CM (eds) Acoustic tumors, vol 1: Diagnosis. University Park Press, Baltimore, p 25–32
232. Houser OW, Baker HL, Rhoton AL, Okazaki H (1972) Intracranial dural arteriovenous malformations. Radiology 105:55–64
233. Huang YP, Wolf BS, Antin SP, Okudera T (1968) The veins of the posterior fossa – anterior or petrosal draining group. AJR 104:36–56
234. Huang YP, Wolf BS (1970) Differential diagnosis of fourth ventricle tumors from brain stem tumors in angiography. Neuroradiology 1:4–19
235. Huete I, Corrales M (1979) Cisternographie computerisée dans le diagnostic des petits neurinomes de l'acoustique. J Neuroradiol 6:335–340
236. Hugosson R, Bergström K (1974) Surgical treatment of dural arteriovenous malformation in the region of the sigmoid sinus. J Neurol Neurosurg Psychiatry 37:97–101
237. Huk W, Schiefer W (1978) Computertomographie bei Prozessen der Schädelbasis und der Orbitae. RÖFO 128:8–11
238. Ignelzi RJ, Bucy PC (1967) Intracranial hypoglossal neurofibroma: Case report. J Neurosurg 26:352–356
239. Jackson CG, Glasscock ME, Hughes G, Simanis A (1980) Facial paralysis of neoplastic origin: diagnosis and management. Laryngoscope 90:1581–1595
240. Jamieson KG (1964) Aneurysms of the vertebrobasilar system. Surgical intervention in 19 cases. J Neurosurg 21:781–797
241. Jerger J, Hartford E, Clemis J, Alford B (1974) The acoustic reflex in eighth nerve disorders. Arch Otolaryngol 99:409–413
242. Johnson DW (1984) Air cisternography of the cerebellopontine angle using high resolution computed tomography. Radiology 151:401–403
243. Johnson DW, Voorhees RL, Wong ML (1985) Virtues and vagaries of high-resolution CT air cisternography in the diagnosis of acoustic neuromas. Otolaryngol Head Neck Surg 93:156–160
244. Johnson EW (1979) Results of audiometry tests in acoustic tumor patients. In: House WF, Luetje CM (eds) Acoustic tumors: vol 1: Diagnosis. University Park Press, Baltimore, pp 209–224
245. Johnson JH, Kline DG (1978) Anterior inferior cerebellar artery aneurysms. J Neurosurg 48:455–460
246. Jordan CE, Newton TH (1975) Internal carotid artery supply to temporal bone chemodectomas. Neuroradiology 8:249–257
247. Jörgensen MB (1962) Intracochlear neurinoma. Acta Otolaryngol (Stockh) 54:227–232
248. Josey AF, Jackson CG, Glasscock ME (1980) Brainstem evoked response audiometry in confirmed eighth nerve tumors. Am J Otolaryngol 1:285–290
249. Kapila A, Chakeres DW, Blanco E (1984) The Meckel Cave: Computed tomographic study. Radiology 152:425–433
250. Kaplan HA, Browder J, Krieger AJ (1975) Venous channels within the intracranial dural partitions. Radiology 115:641–645

251. Kasantikul V, Netsky MG, Glasscock ME, Hayes JW (1980) Intracanalicular neurilemmomas: Clinico-pathologic study. Ann Otol Rhinol Laryngol 89:29–32
252. Kasantikul V, Netsky MG, Glasscock ME, Hayes JW (1980) Acoustic neurilemmoma. Clinicoanatomical study in 103 patients. J Neurosurg 52:28–35
253. Kaseff LG, Perkins R, Hambley WH (1981) Radiological techniques for small acoustic tumors. A re-evaluation. Laryngoscope 91:63–70
254. Kawano H, Kobayashi H, Hayashi M, Tsuji T, Kabuto M, Nozaki J (1984) Trigeminal neuralgia caused by arteriovenous malformation of the cerebellopontine angle – report of two cases. No To Shinkey 36, pp 1175–1179
255. Kaye AH, Hahn JF, Kinney SE, Hardy RW, Bay JW (1984) Jugular foramen schwannomas. J Neurosurg 60:1045–1053
256. Kazner E, Grumme T, Lanksch W, Wilske J (1978) Limitations of computerized tomography in the detection of posterior fossa lesions. Adv Neurosurg 5:166–170
257. Kazner E, Wende S, Grumme T, Lanksch W, Stochdorph O (1981) Computertomographie intracranieller Tumoren aus klinischer Sicht. Springer, Berlin Heidelberg New York
258. Kendall BE, Claveria LE (1976) The use of computed axial tomography (CAT) for the diagnosis and management of intracranial angiomas. Neuroradiology 12:140–160
259. Kendall B, Symon L (1977) Investigation of patients with cerebellopontine angle syndromes. Neuroradiology 13:65–84
260. Kendall BE, Lee BCP (1977) Cranial chordomas. Br J Radiol 50:687–698
261. Kerber CW, Margolis MT, Newton TH (1972) Tortuous vertebrobasilar system: a cause of cranial nerve signs. Neuroradiology 4:74–77
262. Kernohan JW (1971) Tumors of congenital origin. In: Minckler J (ed) Pathology of the nervous system, vol 2. McGraw-Hill, New York, pp 1927–1937
263. Khangure MS, Dolan KD (1983) High resolution CT air cisternography in the diagnosis of small acoustic neuromas. Head Neck Surg 5:489–494
264. Khangure MS, Mojtahedi S (1983) Air CT cisternography of anterior inferior artery loop simulating an intracanalicular acoustic neuroma. AJNR 4:994–995
265. Kim SK, Capp MP (1966) Jugular foramen and early roentgendiagnosis of glomus jugulare tumor. AJR 97:597–600
266. Kingsley DP, Thornton A, Furneaux C, King TT (1984) Transmural passage of subarachnoid metrizamide into a cystic acoustic schwannoma of the cerebellopontine angle: a diagnostic dilemma. Neuroradiology 26:319–321
267. Kingsley DPE, Brooks GB, Leung AW-L, Johnson MA (1985) Acoustic neuromas: evaluation by magnetic resonance imaging. AJNR 6:1–5
268. Kirdani M (1973) The hypoglossal canal. In: Berrett A, Brünner S, Valvassori G (eds) Modern thin-section tomography. CC Thomas, Springfield, pp 123–138
269. Kleinsasser O, Friedmann G (1958) Die Knorpelgeschwülste der Schädelbasis. Dtsch Z Nervenheilkd 177:378–404
270. Kleinsasser O, Friedmann G (1959) Über Neurinome des Nervus facialis. Zentralbl Neurochir 19:49–59
271. Kokunai T, Kuwamura K (1982) Primary sarkoma of the brain with enlargement of the internal auditory canal in a child. Rinsho Hoshasen 27:939–941
272. Kormano M, Dean PB (1976) Extravascular contrast material: The major component of contrast enhancement. Radiology 121:379–382
273. Krainer L (1935) Die Hirn- und Rückenmarkslipome. Virchows Arch Pathol Anat 295: 107–142
274. Kramer RA (1977) Vermian pseudotumor: a potential pitfall of CT brain scanning with contrast enhancement. Neuroradiology 13:229–230
275. Krause F (1903) Zur Freilegung der hintern Felsenbeinfläche und des Kleinhirns. Beitr Klin Chir 37:728–764
276. Krayenbühl H (1936) Primary tumours of the root of the fifth cranial nerve: their distinction from tumours of the gasserian ganglion. Brain 59:337–352
277. Krayenbühl H, Yaşargil MG (1957) Die vaskulären Erkrankungen im Gebiete der Arteria vertebralis und Arteria basialis. Thieme, Stuttgart
278. Krayenbühl H (1959) Das Neurinom des Nervus trigeminus. Bull Schweiz Akad Med Wiss 15:89–100

279. Krayenbühl HA, Yaşargil MG (1965) Die zerebrale Angiographie. Thieme, Stuttgart
280. Krayenbühl H, Yaşargil MG (1975) Cranial chordomas. Prog Neurol Surg 6:380–434
281. Kricheff II, Pinto RS, Bergeron RT, Cohen N (1980) Air-CT cisternography and canalography for small acoustic neuromas. AJNR 1:57–63
282. Kricheff I, Pinto R, Bergeron RT, Cohen N (1980) The diagnosis of small acoustic neuromas by air CT cisternography and canalography. In: Caillé JM, Salamon G (eds) Computerized tomography. Springer, Berlin Heidelberg New York, pp 115–120
283. Kricheff II (1981) Diskussionsbeitrag. In: Felix R, Kazner E, Wegener OH (eds) Contrast media in computed tomography. International Congress Series 561, Excerpta Medica, Amsterdam Oxford Princeton
284. Krol G, Sundaresan N, Deck M (1983) Computed tomography of axial chordomas. J Comput Ass Tomogr 7:286–289
285. Kurze T, Doyle JB (1962) Extradural intracranial (middle fossa) approach to the internal auditory canal. J Neurosurg 19:1033–1077
286. Lagemann K (1975) Pharmakokinetik angiographischer Kontrastmittel unter besonderer Berücksichtigung des extravasalen Raumes. 1. Mitteilung. RÖFO 123:247–252; 2. Mitteilung. RÖFO 123:515–521
287. Laine E, Nyrac P (1948) Hémispasme facial guéri par intervention sur la fosse postérieure. Rev Neurol 80:38–40
288. Laine E, Galibert P, Lopez C, Delahousse J, Delandtsheer JM, Christiaens JL (1963) Anévrysmes artério-veineux intra-duraux (développés dans l'épaisseur de la dure-mère) de la fosse postérieure. Neurochirurgie 9:147–158
289. Lang ER, Watts JW, Jacoby RK, Fox JL (1968) Recent observations on the diagnosis and pathologic anatomy of posterior fossa meningiomas. Johns Hopk Med J 122:336–342
290. Lange S, Steinhoff H, Aviles C, Kazner E, Grumme T (1979) Kontrastmittelkinetik in zerebralen Tumoren. RÖFO 130:666–669
291. Lapayowker MS, Cliff MM (1969) Bone changes in acoustic neurinomas. AJR 107: 652–658
292. Lasjaunias P, Moret J (1976) The ascending pharyngeal artery: normal and pathological aspects. Neuroradiology 11:77–82
293. Lasjaunias P, Théron J (1976) Radiographic anatomy of the accessory meningeal artery. Radiology 121:99–104
294. Lasjaunias P, Théron J, Moret J (1978) The occipital artery. Neuroradiology 15:31–37
295. Lasjaunias P, Moret J, Théron J (1978) The so-called anterior meningeal artery of the cervical vertebral artery. Neuroradiology 17:51–55
296. Lasjaunias P, Menu Y, Bonnel D, Doyon D (1981) Paragangliomes non chromaffines de la tête et du cou. Place de l'angiographie diagnostique et thérapeutique. A propos de 19 cas, entre 1977 et 1980. J Neuroradiol 8:281–299
297. Lassila Y (1937) Über die Resultate der Röntgenuntersuchung bei Acusticustumoren. Nervenarzt 10:448–453
298. Latack JT, Gabrielsen TO, Knake JE, Kemink JL, Graham MD, Gebarski SS, Yang PJ (1983) Facial nerve neuromas. Radiologic evaluation. Radiology 149:731–739
299. Leblanc R, Ethier R, Little JR (1979) Computerized tomography findings in arteriovenous malformations of the brain. J Neurosurg 51:765–772
300. Lecuire J, Dechaume JP (1971) Les méningiomes de la fosse cérébrale postérieure. Neurochirurgie [Suppl] 17, 2:1–146
301. Lee BCP (1979) Intracranial cysts. Radiology 130:667–674
302. Lee SH, Lewis E, Montoya JH, Seelaus JF (1981) Bilateral cerebellopontine angle air-CT cisternography. AJNR 2:105–106
303. Leo JS, Pinto RS, Hulyat GF, Epstein F, Kricheff II (1979) Computed tomography of arachnoid cysts. Radiology 130:675–680
304. Lepoire J, Pertuiset B (1957) Les kystes épidermoides cranioencéphaliques. Neurochirurgie 3:319–322
305. Lévy A, Botelli J (1953) Signes radiologiques des neurinomes de l'acoustique. Arguments statistiques. J Radiol Electrol 34:842
306. Lewander R, Bergström M, Bergvall U (1978) Contrast enhancement of cranial lesions in computed tomography. Acta Radiol [Diagn] 19:529–552

307. Liliequist B (1959) The subarachnoid cisterns. Acta Radiol [Suppl] (Stockh) 185:1–108
308. Liliequist B (1959) Pontine angle tumour. Encephalographic appearances. Acta Radiol [Suppl] (Stockh) 186:1–96
309. Lim GHK (1975) Clivus chordoma with unusual bone sclerosis and brainstem invasion. A case report with review of the radiology of cranial chordoma. Aust Radiol 19:242–250
310. Lin SR, Silverstein H (1973) False positive roentgenologic diagnosis of small intra-canalicular acoustic neurinomas. AJR 118:511–516
311. Lindgren E (1941) Das Rötgenbild bei Tumoren des Ganglion Gasseri. Acta Chir Scand 85:181–194
312. Lindgren E (1949) Some aspects on the technique of encephalography. Acta Radiol 31: 161–177
313. Lindgren E (1950) Encephalographic examination of tumours in the posterior fossa. Acta Radiol 34:331–338
314. Lindgren E, Di Chiro G (1951) Suprasellar tumours with calcification. Acta Radiol 36: 173–195
315. Lindgren E (1954) Röntgenologie. In: Olivecrona H, Tönnis W (eds) Handbuch der Neurochirurgie. vol 1. Springer, Berlin Göttingen Heidelberg
316. Lindgren E (1956) Another method of vertebral angiography. Acta Radiol 46:257–261
317. Linthicum FH, Churchill D (1968) Vestibular test results in acoustic tumor cases. Arch Otolaryngol 88:604–607
318. Linthicum FH, Khalessi MH, Churchill D (1979) Electronystagmographic caloric bithermal vestibular test (ENG): Results in acoustic tumor cases. In: House WF, Luetje CM (eds) Acoustic tumors, vol 1: Diagnosis. University Park Press, Baltimore, pp 237–240
319. Lipkin AF, Jenkins HA (1984) Role of air contrast computed tomography in diagnosis of small acoustic neuromas. Laryngoscope 94:890–895
320. List CF (1933) Die Differentialdiagnose der Kleinhirnbrückenwinkelerkrankungen mit besonderer Berücksichtigung der Tumoren. Z Ges Neurol Psychiat 144:54–95
321. Littleton JT, Shaffer KA, Callahan WP, Durizch ML (1981) Temporal bone: comparison of pluridirectional tomography and high resolution computed tomography. AJR 137: 835–845
322. Lo WWM, Solti-Bohman LG, Brackmann DE, Gruskin P (1984) Cholesterol granuloma of the petrous apex: CT diagnosis. Radiology 153:705–711
323. Loepp W (1940) Die Pathologie der Pyramidenspitze im Röntgenbild. RÖFO 61:205–222
324. Loew F, Tönnis W (1954) Klinik und Behandlung der Neurinome des N. trigeminus. Zentralbl Neurochir 1:32–41
325. Long JM, Kier EL, Schechter MM (1973) The radiology of epidermoid tumors of the cerebellopontine angle. Neuroradiology 6:188–192
326. Lübbers J (1937) Gezwel van het os petrosum met gecombineerede hersenzenuwverlamming (Syndroom van het foramen jugulare (Burger), en gelijkijdig gezwel van glomus caroticum aan de andere zijde). Ned Tijdschr Geneesk 81:2566–2567
327. Luse SA (1960) Electron microscopic studies on brain tumors. Neurology 10:881–905
328. Lysholm E (1928) Contribution to the technique of projection in roentgenological examination of pars petrosa. Acta Radiol 9:54–66
329. Lysholm E (1931) Apparatus and technique for roentgen examination of the skull. Acta Radiol [Suppl] (Stockh) 12:1–120
330. Lysholm E (1941) Skelettveränderungen bei 2 Fällen mit einem, einen Acusticustumor vortäuschenden Brückenwinkelmeningeom. Acta Chir Scand 85:195–197
331. MacCarty CS, Leavens ME, Love JG, Kernohan JWL (1959) Dermoid and epidermoid tumors in the central nervous system of adults. Surg Gynecol Obstet 108:191–198
332. Malter IJ, Roberson G (1972) Angiògraphic demonstration of anterior inferior cerebellar artery aneurysms by the use of the base view. Radiology 103:125–126
333. Mafee MF, Aimi K, Valvassori GE (1984) Computed tomography in the diagnosis of primary tumors of the petrous bone. Laryngoscope 94:1423–1430
334. Mafee MF, Kumar A, Valvassori GE, Dobben GD, Meyer D (1985) Diagnostic potential of CT in neurologic disorders. Laryngoscope 95:505–514
335. Manelfe C, Giraud B, Espagno J, Rascol A (1978) Cisternographie computérisée au metrizamide. Rev Neurol 134:471–484

336. Manelfe C (1980) La cisternographie computérisée gazeuse. Une nouvelle méthode d'exploration tomodensitométrique de l'angle ponto-cérébelleux et du conduit auditif interne. Ann Radiol 23:47–48
337. Manelfe C, Bonafe A (1980) Normal computed tomographic anatomy of the cisterns and cranial nerves. In: Caille JM, Salamon G (eds) Computerized tomography. Springer, Berlin Heidelberg New York, pp 104–114
338. Maniglia AJ, Chandler JR, Goodwin WJ, Parker JC (1979) Schwannomas of the parapharyngeal space and jugular foramen. Laryngoscope 89:1405–1414
339. Mannsell HW (1889) Subtentorial hydatid tumor removed by trephining: recovery. N Z Med J 2:151–156
340. Markham JW, Fager CA, Horrax G, Poppen JC (1955) Meningiomas of posterior fossa, their diagnosis, clinical features and surgical treatment. Arch Neurol Psychiat 74:163–170
341. Marsman JWP (1979) Tumors of the glomus jugulare complex (chemodectomas) demonstrated by cranial computed tomography. J Comput Ass Tomogr 3:795–799
342. Martínez R, Vaquero J, Cabezudo J, Areitio E, Bravo G (1981) Neurinomas of the jugular foramen in children. Report of two cases. J Neurosurg 54:693–695
343. Masson M, Cambier J (1967) Les anévrysmes vertebro-basilaires. La dolichomégabasilaire. Rev Prat 17:2759–2769
344. Mathew GD, Facer GU, Suh KW, Houser OW, O'Brien PC (1978) Symptoms, findings, and methods of diagnosis in patients with acoustic neuroma. Laryngoscope 88:1893–1903
345. Mattern WC, Blattner RE, Werth J, Shuman R, Bloch S, Leibrock LG (1980) Eighth nerve lipoma. J Neurosurg 53:397–400
346. Mazzoni A, Hansen CC (1970) Surgical anatomy of the arteries in the internal auditory canal. Arch Otolaryngol 91:128–135
347. McCormick WF, Boulter TR (1966) Vascular malformations ("angiomas") of the dura mater; report of two cases. J Neurosurg 25:309–311
348. McCoyd K, Barron KD, Cassidy RL (1974) Acoustic neurinoma presenting as subarachnoid hemorrhage. Case report. J Neurosurg 41:391–393
349. McGinnis BD, Brady TJ, New PFJ, Buonanno FS, Pykett IL, DeLaPaz RL, Kistler JP, Taveras JM (1983) Nuclear magnetic resonance (NMR) imaging of tumors in the posterior fossa. J Comput Ass Tomogr 7:575–584
350. McGrew EA (1955) Presentation of case. JAMA 158:183–184
351. Mendelsohn DB, Hertzanu Y, Glass RBJ, Anderson JEM (1983) Computed tomographic diagnosis of basilar artery ectasia. S Afr Med J 64:867–869
352. Mensuy L, Girard P, Bret P (1964) A propos de deux observations de tumeur du trou déchiré postérieur. Rev Otoneuroophthalmol 36:249–254
353. Merland JJ, Tempier P, Rancurel G, Bories J, Buge A (1977) Tentative de traitement par embolisation d'une volumineuse tumeur glomique tympano-jugulaire et rétropharyngée. Ann Neurol 133:491–498
354. Michael WF (1974) Posterior fossa aneurysms simulating tumors. J Neurol Neurosurg Psychiatry 37:218–223
355. Mikhael MA, Mattar AG (1978) Intracranial pearly tumors: the roles of computed tomography, angiography and pneumoencephalography. J Comput Ass Tomogr 2: 421–429
356. Mikhael MA, Ciric IS, Wulff AP (1985) Differentiation of cerebellopontine angle neuromas and meningiomas with MR imaging. J Comput Ass Tomogr 9:852–856
357. Miller EM, Newton TH (1978) Extra-axial posterior fossa lesions simulating intra-axial lesions on computed tomography. Radiology 127:675–679
358. Mironov A (1984) Gegenwärtiger Stand der neuroradiologischen Diagnostik von Kleinhirnbrückenwinkel-Tumoren. Radiologe 24:493–501
359. Mitsumara H, Torii T, Inoue T et al. (1960) An autopsy case of intracranial neurinoma arising from the nervus vagus or glossopharyngicus. J Kyoto Prefectural Univ Medecine 68:1364–1371
360. Möller A, Hatam A, Olivecrona H (1978) Diagnosis of acoustic neuroma with computed tomography. Neuroradiology 17:25–30
361. Möller A, Hatam A, Olivecrona H (1978) The differential diagnosis of pontine angle meningioma and acoustic neuroma with computed tomography. Neuroradiology 17:21–23

362. Moniz E (1927) L'Encéphalographie artérielle, son importance dans la localisation des tumeurs cérébrales. Rev Neurol 2:72–90
363. Moody DM, Ghatak NR, Kelly DL (1976) Extensive calcification in a tumor of the glomus jugulare. Neuroradiology 12:131–135
364. Morelli RJ (1966) Intracranial neurilemmoma of the hypoglossal nerve: Review and case report. Neurology (Minneap) 16:709–713
365. Morello G, Paleari A (1949) I meningiomi della fossa cranica posteriore. Chirurgia 4:239
366. Moret J, Delvert JC, Lasjaunias P (1982) La vascularisation de l'oreille et de l'angle ponto-cérébelleux. Territories vasculaires de la caisse tu tympan. J Neuroradiol 9:215–226
367. Moret J, Delvert JC, Lasjaunias P (1982) Architecture vasculaire des tumeurs glomiques tympano-jugulaires. Application à l'angiographie thérapeutique. J Neuroradiol 9:237–260
368. Morgagni (1761) Quoted by Pribram HFW, Hudson JD, Joynt RJ (1969) Posterior fossa aneurysms presenting as mass lesions. AJR 105:334–340
369. Morley TP, Barr HWK (1969) Giant intracranial aneurysms: diagnosis, course and management. Clin Neurosurg 16:73–94
370. Moscow NP, Newton TH (1975) Angiographic features of hypervascular neurinomas of the head and neck. Radiology 114, 635–640
371. Moseley IF, Holland IM (1979) Ectasia of the basilar artery: The breadth of the clinical spectrum and the diagnostic value of computed tomography. Neuroradiology 18:83–91
372. Mourgues G (1954) Aneurysmen der Arteria basialis als extracerebrale Pseudotumoren. Ärztl Wochenschr 9:417–420
373. Müller H (1858) Über das Vorkommen von Resten der Chorda dorsalis beim Menschen nach der Geburt und über ihr Verhältnis zu den Gallertgeschwülsten des Clivus. Z Rat Med 2:202–230
374. Müller J (1938) Über den feineren Bau und die Formen der krankhaften Geschwülste. G Reimer, Berlin
375. Mündnich K, Frey KW (1959) Das Röntgenschichtbild des Ohres. Thieme, Stuttgart
376. Murray MR, Stout AP (1940) Schwann cell versus fibroblast as origin of specific nerve sheath tumor. Am J Pathol 16:41–60
377. Nadjmi M, Ratzka M, Wodartz M (1978) Giant aneurysms in CT and angiography. Neuroradiology 16:284–286
378. Nadjmi M, Piepgras U, Vogelsang H (1981) Kranielle Computertomographie. Ein synoptischer Atlas. Thieme, Stuttgart New York
379. Nagashima C, Takahama M, Sakaguchi A (1982) Dense cerebellopontine epidermoid cyst. Surg Neurol 17:172–177
380. Nager GT (1954) Origins and relations of the internal auditory artery and the subarcuate artery. Ann Otol Rhinol Laryngol 63:51–61
381. Nager G (1964) Association of bilateral VIII nerve tumor with meningiomas in von Recklingshausen's disease. Laryngoscope 74:1220–1261
382. Nager G (1964) Meningiomas involving the temporal bone. Clinical and pathological aspects. Thomas, Springfield
383. Nager GT (1969) Acoustic neurinomas. Pathology and differential diagnosis. Arch Otolaryngol 89:252–279
384. Nager GT, Masica DN (1970) Meningiomas of the cerebellopontine angle and their relation to the temporal bone. Laryngoscope 80:863–895
385. Naidich TP, Kricheff II, George AE, Lin JP (1976) The normal anterior inferior cerebellar artery. Anatomic radiographic correlation with emphasis on the lateral projection. Radiology 119:355–373
386. Naidich TP, Kricheff II, George AE, Lin JP (1976) The anterior inferior cerebellar artery in mass lesions. Preliminary findings with emphasis on the lateral projection. Radiology 119:375–383
387. Naidich TP, Lin JP, Leeds NE, Kricheff II, George AE, Chase NE, Pudlowski RM, Passalaqua A (1976) Computed tomography in the diagnosis of extra-axial posterior fossa masses. Radiology 120:333–339
388. Naidich TP (1977) Infratentorial masses. In: Norman D, Korobkin M, Newton TH (eds) Computed tomography 1977. University of California, San Francisco, pp 231–242

389. Naidich TP, Leeds NE, Kricheff II, Pudlowski RM, Naidich JB, Zimmermann RD (1977) The tentorium in axial section. I. Normal CT appearance and non-neoplastic pathology. Radiology 123:631–638
390. Naidich TP, Leeds NE, Kricheff II, Pudlowski RM, Naidich JB, Zimmermann RD (1977) The tentorium in axial section. II. Lesion localization. Radiology 123:639–648
391. Naidich TP, Lin JP, Leeds NE, Pudlowski RM, Naidich JB (1977) Primary tumors and other masses of the cerebellum and fourth ventricle: Differential diagnosis by computed tomography. Neuroradiology 14:153–174
392. Naidich TP, Pudlowski RM, Leeds NE, Deck MDF (1978) Hypoglossal palsy: Computed tomography demonstration of denervation hemiatrophy of the tongue associated with glomus jugulare tumor. J Comput Ass Tomogr 2:630–632
393. Naidich TP (1980) Air CT canalography for the evaluation of the internal auditory canals. Laryngoscope 90:526–530
394. Nakada T, St. John JN, Knight RT (1983) Solitary metastasis of systemic malignant lymphoma to the cerebellopontine angle. Neuroradiology 24:225–228
395. Nakamura N, Ishiyama R (1974) Jugular foramen syndrome. Surg Ther 31:645–650 (Jpn)
396. Nakayama N, Wende S (1978) Cerebrale Vergrößerungsangiographie bei Kleinhirnbrückenwinkeltumoren. In: Plester D, Wende S, Nakayama N (eds) Kleinhirnbrückenwinkeltumoren. Diagnostik und Therapie. Springer, Berlin Heidelberg New York, pp 189–195
397. Naunton RF, Proctor L, Elpern BS (1968) The audiologic signs of ninth nerve neurinoma. Arch. Otolaryngol 87:222–227
398. Neely JG, Alford BR (1974) Facial nerve neuroma. Arch Otolaryngol 100:298–301
399. Nieuwenhuys R, Voogd J, van Huijzen C (1978) The human central nervous system. Springer, Berlin Heidelberg New York
400. Nelson RA, House WF (1982) Facial nerve neuroma in the posterior fossa: surgical considerations. In: Graham MD, House WF (eds) Disorders of the facial nerve. Raven Press, New York, pp 403–406
401. New PFJ, Scott WR (1975) Miscellaneous primary neoplasms: medulloblastomas, epidermoids, cavernous hemangioma, choroid plexus papilloma. In: Computed tomography of the brain and orbit. Williams and Wilkins, Baltimore, chap 11, pp 209–226
402. New PFJ, Hesselink JR, O'Carroll CP, Kleinman GM (1982) Malignant meningiomas: CT and histologic criteria, including a new CT sign. AJNR 3:267–276
403. New PFJ, Bachow TB, Wismer GL, Rosen BR, Brady TJ (1985) MR imaging of the acoustic nerves and small acoustic neuromas at 0.6 T: prospective study. AJNR 6:165–170
404. Newton TH, Kramer RA (1966) Clinical uses of selective external carotid angiography. AJR 66:458–472
405. Newton TH, Weidner W, Greitz T (1968) Dural arteriovenous malformation in the posterior fossa. Radiology 90:27–35
406. Newton TH, Gooding CA, Price DC (1970) Opacification of falx and tentorium during cerebral angiography. Preliminary report. Invest Radiol 5:348–354
407. Nick I, Fischgold H, Pertuiset B, Sabouraud O (1955) Etude diagnostique d'un neurinome craniocervical de l'hypoglosse. Intérêt de la tomographie et de la veinographie jugulaire rétrograde. Rev Neurol 93:834–838
408. Nielsen A (1942) Acoustic tumors with special reference to end results and sparing of the facial nerve. Ann Surg 115:849–863
409. Nijensohn DE, Ruben J, Saez J, Reagan TJ (1974) Clinical significance of basilar artery aneurysms. Neurology 24:301–305
410. Novy S, Jensen KM (1975) Filling defects and nonfilling of the internal auditory canal in posterior fossa myelography. AJR 124:265–270
411. Numaguchi Y, Kishikawa T, Ikeda J, Tsukamoto Y, Fukui M, Kitamura K, Matsuura K (1980) Angiographic diagnosis of acoustic neurinomas and meningiomas in the cerebellopontine angle – a reappraisal. Neuroradiology 19:73–80
412. Obrador S, Lopez-Zafra JJ (1969) Clinical features of the epidermoids of the basal cisterns of the brain. J Neurol Neurosurg Psychiatry 32:450–454
413. Obrador S, Soto M, Silvela J (1975) Clinical syndromes of arteriovenous malformations of the transverse-sigmoid sinus. J Neurol Neurosurg Psychiatry 38:436–451

414. O'Connor SM, Sackett JF (1981) Radiologic evaluation of the cerebellopontine cistern and the internal auditory canal. Head Neck Surg 3:193–197
415. Ojemann RG, Montgomery WW, Weiss AD (1972) Evaluation and surgical treatment of acoustic neuroma. N Engl J Med 287:895–899
416. Olivecrona H (1927) Die chirurgische Behandlung der Gehirntumoren. Eine klinische Studie. Springer, Berlin
417. Olivecrona H (1967) The removal of acoustic neurinomas. J Neurosurg 26:100–103
418. Olivecrona H (1967) The surgical treatment of intracranial tumors. Meningiomas of posterior surface of petrous bone. In: Olivecrona H, Tönnis W (eds) Handbuch der Neurochirurgie, vol 4, part 4. Springer, Berlin Heidelberg New York, pp 181–184
419. Olsen A, Horrax G (1944) Symptomatology of acoustic tumors with special reference to atypical features. J Neurosurg 1:371–378
420. Olsen WO, Noffsinger D, Kurdziel S (1975) Acoustic reflex and reflex decay. Occurrence in patients with cochlear and eighth nerve lesions. Arch Otolaryngol 101:622–626
421. Olsson O (1953) Vertebral angiography in the diagnosis of acoustic nerve tumors. Acta Radiol (Stockh) 39:265–272
422. Osborn JD (1975) A comparative study of special petrous views and tomography in the diagnosis of acoustic neuromas. Br J Radiol 48:996–999
423. Osborn AG, Brinton WR, Smith WH (1978) Radiology of the jugular tubercles. AJR 131:1037–1040
424. Ouaknine GE (1981) Microsurgical anatomy of the arterial loops in the pontocerebellar angle and the internal acoustic meatus. In: Samii M, Jannetta PJ (eds) The cranial nerves. Springer, Berlin Heidelberg New York, pp 378–390
425. Palacios E, McGee EE (1972) The radiographic diagnosis of trigeminal neurinomas. J Neurosurg 26:153–156
426. Pardal E, Dichmann GH, Insausti T (1972) Neurinoma perforante en el foramen jugular. Prensa Med Argent 59:336–339
427. Parker SW, Davis KR (1977) Limitations of computed tomography in the investigation of acoustic neuromas. Ann Otol Rhinol Laryngol 86:436–440
428. Pearse AGE (1975) Neurocrestopathy, neuroendocrine pathology and APUD concept. Z Krebsforsch 84:1–18
429. Peeters FLM, Westra D, Verbeeten B (1977) Radiological diagnosis of pontine angle tumors. Radiol Clin (Basel) 46:94–108
430. Penley MW, Pribram HFW (1981) Diagnosis of cerebellopontine angle tumors with small quantities of air. Otolaryngol Head Neck Surg 89:457–462
431. Peron DL, Schuknecht H (1975) Congenital cholesteatoma with other anomalies. Arch Otolaryngol 101:499–505
432. Peterson NT, Duchesneau PM, Westbrook EL, Weinstein MA (1977) Basilar artery ectasia demonstrated by computed tomography. Radiology 122:713–715
433. Petit-Dutaillis D, Daum S (1949) Les méningiomes de la fosse postérieure. Premier memoire. Rev Neurol 81:557–572
434. Petit-Dutaillis D, Daum S (1950) Les méningiomes de la fosse postérieure. Deuxième memoire. Rev Neurol 83:241–245
435. Petit-Dutaillis D, Messimy R, Benhain J (1952) A propos du diagnostic des chordomes sphénooccipitaux. Rev Otoneuroophthal 24:202–206
436. Petit-Perrin D, Aubin ML, Vignaud J (1979) Apport de la scanographie au diagnostic des anevrysms géants intracrâniens. J Neuroradiol 6:317–326
437. Peyton WT, Baker AB (1942) Epidermoid, dermoid and teratomatous tumours of the central nervous system. Arch Neurol Psychiatry 47:890–917
438. Phelps PD, Lloyd GAS (1980) The radiology of cholesteatoma. Clin Radiol 31:501–512
439. Phelps PD, Lloyd GAS (1982) High resolution air CT meatography: the demonstration of normal and abnormal structures in the cerebello-pontine cistern and internal auditory meatus. Br J Radiol 55:19–22
440. Picard L, Friot JM, Roland J, Sigiel M, Wayoff M (1976) L'embolisation des chemodectomes jugulo-tympaniques. Ann Otol Laryngol 93:263–274
441. Pineda A (1964) Submicroscopic structure of acoustic tumors. Neurology 14:171–184

442. Pinto RS, Kricheff II, Butler AR, Murali R (1979) Correlation of computed tomographic, angiographic and neuropathological changes in giant cerebral aneurysms. Radiology 132:85–92
443. Pinto R, Kricheff II, Bergeron RT, Cohen N (1981) The diagnosis of small acoustic neuromas by gas computed tomography cisternography and canalography. In: Felix R, Kazner E, Wegener OH (eds) Contrast media in computed tomography. ICS 561, Excerpta Medica, pp 165–170
444. Pinto RS, Kricheff II, Bergeron RT, Cohen N (1982) Small acoustic neuromas: Detection by high resolution gas CT cisternography. AJNR 3:283–286
445. Pluchino F, Crivelli G, Vaghi MA (1975) Intracranial neurinomas of the nerves of the jugular foramen. Report of 12 personal cases. Acta Neurochir 31:201–221
446. Podlas H, Snyckers FD (1980) Atypical intracranial meningiomas. S Afr Med J 57:85–90
447. Poirier J, Escourolle R, Castaigne P (1968) Les neurofibromes de la maladie de Recklinghausen. Acta Neuropathol 10:279–294
448. Pool JL, Pava AA (1957) The early diagnosis and treatment of acoustic nerve tumors. Thomas, Springfield
449. Pool JL, Pava AA, Greenfield EC (1970) Acoustic nerve tumors: Early diagnosis and treatment. 2nd ed, Thomas, Springfield
450. Poppen JL, King AB (1952) Chordoma. Experience with thirteen cases. J Neurosurg 9: 139–163
451. Porta C (1954) Contributi della stratigrafia alla diagnosis dei tumori della base cranica. Neurone 12:57–71
452. Porter RJ, Eyster EF (1973) Aneurysms in the anterior inferior cerebellar artery at the internal acoustic meatus. report of a case. Surg Neurol 1:27–28
453. Prasher DK, Gibson WP (1983) Brainstem auditory-evoked potentials and electrocochleography: comparison of different criteria for the detection of acoustic neuroma and other cerebello-pontine angle tumors. Br J Audiol 17:163–174
454. Psenner L (1963) Über tumorbedingte Destruktionsprozesse der Pyramiden. Radiologe 3:87–99
455. Psenner L (1963) Das Röntgenbild der Meningiome des Schläfenbeines. In: Diethelm L, Strnad F (eds) Die Röntgendiagnostik des Schläfenbeines. Handbuch der medizinischen Radiologie. Röntgendiagnostik des Schädels II. Springer, Berlin Göttingen Heidelberg, vol VII/2, pp 571–573
456. Pulec JL, House WF, Britton BH, Hitselberger WE (1971) A system of management of acoustic neuroma based on 364 cases. Trans Am Acad Ophthalm Otol 75:48–55
457. Pulec JL (1972) Facial nerve neuroma. Laryngoscope 82:1160–1176
458. Pullen FW (1977) The use of computerized tomography in otolaryngology. Trans Am Acad Ophthalm Otol 84:622–627
459. Pullicino P, Kendall BE, Jakubowski J (1980) Difficulties in diagnosis of intracranial meningiomas by computed tomography. J Neurol Neurosurg Psychiatry 43:1022–1029
460. Ramsey RG, Huckman MS (1977) Computed tomography of porencephaly and other cerebrospinal fluid-containing lesions. Radiology 123:73–77
461. Rand CW, Reeves DL (1943) Dermoid and epidermoid tumors (cholesteatomas) of the central nervous system: report of twenty-three cases. Arch Surg 46:350–376
462. Raney RB, Raney AA, Bayless AE (1954) Tumors of hypoglossal nerve: report of case. Bull Los Angeles Neurol Soc 19:160–165
463. Rao KG, Woodlief RM (1979) CT simulation of cerebellopontine tumor by tortuous vertebrobasilar artery. AJR 132:672–673
464. Rasdolsky L (1936) Zur Frage der Klinik der Meningeome der hinteren Schädelgrube. Z Ges Neurol Psychiat 156:211
465. Rausch FJ (1956) Typische Knochenveränderungen an der Schädelbasis beim Neurinom des Nervus V und XII. Acta Neurochir 4:433–447
466. Rausch F, Rembold F (1956) Zur Röntgendiagnostik der Acusticusneurinome. RÖFO 84:702
467. Reidy J, Lacey GJ, Wignall BK, Uttley D (1975) The accuracy of plain radiographs in the diagnosis of acoustic neuromas. Neuroradiology 10:31–34

468. Remaggi PL (1951) Cordoma primitivo della rocca petrosa a lunghissimo decorso (18 anni), estrinsecatosi verso la mastoide e la regione postero-laterale del collo. Sua evoluzione in sarcoma. Otolaring Ital 19:249
469. Rengachary SS, Watanabe I, Brackett CE (1978) Pathogenesis of intracranial arachnoid cysts. Surg Neurol 9:139–144
470. Rettinger G, Kalender W, Henschke F (1981) Hochauflösungs-Computertomographie des Felsenbeines. Computertomographie 1:109–116
471. Rettinger G, Haid T, Wigand ME (1981) Die computertomographische Frühdiagnostik des Akustikusneurinomes durch Luftfüllung des inneren Gehörganges. Ein Vergleich zur Meatographie mit öligen Kontrastmitteln. HNO 29:73–78
472. Rettinger G, Wigand ME, Kalender W (1984) Computertomographische Darstellung von Nerven und Gefäßen des Kleinhirnbrückenwinkels. Ergebnisse der Luft-Zisternographie im Vergleich zu intraoperativen Befunden. HNO 32:320–325
473. Revilla GA (1948) Differential diagnosis of tumors of the cerebellopontine recess. Bull Johns Hopk Hosp 83:47
474. Rhoton AL, Kobayashi S, Hollinshead WH (1968) Nervus intermedius. J Neurosurg 29:609–618
475. Rice RP, Holman CB (1963) Roentgenographic manifestations of tumors of the glomus jugulare (chemodectoma). AJR 89:1201–1208
476. Riemenschneider PA, Hopple GD, Brewer D, Jones D, Ecker A (1953) Roentgenographic diagnosis of tumors of glomus jugulare. AJR 69:59–65
477. Robbins B, Marshall WH (1978) Computed tomography of acoustic neurinoma. Radiology 128:367–370
478. Roberson GH, Kleefield J, Ellis G, Taveras JM, Davis KR (1977) Metrizamide enhancement of cerebrospinal fluid for computer tomography. Acta Radiol [Suppl] (Stockh) 355:306–313
479. Robertson HJ, Hatten HP, Keating JW (1983) False positive CT gas cisternogram. AJNR 4:474–477
480. Robinson JS, Lopez J, Moody R (1979) Intracranial hypoglossal neurilemmoma. Surg Neurol 12:496–498
481. Rosenbaum AE, Drayer BP, Dubois PJ, Black O (1978) Visualization of small extracanalicular neurilemmomas by metrizamide cisternographic enhancement. Arch Otolaryngol 104:239–243
482. Rosenbloom SB, Carson BS, Wang H, Rosenbaum AE, Udvarhelyi GB (1985) Cerebellopontine angle lipoma. Surg Neurol 23:134–138
483. Rosenwasser H (1945) Carotid body tumor of the middle ear and mastoid. Arch Otolaryngol 41:64–67
484. Roukkula M (1964) Roentgenologic findings in chondromas of the pontine angle. Acta Radiol (Diagn) 2:120–128
485. Rozario RA, Levine HL, Scott RM (1978) Obstructive hydrocephalus secondary to an ectatic basilar artery. Surg Neurol 9:31–34
486. Rubert R, Carteri A (1961) Neurinomi del foramen lacero posteriore. G Psichiatr Neuropatol 89:1099–1128
487. Rubinstein LJ (1972) Tumors of the central nervous system. Atlas of tumor pathology. Second series, Fasc. 6. Armed Forces Institute of Pathology, Washington D.C., pp 206–212
488. Rucker TN (1963) Radiology of glomus jugulare tumors in the temporal bone. Radiology 81:807–816
489. Ruggiero G, Constans JP (1954) L'artériographie vertébrale. Analyses de 48 cas d'artériographie vertébrale percutanée selon la méthode de Lindgren. Rev Neurol 90: 467–502
490. Ruggiero G (1957) L'Encéphalographie fractionnée. Masson, Paris
491. Ruscalleda J, Guardia E, dos Santos FM, Carvajal A (1980) Dynamic study of arachnoid cysts with metrizamide. Neuroradiology 20:185–189
492. Russell DS, Rubinstein LJ (1977) Pathology of tumours of the nervous system. 4th ed. Arnold, London, pp 66–89
493. Russell EJ, George AE, Kricheff II, Budzilovich G (1980) Atypical computed tomographic features of intracranial meningioma. Radiological-pathological correlation in a series of 131 consecutive cases. Radiology 135:673–682

494. Russell EJ, Koslow M, Lasjaunias P, Bergeron RT, Chase N (1982) Transverse axial plane anatomy of the temporal bone employing high spatial resolution computed tomography. Neuroradiology 22:185–191
495. Sacks JG, Lindburg R (1969) Dolicho-ectatic intracranial arteries: symptomatology and pathogenesis of arterial elongation and distention. Johns Hopk Med J 125:95–106
496. Salah S, Bock FW, Perneczky A, Koos WT, Tschabitscher M (1978) Vascular anatomy of the cerebello-pontine angle. In: Koos WT, Bock FW, Spetzler RF (eds) Microneurosurgery. Thieme, Stuttgart, pp 70–71
497. Salama N, Stafford N (1982) Meningioma presenting in the middle ear. Laryngoscope 92:92–97
498. Salamon GM, Gombalbert A, Raybaud C, Gonzalez J (1971) An angiographic study of meningiomas of the posterior fosa. J Neurosurg 35:731–741
499. Salvolini U, Menichelli F, Pasquini U (1978) Cerebellopontine expansive lesions. In: Baert A, Jeanmart L, Wackenheim A (eds) Clinical computer tomography. Head and trunk. Springer, Berlin Heidelberg New York, pp 79–105
500. Sandifort E (1777) Observationes anatomo-pathologicae. Lugduni Batvarovum. Chap IX, pp 116–120
501. Sarwar M, Swischuk LE, Schechter MM (1976) Intracranial chondromas. AJR 127: 973–977
502. Sarwar M, Batnitzki S, Schechter MM (1976) Tumorous aneurysms. Neuroradiology 12:79–97
503. Scanlan RL (1964) Roentgen diagnosis of acoustic neuroma with particular reference of the use of Pantopaque. Laryngoscope 74:999–1003
504. Schadel A, Thiede G, Galanski M (1982) CT-Diagnostik der Glomus-jugulare-Tumoren. RÖFO 136:291–295
505. Schechter MM, Liebeskind AL, Azar-Kia B (1974) Intracranial chordomas. Neuroradiology 8:67–82
506. Schenk JF, Foster TH, Henkes JL et al. (1985) High-field surface coil MR imaging of localized anatomy. AJNR 6:181–186
507. Schisano G, Olivecrona H (1960) Neurinomas of the Gasserian ganglion and trigeminal root. J Neurosurg 17:306–322
508. Schisano G, Tovi D (1962) Clivus chordomas. Neurochirurgia 5:99–120
509. Schlungbaum W (1959) Zur Röntgendiagnostik des Acusticusneurinoms. Radiol Clin (Basel) 28:139–149
510. Schmerler M, Sandok BA, McDonald TJ, Houser W, MacCarty CS (1978) The clinical diagnosis of acoustic neuroma. Neurology 28:361
511. Schmidt C (1930) Neurinom des N. facialis. Zentralbl Hals-Nas-Ohrenheilkd 16:329
512. Schörner W, Felix R, Claussen C, Fiegler W, Kazner E, Niendorf HP (1984) Kernspintomographische Diagnostik von Hirntumoren mit dem Kontrastmittel Gadolinium-DTPA. RÖFO 141:511–516
513. Schubiger O, Valavanis A, Wichmann W (in press) Growth-mechanism of giant intracranial aneurysms: demonstration by CT and MR imaging. Neuroradiology
514. Schubiger O (1976) Die radiologischen Untersuchungen in der Otologie. Schweiz Med Wochenschr 106:677–682
515. Schubiger O, Valavanis A, Hayek J (1978) Computed tomography for small acoustic neuromas. Neuroradiology 15:287–290
516. Schubiger O, Valavanis A, Hayek J (1980) Computed tomography in cerebral aneurysms with special emphasis on giant intracranial aneurysms. J Comput Ass Tomogr 4:24–32
517. Schubiger O, Valavanis A (1982) Die hochauflösende Computertomographie zum Nachweis von Frakturen der Schädelbasis, besonders der Felsenbeine. RÖFO 137: 123–128
518. Schubiger O, Valavanis A, Gessaga E (1983) Dense suprasellar epidermoid cyst. Neuroradiology 24:269–271
519. Schubiger O, Valavanis A (1985) Specific CT-signs of meningioma of the cerebellopontine angle (abstr). Neuroradiology 27:377
520. Schüller A (1905) Die Schädelbasis im Röntgenbilde. RÖFO, Suppl 11
521. Schüller A (1928) Röntgendiagnose der Acusticustumoren. In: Ergebnisse der medizinischen Strahlenforschung. Vol 3, Springer, Berlin

522. Scott M, Wycis HT (1949) Intracranial neurinoma of hypoglossal nerve. Successful removal: Case report. J Neurosurg 6:333–336
523. Scotti G, De Grandi C, Colombo A (1978) Ectasia of the intracranial arteries diagnosed by computed tomography. Megadolichobasilar artery: CT diagnosis. Neuroradiology 15: 183–184
524. Sekhar LN, Janetta PJ (1984) Cerebellopontine angle meningioma. Microsurgical excision and follow-up results. J Neurosurg 60:500–505
525. Selters WA, Brackman DE (1977) Acoustic tumor detection with brain stem electric response audiometry. Arch Otolaryngol 103:181–187
526. Servo A, Porras M, Jääskinen J (1981) Metrizamide cisternography in the diagnosis of acoustic neurinomas. Neuroradiology 21:37–41
527. Shaffer KA, Volz DJ, Haughton VM (1980) Manipulation of CT data for temporal-bone imaging. Radiology 137:825–829
528. Shaffer KA, Haughton VM, Wilson CR (1980) High resolution computed tomography of the temporal bone. Radiology 134:409–414
529. Sheehy JL, Inzer BE (1976) Acoustic reflex test in neurootologic diagnosis: A review of 24 cases of acoustic tumors. Arch Otolaryngol 102:647–653
530. Shiffman F, Dancer J, Rothballer AB, Berrett A, Baum S (1973) The diagnosis and evaluation of acoustic neuromas. Otolaryngol Clin North Am 6:189–228
531. Sicard, Forestier (1922) Méthode générale d'exploration radiologique par l'huile iodée (Lipiodol). Bull Soc méd Hôp Paris 46:463–469
532. Singh KP, Smyth GDL, Gordon DS (1978) The diagnosis of acoustic neurinoma. A retrospective study. J Laryngol Otol 92:1–7
533. Sjögren SE (1953) Percutaneous vertebral angiography. Acta Radiol (Stockh) 40:113–127
534. Skalpe IO (1977) Adverse effects of water soluble contrast media in myelography, cisternography and ventriculography. A special review with reference to metrizamide. Acta Radiol [Suppl] (Stockh) 335:359
535. Sobel D, Norman D, Yorke CH, Newton TH (1980) Radiography of trigeminal neuralgia and hemifacial spasm. AJR 135:93–95
536. Sortland O (1979) Computed tomography combined with gas cisternography for the diagnosis of expanding lesions in the cerebellopontine angle. Neuroradiology 18:19–22
537. Spector GJ, Druck NS, Gado M (1976) Neurologic manifestations of glomus tumors in the head and neck. Arch Neurol 33:270–274
538. Starkman SP, Brown TC, Linell EA (1958) Cerebral arachnoid cysts. J Neuropathol Exp Neurol 17:484–500
539. Steinhoff H, Ambrose J (1981) Neurinome. In: Dietemann L, Heuck F, Olsson O, Strnad F, Vieten H, Zuppinger A (eds) Computertomographie des Gehirns. Handbuch der medizinischen Radiologie, vol 14, part 1B. Springer, Berlin Heidelberg New York, pp 314–318
540. Steinhoff H, Ambrose J (1981) Computertomographie des Gehirns. In: Diethelm L, Heuck F, Olsson O, Strnad F, Vieten H, Zuppinger A (eds) Röntgendiagnostik des Zentralnervensystems. Handbuch der medizinischen Radiologie, vol 14, part 1B. Springer, Berlin Heidelberg New York, pp 305–314
541. Stenvers HW (1917) Roentgenology of the os petrosum. Arch Radiol Electrol 22:97–112
542. Stenvers HW (1928) Röntgenologie des Felsenbeines und des bitemporalen Schädelbildes. Springer, Berlin
543. Stopford JSB (1916) The arteries of the pons and medulla oblongata. J Anat Physiol 50:131–164
544. Strickler JM (1966) New and simple techniques for demonstration of the jugular foramen. AJR 97:601–606
545. Strong RR (1967) Intracranial neurinoma of the hypoglossal nerve. Aust N Z J Surg 37:187–198
546. Sunderland S (1958) The tentorial notch and complications produced by herniations of the brain through that aperture. Br J Surg 45:422–438
547. Sutton D (1971) The vertebro-basilar system and its vascular lesions. Clin Radiol 22: 271–287
548. Suzuki S, Yamaguchi K, Sakai H et al. (1977) Intracranial neurinoma of the jugular foramen. Report of a case and review of references. Its clinical manifestations. Neurol Surg 5:379–384 (Jpn)

549. Svien HJ, Baker HL, Rivers MH (1963) Jugular foramen syndrome and allied syndromes. Neurology 13:797–809
550. Tadmor R, Davis KR, Roberson GH, New PFJ, Taveras JM (1977) Computed tomography in extradural epidermoid and xanthoma. Surg Neurol 7:371–375
551. Takahashi M, Wilson G, Hanafee W (1968) The anterior inferior cerebellar artery: its radiographic anatomy and significance in the diagnosis of extra-axial tumors of the posterior fossa. Radiology 90:281–287
552. Takahashi M, Okudera T, Tomanaga M, Kitamuva K (1971) Angiographic diagnosis of acoustic neurinomas: Analysis of 30 lesions. Neuroradiology 2:191–200
553. Takahashi M (1974) Atlas of vertebral angiography. Urban und Schwarzenberg, Müchen Berlin Wien
554. Takahashi M (1974) The anterior inferior cerebellar artery. In: Newton TH, Potts DG (eds) Radiology of the skull and brain. Mosby, St. Louis, vol 2, Book 2, pp 1796–1808
555. Tans JTJ, de Jongh IE (1977) Computed tomography of supratentorial menigioma. Clin Neurol Neurosurg 80:10–21
556. Tänzer A (1969) Die Veränderungen am Tuberculum jugulare bei raumbeschränkenden Prozessen im Kleinhirnbrückenwinkel. Radiologe 9:484
557. Taveras JM, Ransohoff J (1953) Leptomeningeal cysts of the brain following trauma with erosion of the skull. J Neurosurg 10:233–241
558. Taveras JM, Wood EH (1976) Diagnostic Neuroradiology. 2nd Ed. Williams and Wilkins, Baltimore
559. Taylor S (1982) Petrous temporal bone (including the cerebellopontine angle). Radiol Clin North Am 20:67–86
560. Terbrugge K, Scotti G, Ethier R, Melançon D, Tchang S, Milner C (1977) Computed tomography in intracranial arteriovenous malformations. Radiology 122:703–705
561. Théron J, Lasjaunias P (1976) Participation of the external and internal carotid arteries in the blood supply of acoustic neurinomas. Radiology 118:83–88
562. Thomsen J, Klinken L, Tos M (1984) Calcified acoustic neurinoma. J Laryngol Otol 98:727–732
563. Thomson JLG (1978) Computerised axial tomography in posterior fossa lesions. Clin Radiol 29:233–250
564. Thron A, Bockenheimer S (1979) Giant aneurysms of the posterior fossa suspected as neoplasms on computed tomography. Neuroradiology 18:93–97
565. Tonelli L (1950) I tumori della notocorda. Arch Anat Path 15:471–497
566. Toynbee (1853) Neuroma of the auditory nerve. Transact Path Soc London 4:259
567. Tridon P, Masingue M, Picard L, Briquel F, Roland J (1971) Hémispasme facial et mégadolichobasilaire à symptomatologie pseudotumorale. Rev Otoneuroophthalmol 43:279–286
568. Turner JS, Saudners AZ, Farrell J (1980) Audimetric and radiologic findings in acoustic tumor. South Med J 73:3–5
569. Tytus JS, Pennybacker J (1956) Pearly tumors in relation to the central nervous system. J Neurol Neurosurg Psychiatry 19:241–259
570. Ulrich J (1964) Intracranial epidermoids. A study on their distribution and spread. J Neurosurg 21:1051–1058
571. Ulsø C, Sehested P, Overgaard J (1981) Intracranial hypoglossal neurinoma: diagnosis and postoperative care. Surg Neurol 16:65–68
572. Utne JR, Pugh DG (1955) The roentgenologic aspects of chordoma. AJR 74:593–608
573. Valavanis A, Schubiger O, Wellauer J (1978) Computed tomography of acoustic neuromas with emphasis on small tumor detectability. Neuroradiology 16:598–600
574. Valavanis A (1981) Der Beitrag der Computertomographie zur Diagnostik des Akustikus-neurinomes. Thesis. Juris, Zürich
575. Valavanis A, Schubiger O, Hayek J, Pouliadis G (1981) CT of meningiomas on the posterior surface of the petrous bone. Neuroradiology 22:111–121
576. Valavanis A, Imhof HG, Klaiber R, Dabir K (1981) The diagnosis of solitary primary reticulum cell sarcoma of the posterior fossa with computed tomography. Neuroradiology 21:213–217
577. Valavanis A, Dabir K, Hamdi R, Oguz M, Wellauer J (1982) The current state of the radiological diagnosis of acoustic neuroma. Neuroradiology 23:7–13

578. Valavanis A, Kubik S, Schubiger O (1983) The normal and abnormal Fallopian canal on high-resolution CT. AJNR 4:748–751
579. Valavanis A, Fisch U (1983) The contribution of computed tomography in the management of glomus tumors of the temporal bone. Rev Laryngol 104:411–415
580. Valavanis A, Schubiger O, Oguz M (1983) High-resolution CT investigation of non-chromaffin paragangliomas of the temporal bone. AJNR 4:516–519
581. Valentin G (1840) Über eine gangliöse Anschwellung in der Jacobsonschen Anastomose des Menschen. Arch f Anat Physiol u wissensch Medicin Leipzig 287–290
582. Valvassori GE (1966) The radiological diagnosis of acoustic neuromas. Arch Otolaryngol 83:582–587
583. Valvassori GE (1966) The contribution of radiology to the diagnosis of acoustic neuroma. Laryngoscope 76:1104–1112
584. Valvassori GE, Kirdani HA (1967) The abnormal hypoglossal canal. AJR 99:705–711
585. Valvassori GE (1969) The abnormal internal auditory canal. The diagnosis of acoustic neuroma. Radiology 92:449–459
586. Valvassori GE (1969) The diagnosis of acoustic neuromas. Sem Roentgenol 4:171–177
587. Valvassori GE (1973) The diagnosis of acoustic neuromas. Otolaryngol Clin North Am 6:391–400
588. Valvassori GE (1973) Tomography of the internal auditory canal. In: Berrett A, Brünner S, Valvassori GE (eds) Modern thin-section tomography. CC Thomas, Springfield
589. Valvassori GE, Mafee MF, Dobben GD (1981) Evaluation of the regional blood circulation of the hindbrain by dynamic computed tomography. Laryngoscope 10:1695–1701
590. Valvassori GE, Buckingham RA (1982) Internal auditory canal and acoustic neuroma. In: Valvassori GE, Potter GD, Hanafee WN, Carter BL, Buckingham RA (eds) Radiology of the ear, nose and throat. Part 1: Radiology of the temporal bone. Thieme, Stuttgart New York, pp 95–107
591. Valvassori GE, Buckingham RA (1982) Radiography of the facial canal. In: Valvassori GE, Potter GD, Hanafee WN, Carter BL, Buckingham RA (eds) Radiology of the ear, nose and throat. Thieme, Stuttgart New York, pp 118–123
592. Valvassori GE, Mafee MF, Dobben GD (1982) Computerized tomography of the temporal bone. Laryngoscope 92:562–565
593. Vaquero J, Carrillo R, Cabezudo JM, Nombela L, Bravo G (1981) Arachnoid cysts of the posterior fossa. Surg Neurol 16:117–121
594. Vassilouthis J, Ambrose J (1979) Computerized tomography scanning appearances of intracranial meningiomas. J Neurosurg 50:320–327
595. Verbiest H (1962) Arterial aneurysms and arteriovenous aneurysms of the posterior fossa. Psychiat Neurol Neurochir 65:329–369
596. Vignaud J, Aubin ML, Balériaux-Waha D, Jeanmart L (1980) CT scan diagnosis of lesions causing an angle or internal auditory canal syndrome. J Belge Radiol 63:295–311
597. Virchow R (1858) Das wahre Neurom. Arch Path Anat 13:256–265
598. Vonderrahe AR, Niemer WT (1951) Intracranial lipoma: Report of 4 cases. J Neuropathol Clin Neurol 1:168–178
599. Wackenheim A, Metzger J (1962) Etude radiologique des altérations osseuses des 65 cas de néoformation de l'angle ponto-cérébelleux. J Radiol Electrol 43:860–871
600. Wackenheim A, Braun JP (1978) Angiographie der Kleinhirnbrückenwinkel-Tumoren. In: Plester D, Wende S, Nakayama N (eds) Kleinhirnbrückenwinkel-Tumoren. Diagnostik und Therapie. Springer, Berlin Heidelberg New York, pp 165–188
601. Wackenheim A, Megret M (1981) Die Diagnose der infratentoriellen Tumoren durch die Vertebralisangiographie. In: Diethelm L, Heuck F, Olsson O, Strnad F, Vieten H, Zuppinger A (eds) Röntgendiagnostik des Zentralnervensystems. Handbuch der medizinischen Radiologie, vol 14, part 1B. Springer, Berlin Heidelberg New York, pp 99–140
602. Watt JC, McKillop AN (1935) Relation of arteries to roots of nerves in posterior cranial fossa in man. Arch Surg 30:336–345
603. Weinberg PE, Kim KS, Gore RM (1981) Unilateral enlargement of the internal auditory canal: A developmental variant. Surg Neurol 15:39–42
604. Weitbrecht W-U, Schumacher M, Thoden U, Kleine W (1977) Spindelförmiges Basilarisaneurysma mit Symptomen eines basalen Tumors. Nervenarzt 48:688–691

605. Wellauer J (1969) Jod-Oel-Diagnostik der hinteren Schädelgrube. Radiologe 9:477–481
606. Wells HG (1922) Intracranial aneurysms of the vertebral artery. Arch Neurol Psychiatry 1:311
607. Wende S, Lüdecke B (1971) Technique and value of gas and pantopaque cisternography in the diagnosis of cerebellopontine angle tumors. Neuroradiology 2:24–29
608. Wende S, Nakayama N (1972) Die neuroradiologische Diagnostik des Kleinhirnbrückenwinkeltumors. Z Neurol 203:1–12
609. Wende S, Nakayama N, Schwerdtfeger P (1975) The internal auditory artery (embryology, anatomy, angiography, pathology). Z Neurol 210:21–31
610. Wende S, Nakayama N (1975) The diagnostic value of serial magnification angiography for the representation of vessels in the posterior cranial fossa. In: Kitamara K, Newton TH (eds) Recent advances in diagnostic neuroradiology. Igabu Shoin, Tokyo, pp 71–80
611. Wende S, Nakayama N (1978) Zisternographie mit negativen und positiven Kontrastmitteln. In: Plester D, Wende S, Nakayama N (eds) Kleinhirnbrückenwinkel-Tumoren. Diagnostik und Therapie. Springer, Berlin Heidelberg New York, pp 162–166
612. Wende S (1980) Die kombinierte Anwendung von Computertomographie und Luftzisternographie bei Kleinhirnbrückenwinkeltumoren. RÖFO 132:666–667
613. Wende S (1981) Cerebral computed tomography: Overview. In: Donner MW, Hench FHW (eds) Radiology today. Springer, Berlin Heidelberg New York, pp 377–381
614. Westberg G (1963) Angiographic changes in neurinoma of the trigeminal nerve. Acta Radiol (Diagn) 1:513–520
615. Wickbom I (1953) Angiographic determination of tumour pathology. Acta Radiol (Stockh) 40:529–546
616. Williams JM, Fox JL (1962) Neurinoma of the intracranial portion of the hypoglossal nerve. Review and case report. J Neurosurg 19:248–250
617. Wilner HI, Fenton JL, Eyler WR, Knighton RS (1970) Tomographic evaluation of the internal auditory canal using positive contrast material. Radiology 95:95–99
618. Wilner HI (1970) The neuroradiologist and the ear. AJR 110:190–191
619. Wilner HI, Austin D (1975) Magnification angiography. Identifying the capsular vasculature of acoustic neuromas. AJR 123:31–35
620. Witten RM, Wade CT (1979) Computed tomography in acoustic tumor diagnosis. In: House WF, Luetje CM (eds) Acoustic tumors, vol 1: Diagnosis. University Park Press, Baltimore, pp 253–277
621. Wollschlaeger G, Wollschlaeger PB, Lucas FV, Lopez VF (1967) Experience and results with postmortem cerebral angiography as a routine procedure of the autopsy. AJR 101: 68–87
622. Wolpert SM (1976) Angiography of posterior fossa tumors. Grune & Stratton, New York San Francisco London
623. Wolpert SM, Scott RM (1981) The value of metrizamide CT cisternography in the management of cerebral arachnoid cysts. AJNR 2:29–35
624. Yamaguchi H, Tozuka G, Yoshimoto H et al. (1975) Extension of a jugular foramen neurinoma into the external auditory canal. J Otolaryngol 78:962–963 (Jpn)
625. Yaşargil MG (1957) Vertebralisangiographie, In: Schinz HR, Glauner R, Uehlinger E (eds) Röntgendiagnostik. Ergebnisse 1952–1956. Thieme, Stuttgart, pp 282–306
626. Yaşargil MG, Fisch U (1969) Unsere Erfahrungen in der mikrochirurgischen Exstirpation der Akustikusneurinome. Arch Ohr-Nas-Kehlk-Heilk 194:243–247
627. Yaşargil MG, Fox JL (1974) The microsurgical approach to acoustic neurinomas. Surg Neurol 2:393–398
628. Yaşargil MG, So SC (1976) Cerebellopontine angle meningioma presenting as subarachnoid hemorrhage. Surg Neurol 6:3–6
629. Yaşargil MG (1978) Mikrochirurgie der Kleinhirnbrückenwinkel-Tumoren. In: Plester D, Wende S, Nakayama N (eds) Kleinhirnbrückenwinkel-Tumoren. Diagnostik und Therapie. Springer, Berlin Heidelberg New York, pp 215–257
630. Yaşargil MG, Mortara RW, Curcic M (1980) Meningiomas of basal posterior cranial fossa. Adv Technic Standards Neurosurg 7:3–115
631. Yaskin HE, Alpers B (1944) Aneurysms of the vertebral artery. Report of a case in which the aneurysm simulated a tumor of the posterior fossa. Arch Neurol Psychiatry 51:271–281

632. Yonemitsu T, Niizuma H, Kodama N, Fujiwara S, Suzuki J (1983) Acoustic neurinoma presenting as subarachnoid hemorrhage. Surg Neurol 20:125–130
633. Young IR, Burl M, Clarke GJ, Hall AS, Pasmore T, Collins AG, Smith DT, Orr JS, Bydder GM, Doyle FH, Greenspan RH, Steiner RE (1981) Magnetic resonance properties of hydrogen: imaging the posterior fossa. AJNR 2:487–493
634. Zaunbauer W (1952) Zur Röntgendiagnostik der Acusticustumoren. Wien Arch Psychol 2:166
635. Zimmerman RA, Bilaniuk LT (1978) Computed tomography of vertebrobasilar artery aneurysm. J Comput Tomogr 2:39–48
636. Zimmerman RA, Bilaniuk LT, Bruno L, Rosenstock J (1978) Computed tomography of cerebellar astrocytoma. AJR 130:929–933
637. Zimmerman RA, Bilaniuk LT, Pahlajani H (1978) Spectrum of medulloblastomas demonstrated by computed tomography. Radiology 126:137–141
638. Zimmermann RD, Russell EJ, Leeds NE (1980) Axial CT recognition of anteroposterior displacement of fourth ventricle. AJNR 1:65–70
639. Zimmerman RD, Fleming CA, Saint-Louis FA, Lee BCP, Manning JJ, Deck MDF (1985) Magnetic resonance imaging of meningiomas. AJNR 6:149–157
640. Zülch KJ (1956) Pathologische Anatomie der raumbeengenden intrakraniellen Prozesse. Handbuch der Neurologie, vol 3. Springer, Berlin Göttingen Heidelberg
641. Zülch KJ (1975) Atlas of gross neurosurgical pathology. Springer, Berlin Heidelberg New York

Subject Index

Abducens nerve 100
palsy 100, 138
Accessory nerve 15, 24, 33
neurinoma 30, 117, 121ff.
palsy 33, 107, 121
Acoustic meatus (see internal auditory canal)
Acoustic neurinoma 1, 2, 3, 28, 30, 32ff., 61, 63, 86, 96, 99, 111, 121, 122, 125, 126, 130, 156ff.
intracanalicular 1, 3, 36, 51, 54ff., 63, 127, 156, 163
medial type 2, 34, 35, 51, 54, 63, 65, 99, 125, 137
Acute angle sign 50
Adenoma, pituitary 147
Adhesion 80
Air CT cisternography (see gas CT cisternography)
Anatomy 10ff.
on angiography 21f.
on CT 13ff.
on gas CT cisternography 19
on magnetic resonance imaging 153ff.
on positive-contrast CT cisternography 19
Aneurysm 9, 30, 31, 131f.
giant 99, 132ff., 141
Angiography 1, 2, 3
of acoustic neurinoma 36
of aneurysm 132f.
of arachnoid cyst 89
of arteriovenous malformation 143
of chemodectoma 108, 116, 121
of chordoma 100
of epidermoid 77
of hypoglossal neurinoma 118, 121
of jugular foramen neurinoma 122
of megadolichobasilar anomaly 138, 141
of meningioma 61
of trigeminal neurinoma 95
Antoni-types of neurinoma 45, 55, 118, 156
APUD system 107
Aqueduct 29, 34
Arachnoid cluster cells 60
Arachnoid cyst 6, 30, 78, 86, 89ff., 156
Arachnoiditis 7, 35, 57, 89
Arnold's nerve 107
Arteriovenous malformation 9, 30, 31, 131, 142ff., 170
Artery
anterior inferior cerebellar 2, 4, 13, 15, 19, 21f., 36, 55, 57, 58, 95, 108, 118, 122, 153
ascending pharyngeal 24, 38, 61, 96, 108, 118, 143, 153
auricular 143
basilar 21, 36, 48, 95
internal auditory 32
internal carotid 38, 61, 96, 100, 108, 118, 138, 143
internal maxillary 108
middle meningeal 38, 61, 96, 108, 143
occipital 38, 61, 108, 143
posterior cerebral 36, 95
posterior inferior cerebellar 4, 36, 108, 118, 122
stylomastoid 108
superior cerebellar 95, 96
vertebral 38, 100, 118, 138, 143
Astrocytoma 94, 147
Ataxia 34, 121
Atherosclerosis 138
Atrophy
cerebellar 86
of the masticatory muscles 33
of the tongue 34, 109, 118
peritumoral 38, 42, 65, 136
Audiometry 34

Beam hardening artifact 6, 13, 55
Bell's palsy 126
Bill's bar 23
Bleeding (see hemorrhage)
Blood-brain-barrier 26, 46
Blush (see tumor blush)
Bone erosion 28, 38
in acoustic neurinoma 3, 35, 51ff., 99
in aneurysm 132, 136
in arachnoid cyst 89, 91
in arteriovenous malformation 143
in chemodectoma 108ff., 122, 125
in chordoma 100, 102
in epidermoid tumor 77, 86
in facial nerve neurinoma 127f.

Bone erosion
  in hypoglossal neurinoma 118
  in jugular foramen neurinoma 122, 125
  in meningioma 61, 66, 99, 116, 121
  in metastasis 147
  in trigeminal neurinoma 95f.
Brainstem 28, 80
Bulbar palsy 138

Calcification 4
  in acoustic neurinoma 50, 66
  in aneurysm 132, 133, 136, 137
  in chemodectoma 114
  in chondroma 66
  in chordoma 66, 100, 106, 125, 168
  in epidermoid tumor 77, 78
  in lipoma 86
  in megadolichobasilar anomaly 138, 140
  in meningioma 61, 65f., 74, 116
  in ossifying hemangioma 130
  in trigeminal neurinoma 96
Caloric vestibular testing (see vestibular testing)
Canaliculus tympanicus 107
Capsular vein (see vein, capsular)
Carcinoma
  nasopharyngeal 147
  of the middle ear 147
  squamous cell 77
Carotid canal 24, 100, 109
Caudal nerve neurinoma 116, 117ff.
  (see also hypoglossal neurinoma and jugular foramen neurinoma)
Cauliflower appearance 77, 86
Cerebellar symptoms (see symptoms, cerebellar)
Cerebellum 10, 15, 21, 24, 27, 28, 34, 50, 80, 110, 114, 137, 156
Ceruminoma 30, 147
Chemodectoma 29, 30, 31, 102, 106, 107ff., 118, 121, 125, 147, 170
Cholesteatoma, primary 86f., 126, 147
Cholesterin 77, 78, 84
Chondroma 30, 66, 10
Chondrosarcoma 147
Chorda dorsalis 100
Chordoma 30, 31, 66, 100ff., 116, 125, 147, 168
Choroid plexus (see fourth ventricle)
Cistern
  ambient 13, 28, 39, 73
  cerebellomedullary, lateral 28, 83, 102, 110, 117, 122
    anatomy 13, 15, 24
  interpeduncular 138, 140
  pontocerebellar 27, 30, 32, 35, 50, 56, 60, 80, 89, 95, 102, 107, 117, 120, 126, 140, 153
    anatomy 10ff., 18ff., 21, 22
    obliteration 27, 28, 39
    widening 27f., 39
  prepontine 13, 80, 140
  quadrigeminal plate 26, 29, 73
Classification of
  acoustic neurinomas 38
  aneurysms 131, 132, 136
  arachnoid cysts 91f.
  arteriovenous malformations 143
  caudal nerve neurinomas 117
  chemodectomas 108ff.
  chordomas 100
  facial nerve neurinomas 126
  jugular foramen neurinomas 121
  trigeminal neurinomas 95
Clinoid process 26, 95
Clivus 15, 100, 102
  erosion 91
Cochlear nerve (see vestibulocochlear nerve)
Comma sign 73
Contrast enhancement 4, 22, 26, 28
  in acoustic neurinoma 42ff., 55, 163
  in aneurysm 133, 136
  in arachnoid cyst 89
  in arteriovenous malformation 143
  in cavernous hemangioma 130
  in chemodectoma 102, 106, 108, 114, 121, 170
  in chordoma 102
  in epidermoid tumor 70, 78
  in facial nerve neurinoma 127
  in hypoglossal neurinoma 118
  in jugular foramen neurinoma 122
  in magnetic resonance imaging 156, 163, 168, 170
  in megadolichobasilar anomaly 140
  in meningioma 61, 168
  in trigeminal neurinoma 96
Corneal reflex 33
Corpus callosum 26
Cranial nerve (see nerve, cranial)
Crest
  falciform 23, 35, 51
  inferior vertical 23
Cribriform plate 22, 23
Crow's foot deformity 23, 38
Cyst 38, 46, 66, 118
  entrapment 66

Dandy Walker cyst 89
Deafness (see hearing loss)
Dementia 138
Desmoid fibroma (see fibroma, desmoid)
Dizziness 33
Dumbbell neurinoma
  hypoglossal 117
  trigeminal 95, 99

Dura mater 23, 30, 63, 87, 114, 120, 136
Dynamic CT 8f., 48, 62, 116, 132, 133, 136, 137

Ectasia of the basilar artery (see megadolicho-basilar anomaly)
Edema, perilesional 28, 42, 65, 84, 96, 136, 142
Electronystagmography 33, 34
Embolization 108
Encasement, vascular 77, 83, 86, 100
Encephalography (see pneumoencephalography)
Entrapment cyst (see cyst, entrapment)
Ependymoma 31, 147
Epidermoid tumor 6, 30, 77ff., 94, 99, 137, 168
Epileptic seizure (see seizure, epileptic)
Exostosis 60, 61, 66, 72, 168

Facial canal 128
Facial musculature 33
Facial nerve 4, 7, 13, 19, 21, 22, 23, 33, 55, 59, 72, 74, 152, 153
  neurinoma 30, 58, 126ff.
  palsy 33, 77, 87, 121, 126, 131, 138
Facial spasm (see spasm, facial)
Falciform crest (see crest, falciform)
Falx 26
Fibroma, desmoid 99
Fistula, arteriovenous 143
Flocculus 13, 15, 21
Flow void signal loss 170
Foramen
  lacerum 110
  Magendi 89
  magnum 4, 31, 83, 120
  of Luschka 89
  of Monro 142
  ovale 95, 96, 102
Fourth ventricle 15, 89, 93, 147
  choroid plexus of 15
  compression 34, 39, 72, 91
  dilatation 86
  displacement 28, 38f., 91

Gadolinium-DTPA 156, 163, 170
Gag reflex 33
Gait disturbance 33, 138
Gas CT cisternography 3, 152, 163
  anatomy 7, 19, 21, 22
  in acoustic neurinoma 55ff.
  in aneurysm 132
  in arteriovenous malformation 143
  in cavernous hemangioma 130
  in facial nerve neurinoma 127
  in hemangioma 59
  in meningioma 74
Gasserian ganglion 95, 99
Geniculate ganglion 60, 87, 126, 128
Giant aneurysm (see aneurysm, giant)
Glioma 147
Gliosis 80
Glomus structures 107
Glomus tumor (see chemodectoma)
Glossopharyngeal nerve 15, 24, 33, 107
  neurinoma 30, 116, 117, 121ff.
  palsy 33, 107, 121, 138
Granuloma, intrapetrous 87
Growth
  supratentorial 26
  transincisural 28, 29, 73
  transtentorial 29, 73, 74

Headache 7, 8, 34, 117, 121, 138
Hearing loss 1, 32, 33, 34, 77, 107, 121, 126, 131, 138
Hemangioblastoma 28, 94, 147
Hemangioma 30, 58, 59, 126, 130
  ossifying 130
Hematoma 28
  subdural 86
Hemisphere, cerebellar (see cerebellum)
Hemorrhage
  intratumoral 32, 38, 46, 61
  subarachnoid 46, 131, 132
Herniation, transincisural 38
Herpes zoster oticus 126
Hiatus trigeminus (see porus trigeminus)
High resolution CT 5, 8, 19, 51, 66, 108, 118, 122, 128, 143
Hoarseness 33
Hounsfield artifact 6, 13
Hydrocephalus 29, 34, 38, 39, 72, 84, 89, 137, 138, 141f.
Hygroma 78, 86
Hyperostosis 4, 28, 54, 61, 66, 116
Hypertensive leukoencephalopathy (see leukoencephalopathy, hypertensive)
Hypervascularity 36
Hypoacousis (see hearing loss)
Hypodensity, peritumoral (see edema, perilesional)
Hypoglossal canal 24, 109, 118
  erosion 109
  widening 109, 118, 121
Hypoglossal nerve 34
  neurinoma 116, 117ff., 122
  palsy 34, 117
Hypotympanic bone plate 24, 109
Hypotympanum 24, 109

Incisura tentorii 4, 28, 29, 80, 84
anatomy 26
Inferior vertical crest (see crest, inferior vertical)
Insufficiency, vertebrobasilar 9
Intermediate nerve 13, 19, 21, 22, 33
Internal auditory canal 2, 13, 18, 24, 32, 34, 60, 126, 153
anatomy 22ff.
empty 54
in acoustic neurinoma 35, 50, 51ff., 56ff.
in aneurysm 132
in chemodectoma 110f.
in chordoma 100
in epidermoid tumor 86
in facial nerve neurinoma 128, 130
in jugular foramen neurinoma 122
in megadolichobasilar anomaly 138
in meningioma 61, 66
in trigeminal neurinoma 96
narrowing 23f., 35, 57, 66
widening 1, 35, 51, 54, 61, 66
Internal auditory porus (see porus acusticus internus)
Iodine index 46

Jacobson's nerve 24, 107
Jugular bulb 24, 107, 109
Jugular foramen 15, 60, 102, 108, 109, 110, 117, 147
anatomy 24f.
enlargement 109, 118, 116, 122, 125
erosion 66, 102, 108, 109, 118, 122
neurinoma 117, 121ff., 170
Jugular tubercle 15
erosion 51, 66, 91
Jugular vein (see vein, jugular)

Keratin 78

Leukoencephalopathy, hypertensive 142
Ligament, petroclinoid 26, 95
Lipoma 86, 94
Lymphoma 147

Magnetic resonance imaging 3, 152ff.
Meatocisternography (see Pantopaque meatocisternography)
Medulla 15
Medulloblastoma 31, 147
Megadolichobasilar anomaly 30, 31, 131, 137ff.
Melanoma 30, 99
Meningioma 28, 30, 31, 50, 55, 56, 58, 60ff., 86, 99, 106, 116, 121, 122, 126, 130, 137, 147, 163, 168
Meningitis 77, 84
Mesencephalon 9, 26, 28, 29, 73
Metastasis 28, 30, 31, 58, 99, 106, 116, 121, 147, 168
Metrizamide CT cisternography (see positive-contrast CT cisternography)
Midbrain (see mesencephalon)
Middle ear 24
Multiple sclerosis 77
Mushroom appearance 48

Nerve
cranial 5 (see trigeminal nerve)
cranial 6 (see abducens nerve)
cranial 7 (see facial nerve)
cranial 8 (see vestibulocochlear nerve)
cranial 9 (see glossopharyngeal nerve)
cranial 10 (see vagal nerve)
cranial 11 (see accessory nerve)
cranial 12 (see hypoglossal nerve)
Neurinoma
see acoustic neurinoma
see caudal nerve, neurinoma
see facial nerve, neurinoma
see hypoglossal nerve, neurinoma
see jugular foramen, neurinoma
see trigeminal neurinoma
Neurofibromatosis (see von Recklinghausen's disease)
Neurovascular bundle (see vestibulocochlear and facial nerve)
Notochord (see chorda dorsalis)
Nystagmography (see Electronystagmography)
Nystagmus 58

Obtuse angle sign 50, 63, 99, 168
Occipital condyle 24, 91
Osteoma 106
Otitis media 126

Pantopaque meatocisternography 3, 7, 8, 19, 35, 57, 127, 132, 138
Papilledema 34
Papilloma 86, 147
Paraganglioma (see chemodectoma)
Parasympathetic system 33
Paravertebral space 24, 102
Partial volume phenomenon 5, 155
Petroclinoid ligament (see ligament, petroclinoid)
Petrosal sinus (see sinus, petrosal)
Petrosal vein (see vein, petrosal)
Petrous bone 2, 5, 6, 8
apex 1, 29, 35, 74, 95, 96, 99, 102
infralabyrinthine space 102, 107, 109, 118

posterior surface 7, 10, 13, 15, 18, 22, 23, 27, 29, 50, 60, 66, 77, 86, 89, 96, 102, 122, 136
tumors 30, 31, 60, 66, 116, 126ff., 170
Pituitary adenoma (see adenoma, pituitary)
Pneumoencephalography 1, 2, 18, 27, 28, 77, 86, 89, 100, 141
Pneumoventriculography 1
Pons 9, 10, 13, 15, 18, 21, 27, 28, 50, 73, 110, 137, 156
Porus acusticus internus 13, 21, 22, 23, 35, 51, 55, 60, 132
Porus trigeminus 60, 95, 96
Positive-contrast CT cisternography 3, 6, 7, 19, 86, 91, 153
Precentral cerebellar vein (see vein, precentral cerebellar)
Psammoma body 61
Pseudotumor
flocculi 15
vermis 15
Pterygoid canal 128
Pterygopalatine fossa 128
Pulse sequence 152, 156, 163, 168

Quantum noise 6

Recklinghausen's neurofibromatosis (see von Recklinghausen's disease)
Relaxation time 156, 163
Rhabdomyosarcoma 147

Sarcoma 29, 147
Schwann cell 32
Schwannoma 32
Seizure, epileptic 7
Shunting 93f.
Signal to noise ratio 5, 153
Sinus
petrosal 24, 26, 60, 143
sigmoid 25, 143
straight 26
transverse 25, 26
Soap, calcified 78
Spasm facial 138
Stapedial reflex 34
Statoacoustic nerve (see vestibulocochlear nerve)
Sternocleidomastoid muscle 33, 121
Straight sinus (see sinus, straight)
Stylomastoid foramen 24, 128
Stylomastoid process 24
Supratentorial growth (see growth, supratentorial)
Surface coil 152, 153, 155, 156, 163
Swallowing 33
Symptoms
cerebellar 34, 60, 77, 89, 100, 118, 138
of acoustic neurinoma 1, 32ff.
of aneurysm 131, 132
of arachnoid cyst 89
of chemodectoma 107
of cholesteatoma, primary 87
of chordoma 100
of epidermoid tumor 77
of facial nerve neurinoma 126
of hypoglossal neurinoma 117, 118
of jugular foramen neurinoma 117, 121
of megadolichobasilar anomaly 138
of meningioma 60
of trigeminal neurinoma 95
of vascular lesion 131
vestibular 33

Target sign 136
Taste 33
Temporal horn 29, 73
Temporal lobe 29
Tentorial incisura (see incisura, tentorii)
Tentorium 18, 26, 27, 29, 31, 73
Third ventricle 29, 73, 138, 141, 142
Thrombosis 141
Time-density curve 9, 48, 62, 136
Tinnitus 1, 32, 33, 77, 107, 126
Tomography, pluridirectional 2, 3, 4, 5, 35, 51, 77, 89, 108, 118, 122, 127, 132, 138
Tongue 34
Torcular Herophili 26
Transincisural growth (see growth, transincisural)
Transincisural herniation (see herniation, transincisural)
Transtentorial growth (see growth, transtentorial)
Trapezius muscle 33, 121
Trigeminal hiatus (see porus trigeminus)
Trigeminal nerve 13, 19, 33, 60, 95
neurinoma 30, 95ff.
palsy 33, 77, 100, 138
Trigeminal neuralgia 33, 77
Trigeminal root 95, 96
Tumor blush 36, 38, 55, 61, 100, 118, 122
Tumor capsule 2, 63, 77, 78, 163

Vagal nerve 15, 24, 33, 107
neurinoma 30, 116, 117, 121ff.
palsy 33, 107, 121, 138
Vascular encasement (see encasement, vascular)
Vascular malformation (see arteriovenous malformation)
Vein
capsular 156, 163

Vein
  cortical 143
  jugular 24, 108, 109
  of Galen 26
  of the lateral recess of the fourth ventricle 38
  petrosal 13, 15, 18, 19, 36, 143
  precentral cerebellar 38
Ventriculography 1
Vermis 15, 26
Vertebrobasilar insufficiency (see insufficiency, vertebrobasilar)
Vertex 4
Vertigo 7, 33, 121, 126, 138
Vestibular nerve (see vestibulocochlear nerve)
Vestibular symptoms (see symptoms, vestibular)
Vestibular testing 33, 34, 58
Vestibulocochlear nerve 1, 4, 7, 13, 19, 21, 22, 23, 32, 33, 35, 55, 58, 60, 72, 74, 77, 100, 138, 152, 153, 156
Vomiting 7
Von Recklinghausen's disease 32, 121

MIX
Papier aus verantwortungsvollen Quellen
Paper from responsible sources
FSC® C105338

If you have any concerns about our products,
you can contact us on
ProductSafety@springernature.com

In case Publisher is established outside the EU,
the EU authorized representative is:
Springer Nature Customer Service Center GmbH
Europaplatz 3, 69115 Heidelberg, Germany

Printed by Libri Plureos GmbH
in Hamburg, Germany